ADVANCED NURSING RESEARCH

From Theory to Practice

RUTH M. TAPPEN, EdD, RN, FAAN

Professor
Christine E. Lynn Eminent Scholar in Nursing
Christine E. Lynn College of Nursing
Florida Atlantic University
Boca Raton, Florida

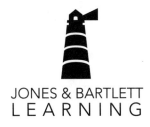

JONES & BARTLETT
LEARNING

World Headquarters

Jones & Bartlett Learning
40 Tall Pine Drive
Sudbury, MA 01776
978-443-5000
info@jblearning.com
www.jblearning.com

Jones & Bartlett Learning
Canada
6339 Ormindale Way
Mississauga, Ontario L5V 1J2
Canada

Jones & Bartlett Learning
International
Barb House, Barb Mews
London W6 7PA
United Kingdom

Jones & Bartlett Learning books and products are available through most bookstores and online book-sellers. To contact Jones & Bartlett Learning directly, call 800-832-0034, fax 978-443-8000, or visit our website, www.jblearning.com.

Substantial discounts on bulk quantities of Jones & Bartlett Learning publications are available to corporations, professional associations, and other qualified organizations. For details and specific discount information, contact the special sales department at Jones & Bartlett Learning via the above contact information or send an email to specialsales@jblearning.com.

The author, editor, and publisher have made every effort to provide accurate information. However, they are not responsible for errors, omissions, or for any outcomes related to the use of the contents of this book and take no responsibility for the use of the products and procedures described. Treatments and side effects described in this book may not be applicable to all people; likewise, some people may require a dose or experience a side effect that is not described herein. Drugs and medical devices are discussed that may have limited availability controlled by the Food and Drug Administration (FDA) for use only in a research study or clinical trial. Research, clinical practice, and government regulations often change the accepted standard in this field. When consideration is being given to use of any drug in the clinical setting, the health care provider or reader is responsible for determining FDA status of the drug, reading the package insert, and reviewing prescribing information for the most up-to-date recommendations on dose, precautions, and contraindications, and determining the appropriate usage for the product. This is especially important in the case of drugs that are new or seldom used.

Production Credits

Publisher: Kevin Sullivan
Acquisitions Editor: Amy Sibley
Associate Editor: Patricia Donnelly
Editorial Assistant: Rachel Shuster
Senior Production Editor: Carolyn F. Rogers
Associate Marketing Manager: Katie Hennessy

V.P., Manufacturing and Inventory Control:
 Therese Connell
Composition: Auburn Associates, Inc.
Cover Design: Scott Moden
Cover Image: © Featherlightfoot/ShutterStock, Inc.
Printing and Binding: Malloy, Inc.
Cover Printing: Malloy, Inc.

Library of Congress Cataloging-in-Publication Data
Tappen, Ruth M.
 Advanced nursing research : from theory to practice / Ruth M. Tappen.
   p. ; cm.
 Includes bibliographical references and index.
 ISBN 978-0-7637-6568-2 (casebound)
 1. Nursing—Research—Methodology. I. Title.
 [DNLM: 1. Nursing Research—methods. 2. Research Design. WY 20.5 T175a 2011]
 RT81.5.T37 2011
 610.73072—dc22

                                                            2010017053

6048
Printed in the United States of America
14 13 12 11 10 10 9 8 7 6 5 4 3 2 1

DEDICATION

In appreciation of the ideas, suggestions, and contributions from family, friends, colleagues, and students. You have greatly enriched the content of this book. Thank you.

Special thanks to Ms. Barbara Blake for her assistance in preparing this manuscript.

CONTENTS

PREFACE

This new textbook on nursing research is written for students, practicing nurses, and nursing faculty who want to learn more about how to conduct a nursing research study. It is written from the perspective of the researcher, beginning with the very first steps of conducting a study and following through each phase of research, all the way to publishing the results and developing a program of research.

CONTENTS OF THE BOOK

The book begins with an Introduction that puts present day nursing research into perspective with a very brief look at the beginnings of nursing research. The first section of the book is concerned with getting started. Chapter 1 provides some guidelines for selecting a topic. Chapter 2 discusses the conduct of literature reviews to learn what is already known on the selected topic, and Chapter 3 discusses use of a theoretical framework for your study.

The next section is the design phase, beginning with that continuing conundrum, quantitative or qualitative research or both? The following chapters address the most frequently used research designs from the true experiment to the many descriptive designs including longitudinal and epidemiological studies, mixed methods, historical research, meta-analysis, and meta-synthesis.Conduct of the study is the focus of the next section. Here, ethical issues, obtaining consent, participant recruitment, quantitative and qualitative data collection, and provision of an intervention are discussed in sufficient detail to prepare the reader to conduct a research study. Interpretation of the data, from data management to basic analysis of quantitative data (including descriptive and inferential analysis) and qualitative data are presented in the fourth section. In the final section, evidence-based practice, presenting and publishing results, preparing proposals, and developing a program of research complete the reader's journey through the exciting and challenging world of nursing research.

Throughout the book, issues of importance to both quantitative and qualitative research are addressed. With the emergence of mixed methodology and growing appreciation of the value of qualitative research within the classic research traditions, it seemed important to include both yet continue to differentiate their foundations, use and unique contributions to nursing knowledge and nursing practice.

USING THIS BOOK

Although each chapter addresses the main points that a beginning researcher should know, it is not possible to provide for in-depth study of the many possible designs, analyses, and issues related to nursing research. There is sufficient information here to become knowledgeable but not to become expert. To become an expert on a particular approach, the reader will need to consult additional resources. The annotations in the reference lists at the end of each chapter (marked by a ✧) provide a guide to some of the most helpful resources related to the practice of research.

Throughout the book, many different research studies are described. They were chosen not only to illustrate an important point but also to introduce the reader to the wide and fascinating array of research that can be done, from a study of foreign nurses trying to understand the culture of the U.S. healthcare system, to the case of a school nurse who deals expertly with student exposure to a rabid bat, to the effect of oral sucrose on infant pain behaviors. There literally is no end to the different topics and different types of research one can conduct under the rubric of nursing research. Surely there is something here to interest every nurse who would like to become involved in research.

A FINAL WORD TO THE READER

It is hoped that you will find this book useful for planning and conducting research and in helping others learn how to do nursing research. Your comments and suggestions for future editions are welcome. You may email me via the publisher at info@jblearning.com.

Ruth M. Tappen, EdD, RN, FAAN

INTRODUCTION

Do you enjoy exploring new ideas? Solving puzzles? Finding new and better ways to care for people? This is what nursing research is all about.

OUR RESEARCH TRADITION

Florence Nightingale, the founder of modern nursing, systematically collected data to demonstrate that the majority of British soldiers fighting in the Crimean War died of preventable problems such as cholera, dysentery, and scurvy, not of war wounds. She even invented diagrams similar to pie charts to better illustrate the data (Gill & Gill, 2005). Back in England, she collated data comparing the death rate of nursing staff to that of all women living in London. She pointed out that "fever and cholera" were responsible for 50% of the nurses' deaths versus 16% of the general population and that the nurses' mortality rate overall was 40% higher than other women. "These figures," she wrote, "prove the very great importance of hospital hygiene" (Nightingale, 1863, p. 21).

Although never abandoned, it took a long time for research to become a prominent activity in nursing. In the 1950s, the Division of Nursing Resources began granting federal money for nursing research studies. Early centers of nursing research activity were located at Teachers College, Columbia University in New York; Wayne State University in Detroit, Michigan; and Walter Reed Army Institute of Research. The journal *Nursing Research* began publication in 1952 (D'Antonio, 1997).

Many early studies focused on nurses and nursing education. Although education always of interest, research on clinical questions received a boost when federal funding was transferred to the newly established National Center for Nursing Research within the National Institutes of Health (NIH) in 1985. The center became an institute of NIH in 1993 and continues to support nursing research and training of nurse researchers today.

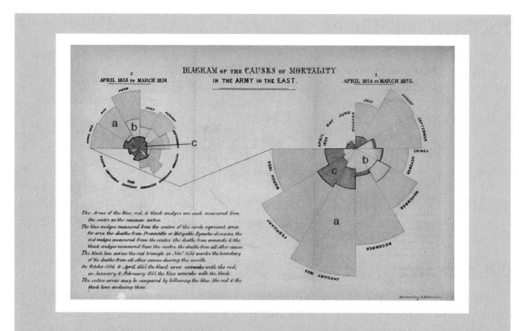

Example of polar area diagram by Florence Nightingale (1820–1910). This "Diagram of the causes of mortality in the army in the East" was published in *Notes on Matters Affecting the Health, Efficiency, and Hospital Administration of the British Army* and sent to Queen Victoria in 1858. This graphic indicates the number of deaths that occurred from preventable diseases (a), those that were the results of wounds (b), and those due to other causes (c).

DEFINING RESEARCH

Research is the systematic collection and analysis of information (data). It is planned, organized, and carefully thought out before being done. The information or data that you collect and analyze may be numeric (quantitative) or verbal (qualitative).

Research studies may be small, simple projects involving just a few participants. Complex studies may involve thousands of people and last more than 5, 10, 20, or even 50 years.

WHAT DOES RESEARCH INVOLVE?

Research is a multidimensional activity that requires conscientiousness, logic, creativity, and active interaction with others.

Conscientious. There are rules to follow in conducting research. Some of these rules are related to the ethics of research, including protection of your participants, whether human or animal. There are also guidelines for collecting and analyzing data systematically. Mistakes, carelessness, and sloppy work are not acceptable. (They're not acceptable in practice, either).

Logical. Research methods were developed to assure that the results are based upon reason and logic. This is done to help us avoid coming to erroneous conclusions. Also for this reason, research reports are often structured as an argument with a conclusion, building fact upon fact to demonstrate how you reached your conclusion. To be persuasive, the argument is expected to be reasonable, rational, and logical. This does not mean, however, that it is cold and unemotional. Most nurse researchers are passionate about their work and deeply committed to it.

Creative. Research is also a voyage of discovery. The discoveries are often the result of a "hunch," i.e. the researcher's intuitive feel for a possible solution to a problem. To advance knowledge, researchers need to be able to see new patterns, to put existing knowledge together in new ways, and to make leaps of understanding that lead to exciting new ideas. These are the "Aha!" moments the media love to write about. Flexibility, intuition, and innovation are as important to research as are logic and reason.

Interactive. Much complex research is done by teams of people with a wide assortment of skills and experience. Even when a study is done by a single person, he or she will benefit from the feedback of fellow researchers as well as the participants in the study and the nurses who might put the results into practice. These multiple perspectives are valuable both in designing and in interpreting research.

IMPORTANCE OF RESEARCH

Research brings us new knowledge that informs our practice. The ultimate goal is to improve the outcomes of care. What is the best ways to take a neonate's temperature? To prevent SIDS? To reduce nausea and vomiting? Control pain? How do you reduce preoperative anxiety? Obesity in diabetes? Prevent adolescent suicide? How are we going to get hospital-acquired drug-resistant infections under control? Prevent global pandemics? There is no end to the numbers of questions we can ask and answer through nursing research.

There are some questions, however, for which research cannot provide an answer. These are questions of right and wrong. Is it right to withhold fluids? Is it wrong to perform an abortion? Should we tell a patient how long he or she has to live? Research studies can tell us how many people agree or disagree, why they disagree, and what the consequences of a decision might be, but research does not directly address questions of right and wrong.

PURPOSE OF THIS BOOK

This book is designed to prepare you to be a beginning researcher, to be able to conduct simple studies on your own, to be an informed member of a research team conducting more complex studies, and to be an informed consumer of research. At the end of each chapter, you will find resources for further learning should you need more in-depth information. Keep in mind, also, that research is an interactive process. Experienced researchers are happy to talk with you about their work and to help you along the way.

Nursing research is challenging, exciting, engaging, and rewarding. Welcome to the wonderful world of nursing research!

REFERENCES

D'Antonio, P. (1997). Toward a history of research in nursing. *Nursing Research, 46*(2), 105–110.

Gills, C. J., & Gill, G. C. (2005). Nightingale in Scutari: Her legacy reexamined. *Clinical Infectious Diseases, 40,* 1799–1805.

Nightingale, F. (1863). *Notes on hospitals.* London: Longman, Green, Longman, Roberts and Green.

PART 1

Planning Phase

CHAPTER 1

Identifying a Research Topic

In this chapter, we address the very first step in conducting a research study: deciding upon the focus or topic of the study. It is a creative process involving thinking, reflecting, reading, and talking with others.

RESEARCH DEFINED

Research is the systematic investigation of phenomena (Kerlinger, 1986). It begins with identification of a problem or an idea. Reading, searching, discussing, and thinking about the idea should follow. What do we know about this? Is there evidence to support this idea, or is more needed? After you have refined, clarified and focused upon a clearly defined question or hypothesis, what was once an idea becomes your research topic. Deciding how to investigate the topic selected is the next step. The decision should be based upon what is already known and what you have decided to investigate. If very little is known, you probably will need to use one of the many qualitative approaches available. If more is known, then you can ask a very specific question or generate a hypothesis about relationships between specific factors. This is the design phase. The design of your study will become the guide for implementation of the study. Next you enter the implementation phase during which you obtain the necessary permissions, recruit subjects, and collect the data. Analysis may begin during the time you are collecting data or it may be done upon completion of data collection, depending upon the study design.

When the study is completed, you share the findings formally or informally with a number of people who were involved in the study and with those, if any, who provided financial support. Finally, the results should be published with attention to how your study contributed to nursing knowledge and nursing practice and what you would do next to continue this line of research (Figure 1-1).

FINDING A TOPIC

Landmark Studies

In 2006, the National Institute of Nursing Research published a report featuring 10 landmark studies that demonstrate the scope and impact of nursing research. To give you an idea of the wide range of topics that can be addressed by nurse researchers, these landmark studies are listed in Figure 1-2.

What is it that leads researchers to such important discoveries? Root-Bernstein (1997) says that these researchers are no more intelligent than other researchers. Neither are they

> · Identify a problem or area of interest
> · Explore this problem or area to find out what is known
> · Define the research topic
> · Generate questions or hypotheses
> · Design the study
> · Conduct the study
> · Analyze the results
> · Report the findings

Figure 1-1 Major stages of a research study.

right more often. Instead, he thinks that they are "simply more curious . . . more persistent, readier to make detours and more willing to tackle bigger and more fundamental problems" (p. 407). He says they also "possess intellectual courage" and "work at the edge of their competency." As they stretch themselves, they stretch science" (p. 408). They are an inspiration to all of us who do research (Figure 1-3).

Idea Sources

Once you learn to spot them, you will find that you encounter possible topics for research every day, even several times a day. To do this, you need to develop the ability to "think research."

Consider the following sources of ideas for research and some fictional examples of each:

- *An intriguing theory or research finding that needs further testing*—Luis read that wearing scrubs several days without laundering them contributed to hospital acquired (nosocomial) infections (McCaughey, 2009). He decided to retrieve the original research report and to study (1) how many hospital personnel actually did this, and (2) if infection rates could be reduced by ending this practice in his facility.

- *A patient care experience that has had an impact on you as well as on your patients or clients*—In 1 week, Roberts lost three young patients to nosocomial infections. He vowed to stamp out these infections on his unit and turned to research to discover how to do this.

- *A gap in the knowledge base*—Is full-time day care injurious to an infant's growth and development? Does it affect adjustment in later life? How do you select a day care facility that has an environment that fosters maternal–infant bonding and infant growth and development?

- *Personal experience*—When Ellis' closest friend experienced severe brain injury from an auto accident, she decided to study interventions that facilitate regaining independence in individuals with closed head injury.

Aiken, L. H., Clarke, S. P., Sloane, D. M., Sochalski, J., & Silka, J. (2002). Hospital nurse staffing and patient mortality, nurse burnout and job dissatisfaction. *Journal of the American Medical Association, 288,* 1987–1993.

Bergstrom, N., Braden, B., Kemp, M., Champagne, M., & Ruby, E. (1996). Multi-site study of incidence of pressure ulcers and the relationship between risk level, demographic characteristics, diagnoses, and prescription of preventive interventions. *Journal of the American Geriatrics Society, 44*(1), 22–30.

Gear, R. W., Miaskowski, C., Gordon, N. C., Paul, S. M., Heller, P. H., & Levine, J. D. (1999). The kappa opioid nalbuphine produces gender- and dose-dependent analgesia and antianalgesia in patients with postoperative pain. *Pain, 83*(2), 339–345.

Grey, M., Davidson, M., Boland, E. A., & Tamborlane, W. V. (2001). Clinical and psychosocial factors associated with achievement of treatment goals in adolescents with diabetes mellitus. *Journal of Adolescent Health, 28*(5), 377–385.

Harrell, J. S., McMurray, R. G., Bangdiwala, S. I., Frauman, A. C., Gansky, S. A., & Bradley, C. B. (1996). Effects of a school-based intervention to reduce cardiovascular disease risk factors in elementary-school children: The Cardiovascular Health in Children (CHIC) Study. *Journal of Pediatrics, 128,* 797–805.

Hill, M. N., Han, H., Dennison, C. R., Kim, M. T., Roary, M. C., Blumenthal, R. S., et al. (2003). Hypertension care and control in underserved urban African American men: Behavioral and physiologic outcomes at 36 months. *American Journal of Hypertension, 16,* 906–913.

Jemmott, J. B., Jemmott, L. S., & Fong, G. T. (1998). Abstinence and safer sex HIV risk reduction interventions for African American adolescents: A randomized controlled trial. *Journal of the American Medical Association, 279*(19), 1529–1536.

Kitzman, H., Olds, D. L., Henderson, C. R. Jr., Hanks, C., Cole, R., Tatelbaum, R., et al. (1997). Effect of prenatal and infancy home visitation by nurses on pregnancy outcomes, childhood injuries, and repeated childbearing. A randomized controlled trial. *Journal of the American Medical Association, 278*(8), 644–652.

Lorig, K., Gonzalez, V. M., & Ritter, P. (1999). Community-based Spanish language arthritis education program: A randomized trial. *Medical Care, 3,* 957–963.

Naylor, M. D., Brooten, D. A., Campbell, R. L., Maislin, G., McCauley, K. M., & Schwartz, J. S. (2004). Transitional care of older adults hospitalized with heart failure: A randomized, controlled trial. *Journal of the American Geriatrics Society, 52,* 675–684.

Figure 1-2   Ten landmark nursing research studies.

Source: National Institute of Nursing Research. (2006). *Changing practice, changing lives: 10 landmark nursing research studies* (NIH Publication Number: 06-6094). Washington, DC: U.S. Government Printing Office.

> · Action (exploring) leads to results, not inaction.
> · Conduct a broad search for ideas; trial and error is often involved.
> · Think big! Study important problems.
> · Ask new questions and look at old problems from a new perspective.
> · "Do what makes your heart leap!" A quote from Jonas Salk, developer of the Salk polio vaccine (p. 410).

Figure 1-3   Strategies leading to cutting edge research.

Source: Adapted from Root-Bernstein, R. S. (1997). *Discovering.* Cambridge, MA: University Press.

- *A line of inquiry that you have already begun*—Chanisse conducted a small pilot study of the effect of video game playing on sleep quality in middle school students. Her results suggested that more than 2 hours a day of video game playing interfered with entering the REM phase of sleep, so she decided to plan a much larger study to retest her results.

- *A branch off the line of inquiry you have already begun*—Chanisse had observed during her pilot study that the students who played video games for several hours a day tended to be overweight. She decided to study the interaction of inactivity, eating habits that may contribute to weight gain, and video game playing in middle school students as well in her larger study.

"THINK RESEARCH"

In each of the examples above, the person had learned how to spot a possible topic for research. The following are some ways to develop the ability to "think research":

- Read as much as you can about your specialty area in journals, in books, and online.

- Reflect on your practice: Why are we seeing so many young women with urinary tract infections? Why do some of my HIV patients seem to be healthy in spite of their infection? Why do some high school students have second, even third pregnancies, when others do not?

- Talk with colleagues about your practice. Seek out thoughtful, reflective, analytical, and curious people to discuss ideas with.

- Develop your sense of curiosity, ask questions, and explore new ideas.

- Instead of accepting what you read, especially in the popular media, follow up on interesting items by checking them out with the original research.

- Practice thinking critically: Instead of accepting what you read and hear from others, critically evaluate what you are told, not only for its logic but also for evidence to back up the conclusions.

It takes a willingness to question authority and to consider new approaches to problems to "think research." Nursing practice is still dominated to a great extent by routine and the opinions of experts. Uncertainty is too often seen as a threat instead of an opportunity (Schon, 1983). The tendency toward "ritualizing and habitualizing" (Hasseler, 2006, p. 221) of practice are real dangers to providing the highest quality, individualized care. Instead, nurses should be prepared to question accepted routines and expert opinions as well as their own actions and to engage in research that informs practice.

Reflecting on one's own practice and the practices of others raises questions that can be addressed through research. Schon notes that practitioners usually know more than they can say, calling it a "knowing-in-practice" which is not ordinarily verbalized. Research, he says, should not be a distraction from practice but a development of it (1983, p. ix). To become more reflective requires the following (adapted from Johns, 2008):

Curiosity—Interest in why things happen

Openness—Willingness to consider novel ideas

Concern—Believing that what you do matters; caring deeply about what happens to one's patients and clients

Commitment—Owning responsibility for what happens to ones' patients and clients

Intelligence—Ability to critically analyze a patient care situation and identify gaps in nursing knowledge

Courage—To think for yourself, to share your ideas with others, to try new approaches

Schon (1983) wrote that when someone "reflects-in-action," he or she becomes a "researcher in the practice context" (p. 68). The following are a few questions you might ask yourself in reflecting on your practice (adapted from Johns, 2005):

- What is it that concerns me about this client or patient situation?
- How could I (we) have responded more effectively?
- What could have been done differently?
- What gaps in our nursing knowledge are evident in this situation?
- What needs to be done to fill these gaps?

GENERATING AN IDEA LIST

It is often helpful to keep a list in a file labeled "Ideas" in a research folder on your computer or server. Alternatively, keep an Ideas list in your calendar or in a notebook. List all the ideas that occur to you as you think, reflect, read, listen, and talk with colleagues. Many but not all of these ideas will be discarded eventually for various reasons:

- Questions of right and wrong: these are ethical questions, not research questions.
- The problem is outside the scope of nursing.
- The problem is a minor one.
- The situation of concern was primarily a political, financial, personality, or power problem, not a gap in knowledge.
- Much is known and understood about this concern although it has not yet been put into practice in your facility (this situation calls for leadership and perhaps a translational research study).
- While it may be important, it is of little interest to you or outside your expertise.

Once you have discarded those ideas that are inappropriate or not of interest to you, you should be left with some promising ideas. From these, try to select a *strong* topic (Fleming, 2009), one that will be worthy of your time and attention.

MAKING A FINAL SELECTION

Once you have discarded those ideas that are not suitable for one or more reasons, which of the remaining ideas may be the right one to choose? Consider the following characteristics of a strong topic in making your final selection.

Innovative: New, novel, creative, not a topic that has been thoroughly and repeatedly studied. For example, we know and have repeatedly demonstrated that caregiving can be burdensome. Simply demonstrating that again does not add much to our knowledge base.

Significant: Will the results be important? Will they contribute to improving care? How much and what kind of a contribution? There are few studies that are completely worthless and insignificant, but given the amounts of time and energy needed to complete a research study, selecting a significant topic makes this investment worthwhile.

Reasonable: You also have to be practical. You may want to find the cure for asthma or spinal cord injuries or solve the problem of drug use in high risk youth, but these goals are likely to be too ambitious for one study. Nevertheless, you can design a study that will produce results that contribute to these worthy goals. Ask yourself also if you have or can obtain sufficient time, money, personnel, and equipment to conduct the study. Finally, do you have sufficient expertise—either yourself or in members of your team—to conduct the study?

Ethical: While it is unlikely that you will devise an unethical study, it is important to consider whether or not participation will put people in jeopardy (for example, asking abused spouses to keep a diary could put them in danger of inciting further abuse if the diary were found), or if a demonstrably effective intervention is being withheld from participants in your study.

Exciting: Completion of a research study requires a relatively long-term commitment on your part. It is much easier, and you'll do better work, if you are passionate about the study.

CONCLUSION

The above is a guide designed to help you select a strong topic for your research study, one that is innovative, significant, reasonable, ethical, and exciting to you personally. Remember, you do not need to accomplish your long-term goal in your first study. Often, it takes a series of studies to address an important research question.

REFERENCES

Fleming, G. (2009). *Choosing a strong research topic: Start smart with preliminary research.* Retrieved May 27, 2009, from http://homeworktips.about.com/od/researchandreference/a/topic.htm

Hasseler, M. (2006). Evidence-based nursing for practice and science. In H. S. Kim & I. Kollak (Eds.), *Nursing theories: Conceptual and philosophical foundations* (pp. 215–235). New York: Springer.

Johns, C. (2005). Expanding the gates of perception. In C. Johns & D. Freshwater (Eds.), *Transforming nursing through reflective practice.* Oxford, UK: Blackwell Publishing.

Johns, C. (2008, October 20). *Reflective practice.* Presentation at the Christine E. Lynn College of Nursing, Florida Atlantic University, Boca Raton, FL.

Kerlinger, F. (1986). *Foundations of behavioral research.* Chicago, IL: Holt, Rinehart & Winston.

McCaughey, B. (2009, January 8). *Hospital scrubs are a germy, deadly mess. Wall Street Journal*, p. A13.

National Institute of Nursing Research (2006). *Changing practice, changing lives: 10 landmark nursing research studies* (NIH Publication Number: 06-6094). Washington, DC: U.S. Government Printing Office.
  ✧ An impressive list of nursing research studies. If you have time, select two or three to read carefully. They are excellent examples of well written research reports as well.

Root-Bernstein, R. S. (1997). *Discovering.* Bridgewater, NJ: Replica Books.

Schon, D. A. (1983). *The reflective practitioner: How professionals think in action.* New York: Basic Books.

University of Michigan-Flint. (2009). *Select a topic to research.* Retrieved February 26, 2010, from http://www.umflint.edu/library/research/selecttopic.htm
  ✧ Written in a very elementary fashion for a general audience, but you may find a useful tip or two here if you are having trouble identifying a topic.

CHAPTER 2

Reviewing the Literature

To design a research study that builds upon existing knowledge and is clearly connected to that knowledge base, a thorough and analytical review of the literature is needed. Both the theoretical literature and the research literature should be reviewed. Your approach to these two different types of information will differ in several ways discussed in this chapter.

There are several phases to conducting a review of the literature: the search, reading what you have found and making notes on important points, and then writing the review.

SEARCHING THE LITERATURE

The goal in searching the literature is to discover what is known about your topic. This means that the search must be *thorough*; that none of the important, influential works are missed.

Beginning researchers often have difficulty doing a thorough search. The following are a few do's and don'ts for conducting a successful search.

The Do List

- Use as many search terms and variations of the terms as you can think of.
- Continue to search until you find no new references, indicating you have exhausted all sources.
- Carefully review information to identify sources of information.
- Search books (monographs) as well as articles.
- Include policy statements, where relevant, to support the importance of your topic.
- Go back as far as 15 or 20 years (maybe even further back) to find the original work on your topic, especially, but not only, theoretical work.
- Investigate the credibility of an unfamiliar source before using it.
- If one is available, ask a health science librarian for assistance.
- Consider consulting with the staff of a writing center if one is available.

The Do Not List

- Select only the articles that are available in full text online (this is far too limiting).
- Include articles that are not data based unless they contribute substantively to the theoretical foundation of the study or justification of the importance of the study.

- Limit the search to the past 5 years or less. The most important theoretical work or original research studies may have been done years before that.

- Limit your search to one or two databases. Important work may have been done in another discipline. If so, you need to know about it.

- Limit your searching strategy to electronic databases. Browse recent issues of the most relevant journals, and check the references in the latest review articles as well (Rau, 2004).

- Ignore publications from other countries.

- Forget to search for books, reports, and other monographs related to your topic.

- Use secondary sources or anecdotal reports unless absolutely necessary.

- Hesitate to ask for help if you are finding very little information. You may not be using the right search terms or the best database for your topic.

- Use Web-based material from an unknown source.

Barroso and colleagues (2003) described several nondatabase search techniques. Berry picking (Bates, 1989; Barroso et al., 2003) is a way to "wander(s) through the information forest, changing directions as needed to follow up on various leads and shifts in thinking" (p. 157), just as you would do if you were picking wild berries. The following are the five berry picking strategies:

1. Footnote chasing or backward chaining: Check the footnotes or references at the end of book chapters and articles for promising sources.

2. Citation searching or forward chaining: Find out who has cited an especially relevant article. This is more difficult to do than the backward chaining and will not work for very recent articles.

3. Journal runs: Hand-search recent issues of the most relevant journals (select just a few).

4. Area scanning: For this you must go to the library, locate important, relevant monographs on your subject and then look on that shelf and neighboring shelves for other books on your topic. You may find a gem doing this!

5. Author searching: Search the names of those few authors who have written the most important books and articles on your topic. Don't forget to search for their dissertations and theses, as these are often rich resources. Don't skip this strategy; it is often fruitful.

Source Credibility

Fortunately, searches have become easier as the variety of online search engines increases. With increased availability, however, comes the responsibility to verify the credibility of the source. Probably the most important principle to follow in assessing the credibility of information is to *know your source*. This is particularly important with online sources. Reputable sources include government agencies, professional organizations, and large private foundations. Be sure you separate policy and advocacy statements from reports of research, and always cite your source. For research, it is important that it has been peer reviewed. If you find mention of a relevant research study in the general media (online or in print), you need to search for the original study and report that as your source, not the general media source. For nursing sources, you will probably want to begin with PubMed/Medline and CINAHL, but there are many others, including PsychArticles, PsycINFO, ERIC, Sociology, ProQuest Dissertation and theses, Health and Safety Sciences Abstracts, and historic documents. For theoretical literature in particular you will also want to look at *Books in Print*. Other important sources are governmental agencies such as the Centers for Disease Control and Prevention, National Institutes of Health, and the Agency for Healthcare Research and Quality. National not-for-profit organizations such as the Arthritis Foundation, Parkinson's Disease Foundation, Robert Wood Johnson Foundation, and the Commonwealth Fund often make important reports and other publications available on their websites. Through your library, you can also access university and public libraries across the country, requesting materials not available at your library through the interlibrary loan system.

Sorting

The result of your thorough search may be a stack of books and very large folder of articles. If so, then it is time for you to look them over and to begin to sort them out. You may find that some of the material is not relevant: these can be set aside. Others may be secondary sources; set these aside also unless the primary source is unavailable. Then do a preliminary sorting of the remaining materials. You may sort first by theory, significance, potential measures (instruments), and related research. Then sort again by relevance to your topic: is the document closely related or probably of marginal interest? (this may change, so do not discard these marginal materials). Then divide by subtopics such as qualitative and quantitative studies, the age of the target population, the setting of the research, the type of measures used, and so forth.

READ CRITICALLY AND MAKE NOTES

You may want to scan the material first, then go back and read it more carefully. This is a matter of personal style. During the careful reading of the material, mark important passages so you can find them later. Think about the following as you read:

- How does this information connect to my research topic?
- Does this change what I planned to study?
- Are there new ideas here or implications for further research?

- Are there new insights here?
- Which of these research studies address my topic most specifically? Do the results support what I plan to do?
- Which theoretical base most closely aligns with my thinking? Does it suggest new directions for my research?
- How will I organize my review of what is already known on this topic?

WRITING THE REVIEW

Personal style (what works for you) dictates how you proceed from here. Ask yourself a few questions if you are not certain what approach works best for you:

1. Do I prefer to compose (write) on paper or on the computer? Which generates the best product for me?

2. Can I create a preliminary outline in my mind, or do I need to put it on screen or on paper?

3. What helps me organize my ideas? Is it talking with others? Drawing diagrams of the interrelationships of ideas? Writing an outline? Sorting into file folders?

4. Do I work best by writing whole sentences right away or by writing down fragments that I then pull together?

5. How can I synthesize what I have read and avoid using too many direct quotes? (See Questions 3 and 4.)

6. How can I show connections between different theories and different research studies? (See Questions 3 and 4.)

There are many different paths that will eventually bring you to the same desired destination: a clear, organized review of existing theory and research on the chosen topic that ends with a summary of current knowledge and potential directions for future research.

Before you begin writing, look over the materials accumulated, and outline what you have found. Use brief terms and general categories. Don't try to include the details at this point. Move the categories around until they begin to form a logical sequence. Then fill in a little more of the details, enough so that you can imagine the flow of the final product.

Galvan (2006) suggests creating tables to organize what by now may be a "mountain" of information on your topic. If your mountain is really only a small hill, you may not have to do this. But if you are overwhelmed by the amount and complexity of what you have found, these tables may be very helpful.

For example, you can begin by listing the most important definitional terms and then adding explanations of what they mean and how they are related to your topic. Be sure to note whatever is a direct quote and to put the reference right next to the definitions and quotes. It can be difficult to find the reference later.

Once the most important terms are defined, create another table for important theoretical work. To do this in a logical fashion, refer to Chapter 3, "Theory," and use a concept tree as your guide.

Next you build tables for related research studies. Begin with the source or reference, then list the type of study (such as a survey or an intervention study), the sample, measures (or information gathering techniques for qualitative studies), and relevant findings.

You may need several tables on different aspects of the work to be comprehensive. For example, if you are writing a review of the research on depression in children, you might divide the research studies into several categories:

- Incidence and prevalence of depression in children

- Effects of childhood depression on the child and family

- Factors related to childhood depression: physiological, interpersonal, situational, intrapersonal, and so on

- Treatment: pharmacological and nonpharmacological

When the tables are done, you can begin writing the narrative. Keep your outline and tables at hand when you do this. Write the narrative from the outline and tables, checking the original sources as you need to.

The end product of this step is your *first draft*. If you have time, set it aside for a day or two, then return to it, reading it critically as if you were reading it for the first time. Some prefer to read their draft aloud, but finding an attentive audience may be a challenge. Once you have revised and corrected the first draft, it is ready for review by a mentor or colleague. Use their comments and a second reading that you have done to polish your work to create a clear, logical, and persuasive argument for your proposed research study.

A few final do's and don'ts, some based on Galvan's (2006) advice, follow.

The Do List

- Summarize the literature.

- Synthesize, showing connections, similarities, and differences, among the studies reviewed.

- Add a small amount of commentary that increases the reader interest and adds depth to your review.

- Use headings and subheadings liberally.

- Summarize your review at the end. Or, if the review is very long, at several points within the review.

- Connect the review with your proposed study.

The Do Not List

- Simply report findings without any critique (that the sample is too small or nonrandom, for example) or synthesis (connections to theory and other studies).

- Use too many abbreviations (BP, HBP, CVA, AD, SCID, NPI, etc.); use only the few most common abbreviations in your topic area and explain them the first time they are used.

- Use lengthy quotes or large numbers of quotes. Instead, paraphrase when you can.

- Fail to recognize the source of ideas if they did not originate with you.

- Use different terms for the same idea. This is not creative writing, it is scientific writing. Strive for accuracy and consistency.

- Use the largest words possible or try to impress with obscure or flowery phrases. Elegant simplicity is your goal.

CONCLUSION

Consider your search of the literature a voyage of discovery. This is your opportunity to gain an in-depth understanding of the theory and research related to your topic. You should be an expert on the topic by the time the review of the literature is completed. You also will likely have gained an appreciation of the work others have done and some very valuable insight into how you should proceed in planning your own study.

REFERENCES

Barroso, J., Gallop, C. J., Sandelowski, M., Maynell, J., Pearce, P. F., & Collins, L. J. (2003). The challenges of searching for and retrieving qualitative studies. *Western Journal of Nursing Research, 25*(2), 153–178.

Bates, M. J. (1989). The design of browsing and berry picking techniques for online search interface. *Online Review, 13*(5), 407–424.

Galvan, J. L. (2006). Writing literature reviews. Glendale, CA: Pyrczak Publishing.
  ✧ A very detailed (almost too detailed), very readable guide to writing a literature review. There are few shortcuts here but the guidelines and suggestions will help you write an excellent review of the literature. The Self-Editing Checklist and examples at the end of the book are especially helpful.

Morrisey, L. J., & DeBourgh, G. A. (2001). Finding evidence: Refining literature searching skills for the advanced practice nurse. *AACN Clinical Issues, 12*(4), 560–577.
  ✧ Some useful guidelines and tips for conducting database searches with an emphasis on evidence-based practice.

Rau, J. L. (2004). Searching the literature and selecting the right references. *Respiratory Care, 49*(10), 1242–1245.
  ✧ Practical guide to using PubMed/MEDLINE.

CHAPTER 3

Theory

Theory is essential to research. It provides the perspective from which you think about the phenomenon under consideration and design the research study. This is not a one-way street: not only does theory inform research, but research also informs theory (Figure 3-1). In fact, some research methods have been specifically designed to generate theory. Glaser and Strauss's (1967) grounded theory, which is described in a later chapter, is one example.

In this chapter, we will first review some important theory-related definitions. Then we will consider the relationship between theory and research, the development level of various theories, and the multiple levels of theory, from the broadest worldviews to the most discrete, specific operational definitions.

IMPORTANT DEFINITIONS

Theory

There are many definitions of theory. Most simply, a theory may be defined as a statement that describes and/or explains phenomena (Barnum, 1990). Caring theory, for example, provides a description of what occurs between nurse and patient within a caring relationship. Stress theory provides descriptions of what stress is, sources of stress, and how stress affects health.

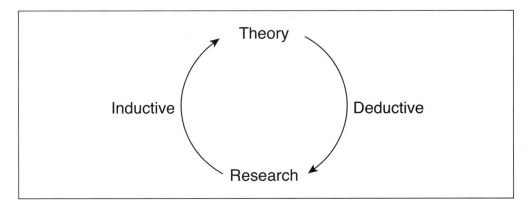

Figure 3-1   The relationship between theory and research.

Here is a more complex but important definition of theory: A set of interrelated concepts and propositions that explain and predict phenomena (Kerlinger, 1986). For example, the six Cs of caring, which are competence, confidence, compassion, conscience, and commitment, describe the caring behaviors of nurses (Roach, 1984). Similarly, Holmes and Rahe (1967) created a list of 43 life changes that they theorized would contribute to stress including trouble with one's boss, pregnancy, and divorce (note that even positive changes are thought to contribute to stress).

Induction and Deduction

Induction and deduction describe the interaction of theory and research. The terms come from ancient Latin words and are used in the study of logic. *Induction* comes from the Latin term meaning "lead in" or "bring into." From logic, induction means drawing a conclusion from particular facts. For our purposes it means developing theory (the conclusion) from the results of research (the particular facts).

Deduction is the opposite. It comes from the Latin term for "lead away." From logic, deduction means reasoning from a known (generally accepted) principle to the as yet unknown or from the general to the specific. For our purposes, it means using theoretical propositions (the known that is generally accepted) to inform our research study (which, until it is done, is the unknown) (*Webster's Unabridged Dictionary*, 1999). You might want to look at Figure 3-1 again to see these relationships illustrated.

Another way to describe the difference between induction and deduction is that induction is the process of theory development, and deduction is the process of theory testing (Fawcett, 1999). You can see, then, that research and theory are highly interrelated. Research may be used to either generate theory or to test it, or both.

DEVELOPMENT STAGES OF THEORIES

Descriptive

At their most basic level, theories simply name, describe and classify phenomena of interest. You may remember from your basic science courses the complex classification and naming conventions for microorganisms such as the A N1H1 swine flu virus. In nursing, the stages of grieving or of a decubitus ulcer are familiar examples. All of these are *descriptive* theoretical statements.

Explanatory

At this next level of development, theories include statements of relationships between phenomena. The relationships are often demonstrated using correlational statistics. For example, high Graduate Record Examination (GRE) test scores have been found to be related to success in graduate school (Brownstein, Green, Hilbert, & Weiner, 1999). Relationships between high levels of stress and a number of health problems have been theorized. Isolation in old age is associated with increased depression. Carotenoids are associated with inhibition of bone breakdown and resorption (Sahni et al., 2009). All of these are at the explanatory or relational stage of theory development.

Predictive

At this highest level of development, theories, predict outcomes given one or more specific inputs. For example, the germ theory of disease predicts that the presence of a sufficient amount of a particular microorganism such as *Streptococcus pneumoniae* (the input) will cause pneumonia (the outcome). Most of these predictions are actually more complex than a single input, however. For example, an individual's level of resistance affects whether or not pneumonia will develop as does the use of prophylactic antibiotics. Likewise, the combination of poor nutrition, immobility, poor circulation, and increased pressure on a bony prominence is predicted to result in a pressure ulcer. Low stimulation is predicted to retard brain development in infants, and inadequate contact is predicted to reduce parent–infant bonding.

USING RESEARCH TO TEST THEORY

Some nursing theorists have put considerable effort into testing their theories and have encouraged others to test them as well.

A number of nurse researchers have tested concepts and propositions derived from King's systems framework for nursing and related midrange theory of goal attainment. For example, Froman (1995) hypothesized that the greater the perceptual congruence between nurse and client, the greater the degree of goal attainment would be achieved (p. 225). She used a researcher-designed Perceptual Congruency Questionnaire to test this hypothesis and found that many perceptions of the nurse and patient respondents were dissimilar. For example, 53% of the nurses did not know what patients believed caused their illness, and 35% were unsure what the patients needed to know to care for themselves at home, suggesting that "validation by nurses with their clients about the means to achieve client goals may occur minimally in actual practice" (p. 235). A moderate relationship between perceptual congruency and satisfaction with care ($r^1 = .43$) was also found providing modest support for the importance of perceptual congruency. Based on King's theory, Hobdell (1995) predicted that perceptual accuracy is affected by mood state. She also found partial support for the hypothesized relationship between chronic sorrow and accuracy of parents' perception of the child's cognitive development in parents of children with neural tube defects, finding it in the fathers but not the mothers. Studies such as these should eventually lead to refinements of King's theory.

$^1 r$ = Correlation coefficient for bivariate analysis.

Kolcaba's work demonstrates the importance of treating theory as dynamic rather than static in nature. In the development and testing of her comfort theory, Kolcaba (2003) used data from testing of her Radiation Therapy Comfort Questionnaire (RTCQ) to determine whether comfort had both state (immediate) and trait (long-term) dimensions as anxiety has been found to have. To do this, Kolcaba and colleagues compared results on the RTCQ at three time points and found that they were not highly correlated, suggesting that comfort is primarily a state characteristic. Relief and ease seemed to be more state specific than did transcendence. Based upon these results, Kolcaba suggests that the characteristic of being able to transcend stressful situations may be a trait (p. 71), but that relief and ease dimensions of comfort are probably state characteristics.

Zeigler and colleagues (2005) reviewed the research support for a number of midrange theories that are familiar to nurses. Here is what they found about several of them:

Aguilera's Crisis Intervention	Research support is limited, but suggests that when the intervention is clearly defined and the interventionists are well trained, crisis intervention may be effective.
Peplau's Interpersonal Relationships	Peplau used an approach similar to grounded theory to develop her interpersonal theory. Primarily qualitative studies and case studies supporting this theory were found. Forchuk (1993) notes that researchers such as Morrison and Shealy (quoted by Forchuk) found that both taking the role of friend and self-disclosure, which are discouraged by Peplau, are frequently used by nurses. Similarly, Williams and Tappen (1999) found the sharing of personal information by the nurse to facilitate development of therapeutic relationships with cognitively impaired individuals. These findings suggest possible modifications to Peplau's theory.
Lewin's Change Theory	Lewin developed action research to evaluate his approach to implementing change, but Zeigler et al. (2005) note that more evidence for its efficacy in practice is needed. Of interest for example, is Semin-Goossens and colleagues' (2003) article, the title of which is particularly informative: "A failed model-based attempt to implement an evidence-based nursing guideline for fall prevention."
Lazarus' Coping Theory	Coping has been frequently studied but is difficult to test experimentally. One reason may be that different people find different strategies suit them best, making generalization difficult.
Erikson's Stages of Growth and Development	These stages were based on Erikson's observations (qualitative data). It is interesting that, while Erikson's focus is primarily on childhood, most of the studies using his stages have been concerned with adults. Some research measurement tools have been based upon Erikson's stages (Zeigler et al., 2005).

USING THEORY TO INFORM RESEARCH

How powerful is the influence of theory on research? Dan Everett, a linguistics professor who studies the languages of remote Brazilian tribes, describes its power quite eloquently, "We ask the questions that our theories tell us to ask" (Colapinto, 2008, p. 27).

We now consider the other half of the research-theory interaction illustrated in Figure 3-1. Every research study has at least an implied worldview, a lens through which the world is viewed and interpreted, even if it is not specifically stated. At the very least, the researcher has elected to use either the scientific methods associated with quantitative research or one of the qualitative approaches with its underlying philosophy (more about this in a later chapter). Most studies also have an implied theoretical base upon which they have been developed. This implied theoretical base may be the germ theory, that infectious organisms cause disease; it may simply be the assumption that humans live in a state of either health or illness or somewhere along the health–illness continuum; or it may be that a combination of biopsychosocial factors affects an individual's health. A few examples follow.

Although not previously well developed according to the researchers, the concept of symptom clusters was the underlying idea for Barsevick, Dudley, and Beck's (2006) secondary analysis of data from an intervention study. They linked this concept (symptom clusters) to Lenz and colleagues' midrange theory of unpleasant symptoms. Barsevick and colleagues evaluated the relationship between two cancer treatment-related symptoms, fatigue and depression, and an important outcome, functional status. They found that their intervention, teaching energy conservation coping skills, changed the relationship between fatigue, depression, and function. In the control group, when fatigue made routine activities difficult to perform, depressive symptomatology increased. This did not occur in the experimental group. They suggested that individuals in the experimental group learned how to prioritize the activities in which they invested their energy, alleviating the depressive reaction.

Limitations and the need for further development of existing concepts, theories, and frameworks are often indicated in the reviews of theory underpinning research studies. For example, Meek and colleagues (2000) noted that existing conceptual frameworks for cancer treatment-related fatigue do not provide specific guidance on factors to include when measuring it. They also note its close association with depression, muscle weakness, and functional status. Also of interest is the idea that fatigue is conceptualized to be a sensation and a self-perceived state and, therefore, should be measured using self-report.

The selection and design of an intervention is also influenced by theory. Carrieri-Kohlman and colleagues (2001) tested a theory-based model for the management of dyspnea. Conceptualizing dyspnea as a symptom that induces anxiety, they hypothesized that monitored exposure to greater than usual degrees of dyspnea during exercise in a safe environment would change the individual's appraisal of this symptom, thereby reducing anxiety and increasing tolerance for dyspnea. This is based upon the concept of desensitization: repeated exposure to a fearful stimulus will reduce the fear and anxiety associated with it. The work of Bandura, Williams, and their colleagues suggested the use of guided mastery, defined for this study as "active guidance with the teaching of coping skills used by a therapist" (Carrieri-Kohlman et al., 2001, p. 137). Their intervention study compared exposure (simple desensitization) to guided mastery, but no differences between the two approaches were found. This necessitated going back to the theory to consider why no difference was found. The researchers suggested several alternative explanations: the classic desensitization theory is sufficient; there may be a learning or practice effect; or the participants may have adapted to the sensation of dyspnea. Note that these explanations are based upon differing but potentially relevant theories.

THE CONCEPT TREE

The terms *theory*, *concept*, and related words are often used loosely, making it difficult for the new researcher to sort out their interrelationships and clarify the theoretical underpinnings of a research study.

In this section, we look closely at the many levels and degrees of specificity of theoretical works, from the broadest worldviews to the narrowest operational definitions. The purpose of creating a conceptual "tree" (it is a tree only in one's imagination) is to help you think more clearly about the theoretical aspects of your research.

The concept tree is an *heuristic*, a guide to thinking about and articulating the theoretical foundation of your research. We begin by looking at an empty tree (Figure 3-2), considering what each level means and how it relates to the levels above and below. The tree illustrates the progression from the concrete to the abstract, from the simple to the complex and from the micro (small, narrow) perspective to the macro (large, broad) perspective. Next we consider a filled-in tree that illustrates how the levels connect to form a comprehensive theoretical base for a research study. The tree diagram can help you organize ideas, but you will have to contribute the ideas from your own knowledge base, your reading, and discussion with colleagues in the field. We will begin at the top of the tree and work our way down to its roots, the empirical indicators.

Conceptual Frameworks

Conceptual frameworks are the broadest of theories. They have been compared to maps or lenses through which we view the world. Conceptual frameworks developed for nursing usually address very broad (metaparadigm) ideas about person, health, and environment (Frey, 1995). Conceptual frameworks guide our exploration of knowledge (i.e., our inquiries) (Newman, Smith, Pharris, & Jones, 2008) and the way in which we interpret our experience.

Conceptual frameworks usually address foundational ideas, both conceptual and philosophical (Kim & Kollak, 2006). For example, King's systems framework assumes that humans are open systems transacting with their environment. Human beings are described as unique, holistic, sentient, social, and purposeful. Concepts within the framework include self, perception, communication, interaction, and so forth (King, 1995).

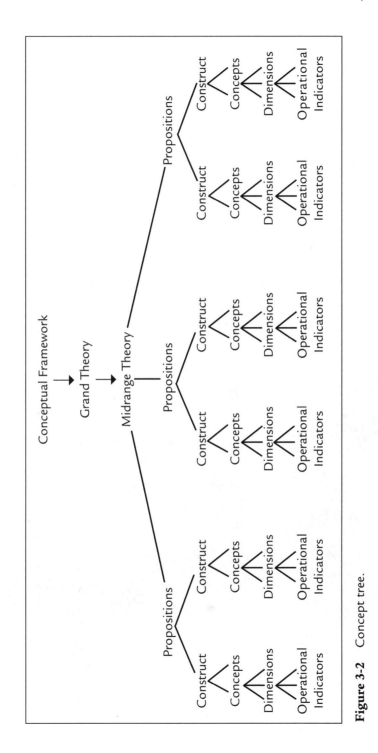

Figure 3-2 Concept tree.

Grand Theory

These are overarching theories that are almost as broad as the conceptual frameworks. In fact, it is not always necessary to identify both a conceptual framework and a grand theory. Grand theories commonly used in nursing research may be derived from theories of other disciplines or developed within nursing. They create a structure to organize knowledge and to define practice (Newman et al., 2008). Rogers' (1970) science of unitary human beings is an example of a nursing-based grand theory. Rogers proposed three principles of homeodynamics that evolved as she continued to elaborate upon her theory. Another example is Leininger's transcultural nursing (Leininger, 1978; Leininger & McFarland, 2002), which focuses on caring and transculturality.

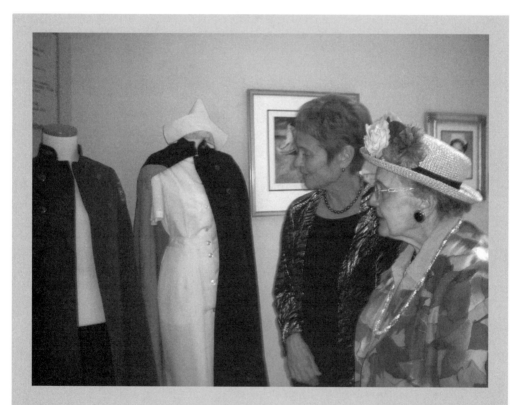

Nurse theorists Dr. Anne Boykin and Dr. Madeleine Leininger shown above at the dedication of the Leininger Collection to be housed in the Christine E. Lynn College of Nursing Archives of Caring in Nursing, Florida Atlantic University, Boca Raton, Florida.

Source: Courtesy of Ruth Tappen, EdD, RN, FAAN.

Midrange Theory

Midrange theories are more focused, less grand theories to which much attention has been given recently in nursing. Middle range theories are sets of related ideas focused on a limited area of knowledge (Smith & Liehr, 2008, p. xvii). These are the workhorses of nursing theory. They connect the grand theories to the constructs and concepts we use in both research and practice. They are far more limited in scope than the grand theories, but they are also more concrete and specific. It is often difficult to bridge the gap between a conceptual framework or grand theory and a research study without midrange theory. Examples of midrange theory include chronic sorrow, unpleasant symptoms, and cultural marginality.

Symptom management is a relatively well-developed midrange theory that includes the symptom experiences, symptom management strategies, and the outcomes of symptom management (Humphreys et al., 2008). The concept of symptom clusters, such as nausea and vomiting, pain and disturbed sleep, or chest tightness, wheezing, and coughing during an asthma attack is a relatively new addition to the theory of symptom management. Quite a few clinical research studies have used this midrange theory, but none so far have tested the theory as a whole (Humphreys et al., 2008).

Propositions

Propositions are statements about a concept or several concepts (Fawcett, 1999). They may describe the characteristics of a phenomenon or predict a relationship between concepts. Propositions may be quite general, or they may refer to very specific situations. For example, a proposition may state that children with attention deficit disorder (ADD) have lower self-esteem than do children without ADD, specifying the relationship between ADD and self-esteem. The proposition that meditation can lower elevated blood pressure predicts the relationship between blood pressure and meditation.

Constructs and Concepts

Because constructs are simply more abstract, more complex, and less observable concepts, they are listed together with concepts. Concepts are frequently called the "basic building blocks of nursing knowledge" (Waltz, Strickland, & Lenz, 2005, p. 22). They are theoretical definitions of phenomena. It is usually not necessary to include both constructs and concepts on a concept tree.

Concepts familiar in nursing vary widely in the degree to which they have matured, in other words, how stable and well defined they are. Morse, Hupcey, Mitcham, and Lenz (1998, p. 76) list criteria for mature concepts:

- Clearly defined
- Distinct (well differentiated from other concepts)
- Coherent

- Systematically related to other concepts
- Applicable to real life practice

A few examples of concepts relevant to nursing include gaze, empathy, dignity, perfusion, balance, dyspnea, REM sleep, and so forth.

Dimensions

Most concepts and constructs have more than one dimension or attribute. Waltz and colleagues (2005) compared the unidimensional concepts of syringe or perfusion (defined as partial pressure of transcutaneous oxygen) with multidimensional concepts such as ADLs (activities of daily living) that generally includes the dimensions of bathing, dressing, toileting, eating, and dressing.

Operational Indicators

Operational or empirical indicators are the means by which the theoretical unit (concept) is measured. They are defined by Dubin (1978, p. 182) as the "operation employed by a researcher to secure measurements of [a given] value" on the theoretical unit. Dubin also notes that many behavioral concepts are somewhat vague, making measurement of them a considerable challenge, calling this a "vexing problem" for researchers.

CONCEPT TREE EXAMPLE

A concept tree created to provide the theoretical foundation for development of a new measure of acculturative stress (E. Millender, personal communication, June 8, 2009) will be used to illustrate use of the concept tree in developing a research study (see Figure 3-3).

Conceptual framework Sir Edward Tylor (1871), a British anthropologist, is credited with the first definition of the term *culture*: "that complex whole which includes knowledge, belief, art, morals, law, custom, and any other capabilities and habits acquired by man as a member of society" (quoted by Andrews & Boyle, 1989, p. 11).

Grand theory Leininger's Transcultural Nursing theory connects culture with the practice of nursing. Leininger (1978) wrote that transcultural nursing is "the subfield of nursing that focuses upon a comparative study and analysis of different cultures and subcultures in the world with respect to their caring behavior; nursing care; and health-illness values, beliefs, and patterns of behavior with the goal of developing a scientific and humanistic body of knowledge in order to provide culture-specific and culture-universal nursing care practices" (p. 8).

Midrange theories Acculturation is the phenomenon that results "when groups of individuals having different cultures come into continuous first-hand contact, with

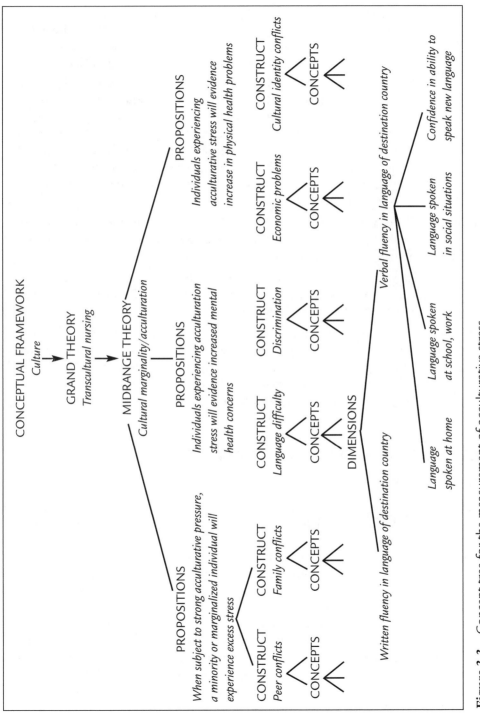

Figure 3-3 Concept tree for the measurement of acculturative stress.

Source of Content for the Concept Tree: E. Millender, personal communication, June 8, 2009.

subsequent changes in the original cultural patterns of either or both groups" (Redfield, Linton, & Herskovits, 1936, p. 149). Cultural marginality is defined as "marginal living while recognizing across-culture conflicts and striving to ease cultural tension" (Choi, 2008, p. 247).

Propositions The three propositions (Figure 3-3) suggest that immigrants to the United States, particularly those who are members of US minority groups, experience cultural marginality and related acculturative stress that affects both mental and physical health. Andrews and Boyle (1999) defined minority as "groups of people who, because of physical or cultural characteristics, receive different and unequal treatment from others in society," and may "see themselves as recipients of collective discrimination" (p. 16).

Constructs The constructs are the problems and conflicts that are frequently linked to acculturation stress. Because they are relatively complex phenomena, they are labeled constructs rather than concepts.

Dimensions Only the dimensions for the language difficulty construct are included in Figure 3-3. These are verbal and written fluency in the dominant language of the host (destination) country.

Operational indicators Several operational indicators are listed. These include the individual preference for his or her original language or language of the host country, actual language use, confidence in ability to speak the new language and actual ability. (Note that language difficulties are experienced primarily by those who come to the United States from non-English speaking countries.)

ISSUES RELATED TO THEORY AND RESEARCH

Confirmation Bias

Greenwald and colleagues (1986) have noted what they call a *confirmation bias* that often occurs in the testing of theory. Particularly, there is always the danger that researchers will see what they expect to see—and this is true for not only qualitative research. For example, Turkel and colleagues (1999) did a phenomenological analysis of nurses' descriptions of their experiences visiting patients at home after discharge from a rehabilitation unit. The interviewed nurses clearly found the home nursing experience to be very different from their usual role and very satisfying. Viewing the nurses' narratives through the lens of caring theory, the researchers concluded it was evident "that developing a caring relationship with patients was essential to nurses feeling rewarded in their work" (p. 11). The nurses interviewed had not used the term *caring relationship*. Was the researchers' conclusion erroneous? Not at all, but it was expressed in the language of caring theory. Had the researchers come from a different theoretical perspective, they likely would have used different language to characterize the nurses' experiences.

Those researchers who are interested in a particular theory are also those who are likely to spend time testing it. They are likely to become strong advocates for the theory, which creates the risk of confirmation bias. Such researchers may report confirming evidence but ignore or discount disconfirming evidence. Their investment in the theory can also blind them to new theoretical formulations. These are cautionary statements, not a call for ignoring theory but for keeping an open mind about the theory used.

The history of cancer research provides an example of the way in which one's paradigm guides research but may also inhibit thinking outside the box. Kevles (1995) describes one such example. Once the existence and disease-producing potential of microorganisms was established, scientists began to look for a connection to cancer but without success. Then a biologist at the Rockefeller Institute injected an extract from an avian breast tumor into healthy chickens who developed sarcomas as a result. Others tried to replicate his work in other healthy animals but failed. Eventually, scientists concluded that these "infectious" cancers did not occur in humans and, as Kevles puts it, "those who held to the theory [publicly] risked their scientific reputations" (p. 76).

A curious finding led researchers back to the infectious theory, though with initial reluctance. In a lab that produced mice with a tendency to develop tumors, John Bittner noticed that the mice developed breast cancer at a high rate if their mother was part of the high-incidence strain but not if only their father was part of the high-incidence strain. At first, they suggested a "milk factor" as the agent, reluctant to use the word *virus*. After years of hiding behind the term *factor*, which alluded to the prevalent genetic theory of causation, and after further research and much debate, the researchers finally recognized the factor for what it was: a mouse mammary tumor virus (Kevles, 1995). The power of theory is evident: it both drove their research and inhibited it, in this case for decades.

Theory is dynamic, not static. In other words, theory should be modified as new evidence to support or refute it is found. It is more troubling when scholars (researchers and theorists) do not change their conclusions than if they propose revisions as they develop their work (Colapinto, 2008).

Nursing or Nonnursing Theory?

There is considerable disagreement within the discipline as to whether a nurse researcher should use only those theories generated within the discipline or use whatever theory, nursing or not, best informs his or her research.

Fawcett (2006) points out that many nurse practitioners and advanced practice nurses base their practice on medical knowledge instead of nursing knowledge, as well as basing their practice on nonnursing research. The nursing profession needs a solid scholarly and scientific foundation (Anderson, 1995). Nursing needs its own scholarship and research, not that borrowed from other disciplines. To accomplish this, Fawcett argues that we "must break the intellectual chains . . . by rejecting nonnursing knowledge . . . and embracing nursing knowledge" (2006, p. 515).

Waltz, Strickland, and Lenz (2005) counter that knowledge is not "owned" by any discipline. Nursing scholars and researchers can use and build on knowledge from other disciplines, but they can do it with a nursing perspective (p. 26).

CONCLUSION

The intimate connection between theory and research should now be evident to you. Research always has at least a worldview or framework underlying it, even if it is only implied. Theories need to be tested, and the results should be used to elaborate upon or to modify the theory, but this has not always been done. Further, our theoretical statements and propositions are often vague or poorly developed, posing some challenges for the researcher. Using the concept tree as an organizer can help clarify these relationships before proceeding with designing your research study.

REFERENCES

Anderson, E. A. (1995). Scholarship: How important is it? *Nursing Outlook, 43*, 247–248.

Andrews, M. M., & Boyle, J. S. (1989). *Transcultural concepts in nursing care*. Philadelphia: Lippincott, Williams & Wilkins.

Barnum, B. J. S. (1990). *Nursing theory: Analysis, application, evaluation*. Glenview, IL: Scott, Foresman/Little Brown Higher Education.

Barsevick, A. M., Dudley, W., & Beck, S. L. (2006). Cancer-related fatigue, depressive symptoms and functional status. *Nursing Research, 55*(5), 366–372.

Brownstein, S. C., Green, S., Hilbert, S., & Weiner, M. (1999). *How to prepare for the GRE with CD-Rom*. New York: Barrons.

Carrieri-Kohlman, V., Gormley, J. M., Eiser, S., Demir-Deviren, S., Nguyen, H., Paul, S. H., et al. (2001). Dyspnea and the affective response during exercise training in obstructive pulmonary disease. *Nursing Research, 50*(3), 136–146.

Choi, H. (2008). Theory of cultural marginality. In M. Smith & P. R. Liehr (Eds.), *Middle range theory for nursing* (pp. 243–250). New York: Springer.

Colapinto, J. (2008). The interpreter. In J. Groopman (Ed.), *The best American science and nature writing 2008* (pp. 9–38). Boston: Houghton Mifflin.

Dubin, R. (1978). *Theory building*. New York: Free Press.

Fawcett, J. (2006). Nursing philosophies, models and theories: A focus on the future. In M. R. Alligood & A. Toomy, *Nursing theory: Utilization and application* (pp. 499–518). St. Louis, MO: Elsevier, Mosby.

Fawcett, J. (1999). *The relationship of theory and research* (3rd ed.). Philadelphia: F.A. Davis.

Forchuk, C. (1993). *Hildegard E. Peplau: Interpersonal nursing theory*. Newbury Park, CA: Sage.

Froman, D. (1995). Perceptual congruency between clients and nurses: Testing King's theory of goal attainment. In M. A. Frey & C. L. Sieloff (Eds.), *Advancing King's systems framework and theory of nursing* (pp. 223–238). Thousand Oaks, CA: Sage.

Frey, M. A. (1995). From conceptual framework to nursing knowledge. In M. A. Frey & C. L. Sieloff (Eds.), *Advancing King's systems framework and theory of nursing* (pp. 3–13). Thousand Oaks, CA: Sage.

Glaser, B. G., & Strauss, A. L. (1967). *The discovery of grounded theory: Strategies for qualitative research*. New York: Aldine de Gruyter.

Greenwald, A. G., Leippe, M. R., Pratkanus, A. R., & Baumgardner, M. H. (1986). Under what conditions does theory obstruct research progress? *Psychological Review, 93*, 216–229.

Hobdell, E. F. (1995). Using King's interacting systems framework for research on parents of children with neural tube defects. In M. A. Frey & C. L. Sieloff (Eds.), *Advancing King's systems framework and theory of nursing* (pp. 126–136). Thousand Oaks, CA: Sage.

Holmes, T. H., & Rahe, R. (1967). The social readjustment rating scale. *Journal of Psychosomatic Research, 2,* 213.

Humphreys, J., Lee, K. A., Carrieri-Kuhlman, V., Puntillo, K., Faucett, J., Janson, S., et al. (2008). Theory of symptom management. In M. J. Smith & P. Liehr (Eds.), *Middle range theory for nursing* (pp. 145–158). New York: Springer.

Johns, C., & Freshwater, D. (2005). *Transforming nursing through reflective practice.* Oxford, UK: Blackwell.
   ◇ Inspiring, thought-provoking essays on mindfulness in nursing practice.

Kerlinger, F. (1986). *Foundations of behavioral research.* Chicago, IL: Holt, Rinehart & Winston.

Kevles, D. J. (1995). Pursuing the unpopular: A history of courage, viruses, and cancer. In R. B. Silver (Ed.), *Hidden histories of science* (pp. 69–114). New York: New York Review of Books.

Kim, H. S., & Kollak, I. (2006). *Nursing theories: Conceptual and philosophical foundations.* New York: Springer.
   ◇ An interesting collection of well researched essays on such fundamental ideas as human needs, interpersonal relations and systems theory by an international group of nursing scholars. Provides a window into the sources and inspiration for many of our nursing theories.

King, I. M. (1995). A system framework for nursing. In M. A. Frey & C. L. Sieloff (Eds.), *Advancing King's systems framework and theory of nursing* (pp. 14–22). Thousand Oaks, CA: Sage.

Kolcaba, K. (2003). *Comfort theory and practice: A vision for holistic health care.* New York: Springer.

Leininger, M. (1978). *Transcultural nursing: Concepts, theories, and practices.* New York: John Wiley & Sons.

Leininger, M., & McFarland, M. R. (2002). *Transcultural nursing: Concepts, theories, research, and practice* (3rd ed.). New York: McGraw Hill.

Meek, P. M., Nail, L. M., Barsevick, A., Schwartz, A. L., Stephen, S., Whitmayer, K., et al. (2000). Psychometric testing of fatigue instruments for use with cancer patients. *Nursing Research, 49*(4), 181–190.

Morse, J. M., Hupcey, J. E., Mitcham, C., & Lenz, E. R. (1998). Choosing a strategy for concept analysis in nursing research: Moving beyond Wilson. In A. G. Gift (Ed.), *Clarifying concepts in nursing research* (pp. 73–96). New York: Springer.

Newman, M. A., Smith, M. C., Pharris, M. D., & Jones, D. (2008). The focus of a discipline revisited. *Advances in Nursing Science, 31*(1), E16–E27.

Redfield, R., Linton, R., & Herskovits, M. J. (1936). Memorandum for the study of acculturation. *American Anthropologist, 38,* 149–152.

Roach, M. S. (1984). Caring: The human mode of being, implications for nursing. *Perspectives in Caring Monograph 1.* Toronto, Canada: Faculty of Nursing, University of Toronto.

Rogers, M. C. (1970). *An introduction to the theoretical basis of nursing.* Philadelphia: F.A. Davis.

Sahni, S., Hannan, M. T., Blumberg, J., Cupples, L. A., Kiel, D. P., & Tucker, K. L. (2009). Inverse association of carotenoid intakes with 4-y change in bone mineral density in elderly men and women: The Framingham Osteoporosis Study. *American Journal of Clinical Nutrition, 89,* 416–424.

Semin-Goossens, A., van de Helm, J. M., & Bossuyt, P. M. M. (2003). A failed model-based attempt to implement an evidence-based nursing guideline for fall prevention. *Journal of Nursing Care Quality, 18*(3), 217–225.

Smith, J. J., & Liehr, P. R. (2008). *Middle range theory for nursing.* New York: Springer.
   ◇ A nice collection of middle range theories developed or applied within the discipline of nursing as well as some helpful chapters related to theory and evaluation of theories.

Turkel, M., Tappen, R. M., & Hall, R. (1999). Moments of excellence. Nurses' response to role redesign in long-term care. *Journal of Gerontological Nursing, 25*(1), 7–12.

Tylor, E. (1871). *Primitive culture*. New York: J. P. Putnam's Sons.

Waltz, C. F., Strickland, O. L., & Lenz, E. R. (2005). *Measurement in nursing and health research*. New York: Springer.

⬧ An excellent, although advanced, text on measurement in nursing.

Webster's Unabridged Dictionary. (1999). (2nd ed.) New York: Random House.

Williams, C. L., & Tappen, R. M. (1999). Can we create a therapeutic relationship with nursing home residents in the later stages of Alzheimer's disease? *Journal of Psychosocial Nursing, 37*(3), 28–35.

Zeigler, S. M. (2005). *Theory-directed nursing practice* (2nd ed.). New York: Springer.

⬧ In this edited book, the authors review 11 mid-range theories frequently used in nursing (only Peplau's theory originated in nursing). Of most interest are the brief summaries of the research support for each of those theories and Appendix C where the author explains why these particular theories were selected.

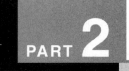

PART **2**

Design Phase

CHAPTER 4

Quantitative or Qualitative Research?

There has been a long-running debate in nursing research between the "quants" and the "quals," that is, between those who primarily do quantitative research and those who do qualitative research. Sometimes the debate is subdued and civil; other times it is quite heated. The arguments are not limited to nurses or to health care. You can find similar debates in education, sociology, communication, international relations, and many other disciplines.

Even the definition of these two major types of research stimulates disagreement. There is also disagreement as to what constitutes research (the definition can be stretched quite far in the qualitative camp): whether research is a craft or a calling, what its purpose is, and the worldview that informs the research.

We will not resolve this argument in this chapter although we will try to find common ground where it is possible. Nor will we try to be comprehensive in covering the subject because it has filled whole books and journals. Instead, the purpose is to inform you, allowing you to choose sides if you wish or to work intelligently with both (there are some who believe this should not be done, by the way). It is important to make informed choices because they will affect the language and methods you use, the funding available for your research, the subjects you study, the questions you ask, and the contribution to nursing knowledge and practice that you can make.

Instead of beginning at the top, or the philosophical level of debate, we will begin at the bottom, briefly considering the name-calling that goes on between the two camps. Then we will turn to more serious matters, reviewing definitions of qualitative and quantitative research, the types of research conducted under each rubric, the philosophical stance behind each, and the substance of the argument for each.

NAME-CALLING

Although usually done in a far more dignified manner than kids in the schoolyard would do, there clearly is some name-calling that occurs between the two camps. Sometimes it is subtle, other times strident, often indicating the strength of the feeling behind the words.

Qualitative research has been called loose, sloppy, subjective, poorly done, uncontrolled, fiction, politicized, art rather than science, useless, and without merit or significance. Some will say that it is not research at all.

Quantitative research, on the other hand, has been called controlled, cold, unfeeling, depersonalized, fragmented, limited, power based, distancing, and nonholistic. It is equated with empiricism and positivism which, for some, have become pejorative (disparaging) words.

Some of the differences between quantitative and qualitative research are reflected in this name-calling.

DEFINING QUANTITATIVE AND QUALITATIVE RESEARCH

The simplest and clearest distinction between quantitative and qualitative research is that quantitative research uses numbers while qualitative research does not (see Table 4-1 for an example). Unfortunately, this is too simple a distinction. On the one hand, qualitative researchers actually do count people, reporting their ages and other numeric values and sometimes quantify (code and count) their results. On the other hand, scientific research can be done without the use of numbers. The well-known litmus test, in which a liquid is dropped on paper treated with a lichen derivative that turns red if the liquid is acid and blue if the liquid is a base, is a basic scientific measure in chemistry but entirely qualitative (number free) (*The Free Dictionary*, 2009). There are many other examples, including the factors affecting the outcomes of collective bargaining negotiations, the effects of losing a child, and symptoms of schizophrenia (Katzner, 1983). Yet investigations of these phenomena are a part of scientific research.

Sandelowski (1986) notes, as we are discovering here, that the term *qualitative research* is not clearly distinguished from quantitative research and that they have overlapping characteristics. Further, some types of research may be either qualitative or quantitative. Historical research and feminist inquiry are two examples of research that may be either quantitative or qualitative.

Quantitative Research

Scientific or *quantitative research* as defined by Kerlinger is the "systematic, controlled, empirical and critical investigation of hypothetical propositions about presumed relations among natural phenomena" (1973, p. 18). The aim is to generate principles and

TABLE 4-1 Comparison of Qualitative and Quantitative Perspectives	
Newborn Baby Tomaselli: Which Column of Information Describes Him Best?	
Qualitative Data	**Quantitative Data**
Muscle tone firm	Weight 3400 g
Cry is vigorous	Length 49.5 cm
Moro reflex present	APGAR score at birth 9
Skin resilient, elastic	Gestational age 38 weeks
Abdominal respirations	Respirations 45/minute
Partial flexion of arms and legs	Pulse 140 beats/minute

propositions that describe and predict phenomena of interest and to be able to generalize to other situations. For example, when staff nurses are concerned about the risk of skin breakdown for an individual patient, they use a set of predictions that have been generated by scientific research on a large number of patients as the basis for creating a care plan. The predictors specify the factors that raise the risk of skin breakdown and need to be addressed to prevent its occurrence.

Qualitative Research

Qualitative research is defined by Creswell (1998) as follows:

> Qualitative research is an inquiry process of understanding, based on distinct methodological traditions of inquiry that explore a social or human problem. The researcher builds a complex, holistic picture, analyzes words, reports detailed views of informants, and conducts the study in a natural setting. (p. 15)

Denzin and Lincoln (2005) offer what they call a generic definition of qualitative research:

> Qualitative research is a situated activity that locates the observers in the world. It consists of a set of interpretive, material practices that make the world visible . . . They turn the world into a series of representations, including field notes, interviews, conversations, photographs, recordings, and memos to the self. (p. 3)

Qualitative researchers, they continue, "study things in their natural settings, attempting to make sense of, or interpret, phenomena in terms of the meanings people bring to them" (p. 3).

Differences

The differences between qualitative and quantitative research begin to emerge from these definitions. Table 4-2 compares some of the characteristics.

TABLE 4-2   Differences Between Qualitative and Quantitative Research

	Qualitative	Quantitative
Ultimate purpose	Discovery	Verification
Criteria for merit	Trustworthiness	Reliability and validity
View of reality	Subjective	Objective
Philosophical perspective	Naturalistic	Positivistic

Source: Based on Sandelowski, 1986.

Even these characterizations are an oversimplication (discovery, for example, occurs also in quantitative research), but they bring us a little closer to understanding qualitative and quantitative research.

Is there a difference in the impact of quantitative versus qualitative health information? Man-Son-Hing and colleagues (2002) compared the effects of qualitative and quantitative information about stroke prevention related to atrial fibrillation in patient decision making. The sample was 198 volunteers aged 60 to 80 who did not have atrial fibrillation. Outcome measures were a decisional conflict scale that measured uncertainty, therapy choices, risk level related to choice of treatment (no treatment, aspirin, or warfarin), knowledge, and how realistic these expectations were. In the qualitative treatment group, terms such as *moderate risk* were used in providing information about stroke risk to the study participants. In the quantitative treatment group, probabilities such as "8 out of 10" were used in providing information about stroke risk. Those who received the quantitative information felt more informed, were better able to estimate their risk and had more realistic expectations, but the two groups did not differ in overall knowledge about atrial fibrillation, its treatment, and other dimensions of the decisional conflict scale.

Next we will consider the types of research conducted under each rubric and then examine the most fundamental source of difference, the philosophical perspectives.

QUANTITATIVE AND QUALITATIVE METHODS

Later in this book there are entire chapters on the research methods of quantitative and qualitative research. Here we will consider the types of research done under each rubric to provide some sense of the scope of each.

Quantitative methods may be divided into experimental and nonexperimental studies. Experimental studies typically test a proposed intervention, comparing it with a placebo intervention or a control group. Here is an example:

> Paul and colleagues (2007) compared the effect of a single dose of honey and honey-flavored dextromethorphan given 30 minutes before bedtime to no treatment on 130 children with respiratory infections. Honey yielded the greatest improvement followed by dextromethorphan; giving no treatment yielded the least improvement.

Nonexperimental or descriptive quantitative studies cover a wide range of possibilities from simple correlational studies such as the relationship of self-efficacy to HgA1C in people with type I diabetes to very complex epidemiological and longitudinal studies such as the following:

- The Centers for Disease Control and Prevention (CDC) (Cisternas, Murphy, Croft, & Helmich, 2009) analyzed state and national total knee replacement (TKR) rates among Medicare enrollees for the years 2000 to 2006 in response to one of the *Healthy People 2010* objectives to reduce racial disparities in rate of total knee replacements among people age 75 and older. They found that rates of TKRs had increased for both blacks and whites. However, the overall TKR rate for blacks was 37% lower than it was for whites in 2000 and 39% lower in 2006. They concluded that little or no progress toward achieving the *Healthy People 2010* objective has been made.

- The Framingham Heart Study (About the Framingham Heart Study, n.d.) began in 1948 with the recruitment of 5209 men and women age 30 to 62 from the town of Framingham, Massachusetts. Since then, members of the second and third generations have been added to this longitudinal study. The initial focus was risk factors for cardiovascular disease: blood pressure, triglycerides, cholesterol, and so forth. More recently, risk factors for dementia and genetic patterns have also been studied. A few of their findings include:
  ○ Cigarette smoking increases the risk of disease.
  ○ High blood pressure increases the risk of stroke.
  ○ High levels of HDL cholesterol reduces risk of death.
  ○ Obesity is found to be a risk factor for heart failure.

This study has continued for over 60 years, providing valuable information about the prevention of stroke, heart disease, and dementia.

There is also meta-analysis, which can be quantitative or qualitative:

Yarcheski and colleagues (2009) conducted a quantitative meta-analysis of 72 studies concerning predictors of maternal-fetal attachment. They searched CINAHL, PsycINFO, MEDLINE, Social Science Index, and Dissertations and Theses for the years 1980 to 2006. They found moderate relationships between maternal-fetal attachment and social support, gestational age, and prenatal testing (the use of ultrasound). They suggest that ultrasound enhances the mother's attachment to her fetus and that that attachment intensifies as the pregnancy progresses. It is also interesting that age, ethnicity, marital status, income, and education had low effect sizes, and that the high-risk pregnancy effect was trivial.

Qualitative methods reflect an even greater variety of studies. The traditional qualitative methods include ethnography, phenomenology, grounded theory, case studies, and historical research. But this list just begins to give you an idea of what can be done with qualitative research. There is also content analysis, action research, feminist studies, queer theory, critical methodologies, and indigenous inquiry (Denzin & Lincoln, 2005; Denzin, Lincoln, & Smith, 2008).

Gance-Cleveland (2004) used ethnographic participant observation, interviews, and focus groups to study school-based support groups for adolescents with a chemically dependent parent. The researcher acted as cofacilitator of the groups. Audiotapes were transcribed verbatim. Features, functions, benefits, and weaknesses of the groups were the focus of this limited ethnography. The program manual for these support groups states that "The group experience aims to break down the unspoken family rules of don't talk, don't trust, and don't feel" (p. 382). Participants shared secrets and supported and challenged each other. Limitations included lack of access to school performance data and students who declined to participate or dropped out of the group. No individual interviews were conducted with any male students.

Fleming and Morse (1991) used grounded theory to address the male experience of physical changes during puberty. They interviewed 14 boys age 14 to 18 and eight teachers, parents, and other adults, two of whom were female. Interviews were tape recorded and transcribed. A male interviewer was used. A basic social psychological process of minimizing embarrassment was identified. This process was related to the boys feeling different about themselves, worrying about being different, and concealing these differences. Also identified were the stages of change: waiting for them, noticing them, dealing with them, and becoming comfortable with them (p. 215).

Kozuki and Kennedy (2004) reviewed 30 records from a bilingual (English-Japanese) private psychotherapy practice in the Pacific Northwest of the United States for a multiple case study research project. Of these, eight met criteria for selection. All were bilingual Japanese Americans and were interviewed at the time of referral to the Japanese therapist. The researchers found that cultural stereotypes hampered treatment (p. 34). Themes of cultural incommensurability were found, frequently resulting in misdiagnosis by Western therapists. For example, the psychological effects of immigration, especially alienation, were minimized by the Western therapists and culturally unique meanings were misunderstood:

> In Japanese culture, her somatic delusions such as "body is rotting from inside," "plum-shaped rashes," and "washing out body from inside out by taking lots of liquids," indicated her belief[s] that having an affair [actually an incident of rape] taints one's own body . . . the family name . . . and that she was infected by syphilis (plum disease). (pp. 34–35)

Dunphy (2001, 2003) conducted a historical study of the iron lung, also called a "steel cocoon." Iron lungs encased the patient's entire body using negative pressure body ventilation to breathe for the patient, most of whom had contracted polio before the 1955 introduction of an effective vaccine. The nursing challenges of caring for someone in an iron lung were many:

- Preventing skin breakdown
- Preventing aspiration
- Managing dysphagia
- Addressing the fear and anxiety of the patient
- Maintaining the machine

The real innovations in care came from the nurses on the job, not textbooks. For example, a patient recalled a nurse who "brought peas in with straws to see if we could hit

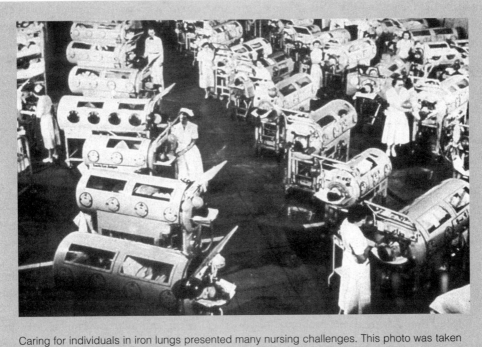

Caring for individuals in iron lungs presented many nursing challenges. This photo was taken on an iron lung ward at Rancho Los Amigos Hospital in California, c. 1953.

Source: Courtesy of the Centers for Disease Control and Prevention.

the ceiling (and increase our vital capacity)" (2003, p. 64I). In health-related disciplines, qualitative studies have gained increasing acceptance in recent years.

How important is qualitative research in nursing? Borreani and colleagues (2004) searched Medline and PsycINFO for qualitative research related to oncology and palliative care from 1989 to 2002. They found 411 articles of which 351 abstracts and 26 full papers met criteria and were reviewed. An astonishing 43% of the articles published before 1999 were found in nursing journals. More than half of the research studies used interviews. The largest percentage (17% to 22%) focused on the illness experience. A substantial proportion of the abstracts did not specify the design, data collection method, or sample size, although the number that did this did improve over time. The authors noted the wider acceptance of qualitative research over time, particularly the increased number appearing in medical journals.

PHILOSOPHICAL UNDERPINNINGS

A research paradigm is an accepted model or pattern of inquiry (Kuhn, 1996, p. 23). This model is shared by a community of scholars and researchers. In science, the model would include the laws, theories and propositions tested, the measurements used, and the research design, all of which are common to a community of researchers and scholars. This may be a community of physicists, sociologists, psychologists, physicians, or nurses.

Patton defined *paradigm* as "A worldview, a general perspective, a way of breaking down the complexity of the real world. As such, paradigms are deeply embedded in the social-ization of adherents and practitioners: paradigms tell them what is important, legitimate, and reasonable" (1978, p. 203, quoted by Munhall, 2007, p. 44).

Although there are many different research paradigms known to nurse researchers and used by them, the two primary ones are the quantitative and qualitative paradigms (Munhall, 2007). There are other ways to classify these inquiry paradigms. For example, Parse divided them into the empirical and interpretive paradigm, which are parallel to the quantitative and qualitative paradigms. Newman and colleagues (2008) divided the para-digms into the particulate/deterministic, interactive/integrative, and unitary/transforma-tive (Racher & Robinson, 2002). Guba and Lincoln (2005) address five major inquiry paradigms: positivism, postpositivism, critical theory and related approaches, construc-tivism, and the participatory paradigm.

Neomodernism offers the means for clinical nurses to use their experience in building new knowledge: "Both the practice of nursing and the practice of science are considered essential to and synergistic in building disciplinary knowledge" (Reed, 2006, p. 37).

Reed (2006) distinguishes modernism, postmodernism, and neomodernism:

- Modernism is based upon Popper's (1968) privileged view of scientific knowledge.
- Postmodernism disputes the modernist idea of the unchanging nature of truth.
- Neomodernism sits between modernism and postmodernism recognizing mul-tiple ways of producing knowledge (Reed, 2006).

The philosophical arguments in support of the two predominant nursing research par-adigms are complex and sometimes arcane. For our purpose, which is to understand how and why they are different, a very simplified description is presented here.

THE QUANTITATIVE PARADIGM

Positivism

The origins of positivism date back hundreds of years. Comte coined the word *positivism* in the early 1800s (1957). "Positive sciences," he wrote, "may deal either with objects them-selves as they exist, or with the separate phenomena that the objects exhibit" (p. 42). "The object [goal] . . . is to present a systematic view of human life, as a basis for modifying its imperfections" (p. 8).

Some of the current literature makes positivism sound like the "bad guy" of the two paradigms. But positivism was actually an improvement over previous approaches to knowledge development, especially in regard to knowledge in the physical and social sci-ences where dependence had been on history, tradition, and theology, which are other sources of knowledge but are not designed to test propositions and produce substantiated generalizations. Kuhn (1996) provides an example of what came before positivistic scientific inquiry:

> What is light? Is it something that emanates from the eye? Or does it emanate from the objects we see? If the object observed is a human body the answer is neither. Our bodies generate heat that can be seen in the infrared range but if you turn off or block all sources of light (sun, stars, fire, electric lights) you cannot see a human body with the naked eye. Likewise, the moon, although quite bright some nights, does not emanate light but reflects it from the sun.[1]

What is our present understanding of what light is? Light is electromagnetic radiation (a type of energy) that has a wavelength within the range that can be seen by the human eye (*The Free Dictionary*, 2009). Ultraviolet light is just above the visible range in frequency and infrared is just below the visual range.

Empiricism

Reality, to positivists, is what can be observed, that is, whatever can be detected by our senses (which can be extended by the use of various measuring instruments). Sensory data are considered the ultimate source of knowledge in empirical inquiry. The realist's viewpoint is contrasted to the viewpoint of the idealist who questioned the application of empiricism to the understanding of humans (Munhall, 2007). Idealists on the other hand, argued that the mind was the creator and source of knowledge. This is one of the core differences between the quantitative and qualitative research paradigms.

Logic, which guides reasoning, and mathematics, provides the symbols (measurements) that represent the sensory data, are fundamental to empirical inquiry. Physical science, chemistry, biology, and eventually the social sciences adapted empirical inquiry as their primary research paradigm (Zammito, 2004).

In the most extreme form, logical positivism and the empirical inquiry that is its outgrowth left no room for imagination, creativity, or interaction. Worse, it assumed an entirely predictable, explainable natural world. Recent thinking has moved well away from any idea of finding absolute truths or assuming that a part of a phenomenon can be studied and understood without considering the whole.

The *experiment* is the ideal research design within the empirical, quantitative inquiry paradigm. The elements of this design have been clearly defined. These include:

- *Control* of extraneous factors that may affect the outcome of the experiment such as the temperature of the room, excess noise, and so forth

---

[1]Note that while all of this is positivist thinking, none of it is quantitative.

- *Treatments* or independent variables that can be *manipulated* (added, subtracted, or modified)
- A no-treatment group the treatment can be compared with.
- Random assignment to treatment or no treatment to help rule out alternative explanations due to extraneous factors including characteristics of the subjects
- Objective outcome measures (Cook & Campbell, 1979)

All of these elements are necessary to allow the research to demonstrate a relationship between the cause (the treatment) and effect (the outcome), in other words, to answer the question, does the experimental treatment make a difference? In addition, most quantitative researchers are interested not just in the people, objects, or other phenomena actually being tested but also in similar people, objects, or phenomena. This is the issue of *generalizability* that asks which populations, settings, treatments, and outcomes can the results be generalized to (Campbell & Stanley, 1963, p. 5).

Cook and Campbell (1979) have added some qualifications to the demonstration of cause and effect through experimental research that are especially relevant to clinical studies:

- Multiple causes are possible. For example, heart disease has a number of contributing causes, not a single cause.
- Given the challenges of controlling all possible extraneous factors that may influence the outcome, any outcome found is considered probable, not absolute.
- Cause and effect may either occur simultaneously or the effect may occur after the cause.
- Not all "treatments" can be manipulated.
- Causation cannot be inferred from observed relationships or patterns. For example, night regularly follows day but cannot be said to be caused by day. In fact, a third factor is responsible for both day and night.

Discovery Stage

There's another aspect to the empirical/quantitative paradigm that is frequently overlooked. This *discovery stage* actually precedes what has just been described, the experimental or verification stage. Here is where the researcher first conceives of a new treatment or invents a new device, procedure, vaccine, or drug that is then examined theoretically and tested in the experimental stage. Popper (in Miller, 1985) quotes Einstein's description of the discovery stage:

> There is no logical path leading to these laws [ideas]. They can only be reached by interaction, based upon something like an intellectual love (*Einfühlung*) of the objects of experience. (pp. 134–135)

What this quote does not add is that it is *informed* intuition that produces an idea; it is *informed* intuition that springs from an ability to see new patterns, make new connections, and make intellectual leaps from the known to the unknown.

Limitations

Limitations of empirical/quantitative paradigm have been thoroughly reviewed by many nursing scholars and qualitative researchers. For example, it is particularly difficult to ascertain the meaning of health and illness experiences with quantitative measures. The uniqueness of the individual is lost when data are aggregated. The context in which the experience occurs is also difficult to incorporate into a quantitative analysis. Although advanced quantitative analyses can incorporate multiple factors, there is still a more fragmented quality to the quantitative analysis than there is to a qualitative analysis (see Table 4-3).

We turn now to consideration of the qualitative research paradigm.

THE QUALITATIVE PARADIGM

As with the quantitative paradigm, we will briefly consider the emergence of the qualitative paradigm and then review the fundamental characteristics of qualitative inquiry. Dombro's (2007) review of the development of qualitative research begins in the 1700s with Kant and other idealist (as opposed to realist) philosophers who believed that we

TABLE 4-3   Comparison of the Two Predominant Nursing Research Paradigms

	Quantitative	Qualitative
Philosophical viewpoint	Realist	Idealist
	Positivism	Naturalism
	Reductionist	Holistic
Purpose or goal	Objectivity	Subjectivity
	Causal explanation	Interpretation
	Generalizability	Understanding
	Search for Truth	Meaning
	Universal laws, propositions	Social, political goals
Approach	Deductive	Inductive
	Experimental	Descriptive
	Observe and test subjects	Engage participants
	Empirical	Multiplicity of voices
	Statistical analysis	Multiplicity of views

filter all of our experiences and impose an order on them in our minds. Dombro then quotes Wordsworth to reflect the emphasis on creative imagination that is a reaction to the rationalism of the quantitative paradigm:

> Enough of Science and of Art,
> Close up those barren leaves;
> Come forth, and bring with you a heart
> That watches and receives. (2007, p. 111)

In the 1800s, Dilthey made clear the difference between the natural sciences and the human sciences: The natural sciences focused on the physical world, objects, natural events, and their behavior. The human sciences, on the other hand, focused on "beings that have 'consciousness' and that 'act purposefully' in and on the world by creating objects of 'meaning' that are 'expressions' of how human beings exist in the world" (van Manen, 1990, p. 4). Instead of testing and verifying phenomena, qualitative inquiries seek to understand the phenomena and to find meaning. "To do research is always to question the way we experience the world, to want to know the world in which we live as human beings" (van Manen, 1990, p. 5). Knowing the world requires intentionally immersing ourselves in it as we consciously study, question, theorize, and write about it.

At about the same time, early Western anthropologists were studying the peoples of newly (to them) discovered portions of the world, exploring diverse cultures through the 17th, 18th, and 19th centuries. Anthropologists described details of distant societies that expanded our understanding of the influence of culture. Although much of this work is now labeled critically as "colonial" in its perspective (Denzin & Lincoln, 2005; Gobo, 2008), it marks the beginning of one of the great traditions in qualitative research. Classic anthropological field work is exemplified by the pioneering work of Malinowski (1922) in New Guinea and the Trobriand Islands. He is widely quoted even today, particularly for his emphasis on learning the indigenous person's point of view, "to realize *his* vision of *his* world" (1922, p. 25, quoted by Spradley, 1979, p. 3). Field work is the imprimatur of cultural anthropology. Spradley (1979) emphasizes that the purpose is not just to describe behavior but to understand others' way of life, that is, the insider's view. To do this requires beginning with a "conscious attitude of almost complete ignorance" (p. 4). In a sense, the researcher becomes the student, and the participants become the teachers.

Fieldwork was also adopted in sociology and brought back to Western cultures: Whyte (1984) used semistructured interviewing and participant observation to learn about street gangs in the United States. He writes that he did this to learn about the people, which he could not accomplish with just statistics such as the income, household size, or land values of the inner city slums. In anthropological terms, this is attention to the *emic* perspective, the participant's point of view as opposed to the *etic* or outsider's (researcher's) point of view, a hallmark of qualitative research (Morse, 1992).

More recently, an "explosion" of new methodologies has occurred in reaction to the colonial overtones of early cultural anthropology and ethnographic studies of the poor, minorities, and oppressed people. A combination of critical theory, cultural critique, participatory action research, a new generation of indigenous scholars, and related forces and interests brings new perspectives and approaches to this important branch of qualitative research.

We turn back now to the other important branch, that which has grown out of the philosophical debate of the last hundred years or so. For this, we look especially to the two main branches of phenomenological research. Spiegelberg (1975) defines phenomenology as "a philosophical movement whose primary objective is the direct investigation and description of phenomena as consciously experienced, without theories about their causal explanation and as free as possible from unexamined preconceptions and presuppositions" (p. 3). Note the emphasis on taking a new look at what is familiar without preconceived ideas about what may be found. This is very different from the use of a hypothesis regarding expected outcomes in quantitative research. *Eidetic* phenomenology emphasizes the description of essential features of a phenomenon (naming); *hermeneutics* emphasizes the interpretive (explaining) element (van Manen, 1990). A few of the most important contributors to this branch are the following (Dombro, 2007; Scheurich & McKenzie, 2005; Spiegelberg, 1975; van Manen, 1990):

- Husserl (1858–1938): Descriptive phenomenology; study of the immediate life world of individuals (Spiegelberg, 1975). Consciousness as the source of our knowledge.
- Heidegger (1899–1976): Interpretive phenomenology (hermeneutics); interpreting the human condition and being-in-the-world (Spiegelberg, 1975).
- Gadamer (1900–2002): "Experience, culture, and prior understanding render the scientific ideal of objectivity impossible" (Dombro, 2007, p. 115).
- Merleau-Ponty (1908–1961): "We access the world physically and through perception come to know our interior and exterior worlds" (Dombro, 2007, p. 116).
- Foucault (1926–1984): Opposed authority as determiner of truth, critiqued existing social forms in which we live (Scheurich & McKenzie, 2005).
- Habermas (born 1929): Critical theory—empirical science expresses our technical interests, hermeneutics expresses practical interests, and critical theory addresses our emancipatory interests (van Manen, 1990, p. 176).

It is interesting to see that attention to issues of oppression and emancipation characterize recent outgrowths of both of these major branches of qualitative research.

CHARACTERISTICS OF QUALITATIVE RESEARCH

The heterogeneity of approaches within the qualitative research paradigm makes it difficult to accurately identify their commonalities. It is important to note that the following is a general list of common characteristics. Not every characteristic will be found in every approach. Together, however, they characterize the qualitative paradigm and illustrate the extent to which qualitative research is, as Lincoln and Guba have said, virtually the reverse of the quantitative paradigm (1985, p. 29). The following is a compilation drawn primarily from Lincoln and Guba (1985), Patton (2002), van Manen (1990), and Denzin and Lincoln (2005):

- Qualitative study, as Spradley (1979) noted, usually begins with a conscious effort to avoid or bracket preconceived ideas about possible outcomes. In other words, the researcher begins without suppositions about what he or she will find. No *a priori* theory is used as the foundation for the study.

- Qualitative research is generally inductive, leading from the particular to the general (see Chapter 3).

- It is assumed that research can be neither context nor value free. Instead, the perspectives (including values) of the researcher are important to consider as is the context in which the study is done.

- The researcher is the instrument. Instead of using external means for collecting data such as questionnaires or physical measures, the qualitative researcher primarily employs the self as observer, interviewer, and participant.

- Natural settings, rather than artificial settings such as laboratory or examination room, are used. This is often called *fieldwork*. Further, neither control nor manipulation is used.

- Purposive or purposeful sampling rather than the random sampling is used.

- Realities are multiple, constructed, and holistic. There is no absolute truth and no single reality or view of the world or of people's experiences in the world.

- The data obtained should be rich, thick, and descriptive, not thin, limited, or superficial (Geertz, 1973).

- The plan for the study (its design) may evolve (change) as understanding increases and deepens. Research is not a linear process but a circular one; new insights inform both the data collection and the analysis, which may occur simultaneously.

- A holistic perspective is adopted; fragmentation is avoided.

- The goal is to capture the insider (*emic*) perspective, not the outsider's (*etic*) perspective.

- The uniqueness of each person (or case) is recognized, although universal meaning is also sought.

- The final result may be a creative synthesis that makes use of multiple sources of data including art, poetry, and other forms of story and literature. Writing the narrative is considered a part of the research effort, not a separate post-research task. Both description and interpretation are goals.

- A dynamic interaction occurs between researcher and participant. Outcomes may be the result of input from participants as well as the researcher and may be negotiated as part of the research process.

- Insight and creativity in the writing are valued. Reflexivity is also valued. The researcher brings his or her perspective to the study and acknowledges it in the writing. The ability to be self-analytical and to think critically are also valued.

- Authenticity is essential to the work. The voices of both the researcher and the participants are reflected in the writing.

CONCLUSION

It should be clear now that the quantitative and qualitative research paradigms are very different, even polar opposites at times. While most effort has been directed toward emphasizing the differences, there have also been some attempts to find common ground, to bridge the differences (Munhall, 2007) even to combine them in mixed methods research. Philosophically these paradigms are not interchangeable and, for some, it is difficult to justify straddling both camps (Rolfe, 2005).

Each research paradigm has its strengths and its shortcomings. Quantitative research does not address the meaning of life experiences in the depth that qualitative research can. Qualitative research does not offer the control and objectivity desired when evaluating a new treatment. We need both kinds of research to inform our practice. The alternative to interchanging or bridging the two paradigms is to ensure that the method selected matches the question that is asked (Patton, 1999). This is often done in nursing research studies using mixed methods. For example, a count of males vs. females, ages of participants, income levels, survey opinions, and the like may be added to a qualitative study. Likewise, open-ended questions may be added to quantitative study questionnaires to give participants an opportunity to explain and elaborate upon their answers. The caveat is that the researcher must be skilled in the method selected. This is always an important consideration in planning a research study. Collaboration between quantitative and qualitative researchers is often an effective way to address this concern.

REFERENCES

About the Framingham Heart Study. (n.d.) Retrieved August 2, 2009, from http://www.framinghamheart study.org/about/index.html
    ◇ Of special interest on this website for the Framingham Study are the risk score profiles for congestive heart failure, stroke and coronary heart disease.
Borreani, C., Miccinesi, G., Bunelli, C., & Lina, M. (2004). An increasing number of qualitative research papers oncology and palliative care: Does it mean a thorough development of the methodology of research? [Electronic version]. *Health and Quality of Life Outcomes, 2*(7), Published online 2004 January 23. doi: 10.1186/1477-7525-2-7.
Campbell, D. T., & Stanley, J. C. (1963). *Experimental and quasi-experimental designs for field settings*. Boston: Houghton Mifflin.
Cisternas, M. G., Murphy, L., Croft, J. B., & Helmich, G. G. (2009). Racial disparities in total knee replacement among Medicare enrollees—United States, 2000–2006. *Morbidity and Mortality Weekly Report, 58*(6), 133–134.
Comte, A. (1957). *A general view of positivism* (Centenary ed.). New York: Robert Speller and Sons.

Cook, T. D., & Campbell, D. T. (1979). *Quasi-experimentation: Design and analysis issues for field settings.* Boston: Houghton Mifflin.

Creswell, J. W. (1998). *Qualitative inquiry and research design: Choosing among five traditions.* Thousand Oaks, CA: Sage.

Denzin, N. K., & Lincoln, Y. S. (2005). *The Sage handbook of qualitative research* (3rd ed.). Thousand Oaks, Sage.

Denzin, N. K., Lincoln, Y. S., & Smith, L. T. (2008). *Handbook of critical and indigenous methodologies.* Los Angeles: Sage.

Dombro, M. (2007). Historical and philosophical foundation of qualitative research. In P. L. Munhall (4th ed.), *Nursing research: A qualitative perspective* (pp. 99–126). Sudbury, MA: Jones and Bartlett.

Dunphy, L. M. (2001). The "steel cocoon." Tales of the nurses and patients of the iron lung: 1929–1955. *Nursing History Review, 9,* 3–33.

Dunphy, L. M. (2003). Iron Lungs: Nurses remember the polio epidemic and medical technology. *American Journal of Nursing, 103*(5), 64I.

Fleming, D., & Morse, J. N. (1991). Minimizing embarrassment: Boys' experiences of pubertal changes. *Issues in Comprehensive Pediatric Nursing, 14,* 211–230.

Gance-Cleveland, B. (2004). Qualitative evaluation of a school-based support group for adolescents with an addicted parent. *Nursing Research, 53*(6), 379–386.

Geertz, C. (1973). The interpretation of cultures. New York: Basic Books.

Gobo, G. (2008). *Doing ethnography.* Los Angeles: Sage.

Guba, E. G., & Lincoln, Y. S. (2005). Paradigmatic controversies, contradictions and emerging confluences. In N. K. Denzin and Y. S. Lincoln (Eds.), *The Sage handbook of qualitative research* (3rd ed., pp. 191–215). Thousand Oaks, CA: Sage.
 ✧ Tables in this chapter outline the primary differences between positivism, postpositivism, critical theory, constructivism and the participatory paradigm.

Katzner, D. W. (1983). *Analysis without measurement.* Cambridge, UK: Cambridge University Press.

Kerlinger, F. N. (1973). *Foundations of behavioral research.* New York: Holt, Rinehart and Winston.

Kozuki, Y., & Kennedy, M. G. (2004). Cultural incommensurability in psychodynamic psychotherapy in Western and Japanese traditions. *Journal of Nursing Scholarship, 36*(1), 30–38.

Kuhn, T. S. (1996). *The structure of scientific revolution* (3rd ed.), Chicago: University of Chicago Press.

Lincoln, Y. S., & Guba, E. G. (1985). *Naturalistic inquiry.* Newbury Park, CA: Sage.

Malinowski, B. (1922). *Argonauts of the Western Pacific.* London: Rutledge.
 ✧ "Chapter 1: Postpositivism and the Naturalist Paradigm" is an excellent review of the basis of postpositivism that is quite readable.

Man-Son-Hing, M., O'Connor, A. M., Drake, E., Biggs, J., Hum, V., & Laupacis, A. (2002). The effect of qualitative vs. quantitative presentation of probability estimates on patient decision-making: A randomized trial. *Health Expectations, 5,* 246–255.

Miller, D. (1985). *Popper selections.* Princeton, NJ: Princeton University Press.

Morse, J. M. (1992). *Qualitative health research.* Newbury Park, CA: Sage.

Munhall, P. L. (2007). Language and nursing research. In P. L. Munhall (4th ed.), *Nursing research: A qualitative perspective* (pp. 37–70). Sudbury, MA: Jones and Bartlett.
 ✧ Readable chapter about the quantitative and qualitative research paradigms with an emphasis on the qualitative.

Newman, M. A., Smith, M. C., Pharris, M. D., & Jones, D. (2008). The focus of a discipline revisited. *Advances in Nursing Science, 31*(1), E16–E27.

Patton, M. Q. (1999). Enhancing the quality and credibility of qualitative analysis. *HSR: Health Services Research, 345*(Part II), 1189–1209.

Patton, M. Q. (2002). *Qualitative research and evaluation methods.* Thousand Oaks, CA: Sage.

Paul, I. M., Beiler, J., McMonagle, A., Shaffer, M. L., Duda, L., & Berlin, C. M. (2007). Effect of honey, dextromethorphan and no treatment on nocturnal cough and sleep quality for coughing children and their parents. *Archives of Pediatric and Adolescent Medicine, 161*(12), 1140–1146.

Popper, K. R. (1968). *The logic of scientific discovery.* New York: Harper Torchbooks.

Racher, F., & Robinson, S. (2002). Are phenomenology and postpositivism strange bedfellows? *Western Journal of Nursing Research, 25*(5), 464–481.

Reed, P. G. (2006). Commentary on neomodernism and evidence-based nursing: Implications for the production of nursing knowledge. *Nursing Outlook, 54*(1), 36–38.

Rolfe, G. (2005). Evidence memory and truth towards a reconstructive: Validation of reflective practice. In C. Johns & D. Freshwater (Eds.), *Transforming nursing through reflective practice* (pp. 13–26). Oxford, UK: Blackwell.

Sandelowski, M. (1986). The problem of rigor in qualitative research. *Advances in Nursing Science, 8*(3), 27–37.

Scheurich, J. J., & McKenzie, K. B. (2005). Foucault's methodologies: In N. Denzin and Y. Lincoln (Eds.), *The Sage handbook of qualitative research* (3rd ed., pp. 841–868). Thousand Oaks, CA: Sage.

Spiegelberg, H. (1975). Doing phenomenology: Essays on and in phenomenology. The Hague, Netherlands: Martinus Nijhoff.

Spradley, J. P. (1979). *The ethnographic interview.* New York: Holt, Rinehart and Winston.

The Free Dictionary. (2009). Retrieved July 27, 2009, from http://www.thefreedictionary.com

van Manen, M. (1990). Researching lived experience: Human science for an active pedagogy (2nd ed.), Albany, NY: State University of New York Press.

Whyte, W. F. (1984). *Learning from the field.* Beverly Hills, CA: Sage.

Yarcheski, A., Mahon, N. E., Yarcheski, T. J., Hanks, M. M., & Cannella, B. L. (2009). A meta-analytic study of predictors of maternal-fatal attachment. *International Journal of Nursing Studies, 46*, 708–715.

Zammito, J. H. (2004). *A nice derangement of epistemes.* Chicago: University of Chicago Press.

CHAPTER 5

Experimental Research Designs

If there is an ideal against which all quantitative designs are compared, it is the *true experiment*. In health-related research, including studies of screening tests, diagnostics, prevention, and therapeutic interventions (DeMets & Fisher, 2008), this takes the form of the randomized clinical trial (RCT). There are many instances, however, in which employing the experimental design is difficult or impossible, premature, or unethical. For this reason, there are a variety of what are called quasi-experimental designs as well as descriptive and observational designs that are discussed in the next chapter. The experimental and quasi-experimental designs, along with their strengths and drawbacks, are discussed in this chapter.

EXPERIMENTAL DESIGN

Regular use of control groups in psychosocial and educational research dates back to about 1908. This is quite a bit later than its first use in the physical and biological sciences. Boring (1954) traced the recorded use of experimental controls back to experiments by Pascal in 1648 in France:

> Wanting to test the relationship of a column of mercury to atmospheric pressure, Pascal arranged for simultaneous measurements using exactly the same procedure to be done at the foot of a mountain, which was 1800 feet above sea level, and at the top of the mountain, which was 4800 feet above sea level. At the top of the mountain, they took measurements inside and outside of a shelter as well on one side of the mountain and the other side, to check for possible influences from other factors.
>
> On the way down the mountain, they took an additional measurement of the column of mercury finding the measurements at the three sites to be the following:
>
> | | |
> |---|---|
> | Top of the mountain | 24.71 inches |
> | Intermediate altitude | 26.65 inches |
> | Foot of the mountain | 28.04 inches |
>
> There were no differences in the measurements taken inside or outside the shelter or on one side of the mountain compared to the other side. Their findings demonstrated the difference in atmospheric pressure at different altitudes.

Research Design

A research design includes the structure of a study and the strategies for conducting that study (Kerlinger, 1973). This plan, at minimum, spells out the variables that will be studied, how they will be studied, and their anticipated relationship to each other (Spector, 1981).

Experimental designs have been developed to reduce biases of all kinds as much as possible. We will review the major sources of bias in the section on threats to internal and external validity.

The primary difference between the true experiment and quasi-experimental designs is the degree of control that the researcher has over the subjects and variables of the study. Control is much easier to achieve in the laboratory than in the field. In nursing research, the "field" includes homes, hospitals, clinics, schools, the workplace, or wherever we find people with health concerns outside a facility that is specifically designed for the conduct of research such as a sleep lab.

Before considering the basic experimental designs, we will consider some additional ideas that underlie the experimental design.

Causation

In everyday conversation, the word *cause* is used frequently, sometimes casually. In research, however, we need to be careful how we use this term. Although we often hope to identify causes of health problems, many of our studies are not designed to do this.

The basic principle behind identifying a cause is based upon the time sequence of variables. Davis (1985) calls this the "great principle of causal order: after cannot cause before" (p. 11). An example may make this clearer:

- Client A visited a sick friend the day *after* he began coughing and had an elevated temperature.

- Client B visited a sick friend the day *before* he began coughing and had an elevated temperature.

- Both blamed their illnesses on their sick friends. Are they both correct?

The principle of causation says *no*, Client A cannot have caught that cold from his friend. Client B, however, *may* have caught his cold from his sick friend. The time sequence, visiting the friend after becoming ill, rules out Client A's hypothesis on the basis of the principle of causation. The cause cannot come after the effect. The indefinite answer to Client B's hypothesis, as you probably have surmised, is because there are many other possible sources of infection (family and coworkers to name just a few), not just Client B's sick friend.

Multiple causes, indirect effects, and spurious effects occur frequently. These potential effects add considerable complexity to many of our research designs. Davis (1985) uses the example of height within a family to illustrate a spurious effect. If mother and father are both tall, this influences the height of their son and daughter genetically, a direct cause and effect relationship. However, the height of the son does not affect the daughter's height or vice versa, although it may appear to because of the high correlation. This apparent but false direct effect between the heights of the son and daughter is a *spurious* effect.

Indirect effects are likened by Davis (1985) to ripples on a pond. A chain of events or factors may lead to the ultimate effect (outcome):

> A couple are arguing with each other on their way home from a party. Brenda has accused Bart of drinking too much and acting very foolish in front of their friends. Bart denies both accusations. Their argument is escalating as Bart drives up the ramp into heavy traffic. As he turned to Brenda to tell her that she had also been acting foolishly, the car in front of him slowed to avoid hitting a tire that fell off a truck. Bart's response was delayed just enough that he slammed into the car in front of him. Bart's speed, following too closely, and the errant tire were *multiple causes* of the accident. The argument was an *indirect effect* as it contributed to his speeding and following too closely. Using cell phones and text messaging while driving could have an effect similar to the argument.

Threats to Internal and External Validity

Internal validity is concerned with minimizing the effects of extraneous or confounding factors that may interfere with interpretation of the results of the experiment. Campbell and Stanley (1963) listed eight threats to internal validity:

1. *History:* What is happening at the same time the experiment is being conducted? Seasonal effects, patient transfers to different units, staff changes, reorganization, a natural disaster, even the beginning of a new school term can affect nursing research studies. For example, a study that is testing the effect of new infection control policies on patient mortality can be confounded by a peak in the incidence of a particularly virulent influenza that raises the death rate of very young and very old patients.

2. *Maturation:* The effect of changes that occur naturally over time. These may include growth and development, growing older, or getting tired, hungry, or bored. For example, infants enrolled in a stimulation study will be experiencing natural development of various cognitive abilities without the added stimulation. These developmental changes may confound the effects of the stimulation intervention.

3. *Testing:* The use of the same questions on pretest and posttest may affect how well subjects do at the second testing. For example, a questionnaire on attitudes toward people who are substance abusers may increase sensitivity to their problems. Likewise, nurses given a drug calculation test at the beginning of a study may practice on their own before the posttest is administered; keeping a food diary may change people's behavior by alerting them to poor eating habits, and so forth.

4. *Instrumentation:* Changes in the way examiners complete observation or rating scales and in the instruments being used may directly affect the quality of the data obtained. This is primarily a question of reliability, which is discussed in detail in a later chapter.

5. *Statistical regression:* The phrase *regression to the mean* describes the likelihood that subjects chosen because they score very high or very low on a particular test are likely to move closer to the mean (average) on subsequent tests without any intervention.

6. *Selection bias:* There may be differences, often subtle ones, in the way people are selected for the experimental treatment group and the comparison or no-treatment group. For example, people who are eager to exercise are easier to recruit for an exercise study, especially for the intervention group, than are people who do not want to exercise.

7. *Experimental mortality:* Differences may occur in the loss of subjects in the treatment group versus the control group. For example, the eager exercisers are more likely to complete a 6-week exercise program than an attention central educational program.

8. *Selection—maturation interaction:* Changes that are due to the interactive effect of selection bias and maturation may be mistaken for the effect of the experimental treatment. For example, a study of school-age children participating in a fitness program may be confounded by maturation in physical ability over time as well as the greater enthusiasm for fitness of those who complete the fitness program.

External validity is concerned with the degree to which the results of the study can be generalized to others. Campbell and Stanley (1963) listed four threats to external validity.

1. *Testing effect:* The effects of having been pretested may be sufficient to make the groups quite different from untested people to whom the results of the study will be generalized.

2. *Selection effect:* The criteria used to select subjects may limit generalizability. For example, in many pharmacological studies the subjects cannot have any illness other than the one for which the drug is intended. While this eliminates the confounding effects of these other illnesses, it also does not represent the reality of multiple comorbidities, especially in older people.

3. *Experiment effect:* Being involved in a carefully designed and implemented experimental study can be a very different experience from receiving the same treatment in ordinary care settings.

4. *Multiple treatment effect:* This threat occurs when the same subjects are exposed to more than one treatment (using the subjects as their own comparison group, for example). Campbell and Stanley (1963) comment that "the effects of prior treatments are not usually erasable" (p. 6).

There is no simple formula for addressing these threats to internal and external validity of an experimental design. Each research study poses different challenges that require thoughtful, often creative solutions.

The True Experiment

Although refinements are continuously being developed, the basic experimental design has remained consistent for quite some time. There are many elaborations on these basic designs as well; the most common of these will be explained.

Basic Experimental Designs

The simplest experimental design tests just one treatment that is compared with a no-treatment condition. Subjects (or *participants*, a term preferred by those who dislike the idea of people being *subjected* to an experiment) are randomly assigned to either the treatment or control (no-treatment) group and are measured or tested both before and after the experimental treatment is implemented.

This simple but elegant design is the basis for most of the variations on the experimental design in research involving human subjects. It can be represented by a set of symbols (Campbell & Stanley, 1963, p. 13):

	Pretest	Treatment	Posttest
R	O_1	X	O_2
R	O_3		O_4

R = randomized, that is subjects are randomly selected and randomly assigned to treatment group

O = observation or testing
X = the treatment

Note that subjects are randomly selected and randomly assigned to the treatment or control group. In addition, if examiners are used, they should be *blinded* to treatment group assignment. In other words, the examiners should not know if a person is part of the experimental or control group.

Technically, if subjects are randomly selected and assigned to treatment or control groups, it should not be necessary to pretest them because the groups are, by definition, equivalent due to randomization. The symbolic representation of this posttest-only design is (Campbell & Stanley, 1963, p. 25):

	Treatment	Posttest
R	X	O_2
R		O_4

In reality, however, when relatively small numbers of subjects are involved, randomization may not produce exactly equivalent groups. One group may be a little older, for example, or have a higher average pretest weight. If known, these differences can be controlled statistically. If not known, a difference at posttest may be attributed to the experimental treatment although it really reflects the failure of randomization to produce equivalent groups.

Given the two concerns about the effect of pretesting and about the possibility that randomization may fail to produce equivalent groups, there is a more complex (and more resource-consuming) design that addresses them. This is the Solomon four-group design that uses two treatment groups, one pretested and the other not pretested, and two no-treatment control groups, one pretested and the other not pretested. Using the same symbols, the Solomon four-group design looks like this (Campbell & Stanley, 1963, p. 24):

	Pretest	Treatment	Posttest
R	O_1	X	O_2
R	O_3		O_4
R		X	O_6
R			O_8

If you want to test both immediate posttreatment outcomes and long-term (3 or 6 months posttreatment, for example) outcomes, there is a nice design that controls for the effect of immediate posttesting (Campbell & Stanley, 1963, p. 32):

	Pretest	Treatment	Immediate Posttreatment	3 Months Posttreatment
R	O_1	X	O_2	
R	O_3		O_4	
R	O_5	X		O_6
R	O_7			O_8

There are many instances in which this long-term effect is equally or even more important than the immediate effect. Maintaining the weight loss of people who had been obese would be an example.

Additional treatment groups may be added as well. You might recall the study described in Chapter 4 comparing honey, dextromethorphan, and no treatment for coughs due to upper respiratory infections in children. This study used two experimental treatments, honey and the ingredient common to many over-the-counter cough medications, and a control group that received nothing for their cough. A study using two experimental treatment groups with randomization and posttesting only would be diagrammed as follows:

	Treatment	Posttest
R	X_1	O_2
R	X_2	O_4
R		O_6

Randomized Clinical Trials

A clinical trial is "an experiment in which a group of individuals is given an intervention and subsequent outcome measures are taken" (Cook & DeMets, 2008, p. 10). Outcomes for the individuals receiving the intervention are compared with outcomes for individuals who did not receive the intervention.

In a *randomized* clinical trial, individuals are randomly assigned to intervention or no intervention groups or "arms" of the study. In a *randomized blinded* clinical trial, the raters or examiners who conduct the pretesting and posttesting are completely ignorant of treatment group assignments. Even more control is achieved if the study uses a *double blind* design where neither the researchers, the examiners, nor the subjects know who is receiving active treatment and who is receiving an inactive placebo that appears the same as the actual treatment. Achieving double blind control is obviously much easier when testing a medication or device that delivers treatment without researcher intervention. Behavioral interventions are difficult to cloak in an effective manner. If, for example, you are comparing two types of therapy, the subject may be blinded as to whether or not it is the experimental therapy being received, and independent raters may also be blinded. Those who are providing the treatment, however, cannot be blinded although they can be kept ignorant of the study hypothesis.

Nurses, physicians, and other healthcare providers employ a number of practices that lack research-based evidence to support their use. Although we will explore this further in a later chapter, a few examples cited by DeMets and Fisher (2008) demonstrate the potentially powerful impact of a well-designed clinical trial on patient care practices:

> The story of the use of high-dose oxygen for premature infants has been told often but bears repeating. Given the respiratory challenges in many preemies, it seemed reasonable to treat them with high doses of oxygen. This became standard practice, but it was eventually noted that retrolental fibroplasia was also increasing, leading to blindness in many of these infants. A review of patient records indicated that it particularly affected the infants who had received the high doses of oxygen. But this evidence did not convince practitioners. In fact, in one trial where infants were randomized to high- or low-dose oxygen, the nurses increased the oxygen setting at night for the infants randomized to the low-dose group because they believed this was the better treatment. You can see why a randomized clinical trial comparing administration of high- and low-dose oxygen to premature infants was a challenge both in terms of research ethics and in its implementation. A later clinical trial in which 800 premature infants were randomized to low-dose or high-dose oxygen produced convincing evidence: 23% of the infants in the high dose group were blinded versus 7% in the low-dose group. DeMets and Fisher (2008) note that as many as 10,000 infants were probably blinded during the time that high-dose oxygen was the accepted treatment. "A widely used but untested intervention," they concluded, "was ultimately shown to be harmful" (p. 16).

There are a number of stories like this. Just two more:

1. IPPB (intermittent positive pressure breathing) used a relatively complex and expensive device to deliver bronchodilators to the lungs. When compared to use of a much cheaper, simpler, handheld nebulizer, the clinical effect was found to be the same.

2. When a trial of coronary artery bypass graft (CABG) was undertaken, many surgeons were hesitant to have their patients randomized to the medical (nonsurgical) treatment group. The randomized clinical trial demonstrated that CABG was not superior to medical therapy in people with less advanced disease and fewer occluded coronary blood vessels (DeMets & Fisher, 2008).

It is interesting to note the reluctance to give up an accepted practice that is evident in two of these three examples. Once a practice is accepted, it takes a large, well-designed (i.e., difficult to argue against) study to reverse an entrenched practice. The first example also illustrates the thinking and nonexperimental research that often precede use of an experimental design. This is the discovery phase mentioned in Chapter 4 in which observation (an increase in blindness in premature infants, for example), development (an easy to use nebulizer), or astute questioning of expensive or untested practices preceded the experimental study. It is not at all unusual for a considerable amount of preliminary work to have been done before conducting a clinical trial.

Variations of the Randomized Clinical Trial

There are several common variations of the basic randomized clinical trial. These are the parallel groups, randomized block design, stratified random sample, paired or matched comparisons, and the crossover design. Each of these is explained below (Fleiss, 1999; Piantadosi, 1997).

Parallel Groups
The simplest and most commonly used design, this is the basic true experiment described earlier.

Randomized Block Design
This is a form of directed or constrained randomization of assignment to treatment group that ensures that equal numbers of subjects are assigned to each of two or more treatment groups. For example, if you use 6 subjects per block to create a final sample of 60, you need 10 blocks altogether. Within each block of 6, you then create a randomized sequence of equal numbers of treatment and no-treatment assignments for the subjects. Each block would have a different, random sequence: treatment, no treatment, no treatment, treatment, treatment, no treatment, for example.

Stratified Random Sample

Certain characteristics of subjects can be expected to affect their response to the experimental treatment. Males may lose weight more easily than females, younger people may complete rehabilitation more quickly than older people, and individuals with severe allergies may have a higher level of motivation to implement allergen control measures than those with mild seasonal allergies. There may be good reasons for ensuring that equal numbers of males and females, smokers and nonsmokers, or other groupings of people are assigned to each treatment group. This can be done by using a stratified random sample in which subjects are randomly selected in equal numbers from each *stratum*, or group, such as males and females. Randomized blocks and stratification are often combined in a single design.

Paired or Matched Comparisons

In some studies, matched pairs of individuals are randomized to treatment and no-treatment control groups. People can be matched on any of a number of characteristics: gender, age, ethnic group, income, severity of illness, functional impairment, and so forth.

Crossover Designs

Each subject serves as his or her own control in this design. Subjects receive each of the treatments to be tested, one at a time, sometimes with a *washout* period in between to reduce the possibility of carryover of the effect of the first treatment on the second treatment, and so forth. An example of a crossover study would be to test infants' tolerance of three or four different formulas, one formula at a time. Do not confuse crossover designs with cross-sectional designs, discussed in the next chapter.

Types of Control Groups

In the design of clinical trials, there are several different ways to construct the control or comparison group. The true experiment model uses a no-treatment control group. This is a group of individuals who are enrolled in the study but who will only be involved in the pretesting, if done, and the posttesting.

When the individuals are patients or clients of a healthcare facility, withholding care usually cannot be done for ethical reasons. Instead, they may receive the usual or customary care, becoming part of a comparison group rather than a no-treatment control group.

Both the control and comparison groups are usually concurrent groups, that is, groups are tested or observed within the same time frame as the treatment group. This is important when the temporal factor is likely to affect outcomes.

An alternative to the concurrent control or comparison group is the *historical control* group (Piantadosi, 1997). The data on a historical control group are obtained from previous studies of individuals who did not receive the experimental treatment (DeMets & Fisher, 2008). An example would be the use of known mortality rates for people with certain advanced cancers. The results of a treatment that dramatically increases survival rates can be compared to these known mortality rates.

Hypothesis vs. Research Question

Randomized clinical trials are designed to be hypothesis-testing research studies. A hypothesis is a statement that specifies the population of interest, the intervention to be tested, and the outcome that is expected. The following are examples based on nursing studies:

- Middle school students who receive an individually tailored physical activity program and nurse counseling will increase their reported physical activity more than those who receive printed information on physical activity (based upon Robbins et al., 2006).

- Use of a culturally appropriate Spanish language home-based educational intervention will improve knowledge, attitudes, and preventive practices of urban Latino households (based upon Larson et al., 2009).

The *null* hypothesis states that no difference will be found between the treatment and control groups, that the treatment has had no effect. Technically, this is the hypothesis that is tested statistically.

Research questions generally do not specify the expected outcomes of the study although they should otherwise be as specific as possible. They are more appropriate for nonexperimental studies. A few examples include "What are the factors affecting the rate of influenza vaccination in low-income urban Latino families?" and "What is the average number of hours of physical exercise of middle school students in low-income urban neighborhoods?"

QUASI-EXPERIMENTAL DESIGNS

There are many instances where you cannot use a true experiment design or meet the criteria for a randomized clinical trial. The following are some examples:

- When your treatment (intervention) cannot be simultaneous with the no-treatment data collection period but has to follow it. For example, a sweeping change in the responsibilities of nursing assistants cannot be contained within the experimental units of an organization if nursing assistants float to other units and/or if nursing assistants ever talk with their colleagues on other units. So preintervention data must be collected before the intervention is implemented.

- When pretesting may have a strong effect on individuals in the no-treatment group. For example, doing poorly on tests of endurance and balance may in itself convince subjects that they need to become more active, so no-treatment controls may also improve their fitness. In some cases, omitting the pretest may be the only solution to this design problem.

- Randomization may fail when participants refuse assignment to a less desirable intervention. For example, individuals with mild cognitive impairment were invited to participate in a study of the effect of art therapy compared with therapist-led talk sessions and passive listening to music. The individuals who agreed to participate were eager to be involved in "something that might do me some good" and were so disappointed if they were assigned to the music group that several dropped out of the study, leaving the researcher with nonequivalent groups.

BASIC QUASI-EXPERIMENTAL DESIGNS

There is an almost endless variety of quasi-experimental designs. Some of these variations are very weak; others are relatively strong if used and interpreted appropriately. We will consider four progressively weaker designs that are commonly used. All are based on descriptions by Cook and Campbell (1979) and are represented symbolically with the same notation used for the experimental designs. If you keep in mind the threats to internal and external validity described earlier in this chapter, you will be able to recognize the weaknesses of these designs.

The first quasi-experimental design employs all the elements of the experimental design except randomization. The control group design with a pretest and posttest includes an intervention (X), pretesting and posttesting (O), and a no-treatment control group (Cook & Campbell, 1979, p. 104).

Pretest	Treatment	Posttest
O_1	X	O_2
O_3		O_4

The primary weakness in this very common design is that the two (or more if multiple interventions are tested) groups may not be equivalent. Even more difficult to address is the fact that they may be different in ways that are not known to the researcher and, therefore, will not be measured in any way. Known differences in the two groups such as differences in mean age or income may be controlled statistically. However, many unknown sources of bias may still be present. If, for example, the first 50 volunteers are placed in the experimental group and the second 50 volunteers are placed in the control group, then you may have more eager participants in the experimental group, or more people who get up early, or more people who are assertive, have more initiative, and so forth. These characteristics may influence willingness to try a new intervention.

Cook and Campbell (1979) devote many pages to the variety of outcomes that may be encountered when using this quasi-experimental design. We will consider just two to touch on the types of concerns that may arise given the direction of the outcome.

The first pattern is one that looks good initially, but there are reasons to be skeptical about the contribution of the experimental treatment to the better outcome for the treatment group. As you can see in Figure 5-1, the control group began at a lower level and progressed

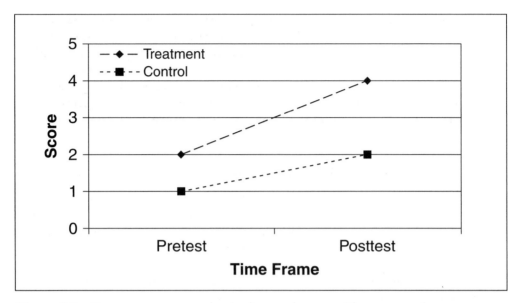

Figure 5-1 First pattern: nonrandomized control group with pretest and posttest design.

Source: Adapted from Cook and Campbell, 1979, p. 106.

only 1 unit by posttest while the treatment group began at a higher level and progressed 2 units by posttest. (The units are scores on the primary outcome measure, which could be an improvement in function measured by degree of assistance needed or an increase in lung capacity or fewer depressive symptoms, and so forth.) It appears that the experimental treatment group progressed at twice the rate than did the control group. Does this mean that the experimental treatment was effective? Not necessarily. Cook and Campbell (1979) point out that the individuals given the experimental treatment (not randomly assigned in this quasi-experimental design) may well have been improving at a faster rate before the study began. This is an example of the selection-maturation interaction threat to internal validity.

Another pattern is more promising. In this pattern (Figure 5-2) there is a crossover of the experimental treatment group and control group means from pretest to posttest: the experimental treatment group began at a lower level but ended at a higher level than the control group, which did not change at all. In other words, the experimental treatment group has "overtaken" the control group (Cook & Campbell, 1979, p. 111).

The tentative conclusion that this is due to the intervention itself is more plausible than in most other patterns for several reasons:

- There is no apparent ceiling (the highest either group could achieve) or basement (the lowest score possible) effect evident here.

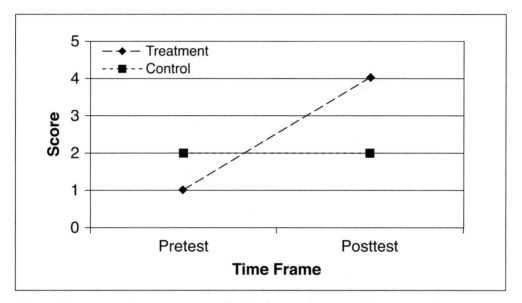

Figure 5-2 Second pattern: nonrandomized control group with pretest and posttest.

Source: Adapted from Cook and Campbell, 1979, p. 111.

- Selection-maturation does not explain the difference because the control group means did not change; few maturation patterns (child growth and development patterns for example) match the pattern in Figure 5-2.
- It also does not appear that a regression to the mean has occurred.

Although this second pattern is more supportive of the hypothesis that the experimental treatment had a substantive effect on the outcomes, this conclusion still remains far weaker without randomization.

The second quasi-experimental design also has an experimental treatment and a control group (that is, two nonequivalent groups) but lacks randomization or pretest information on either group (Cook & Campbell, 1979, p. 98):

Treatment	Posttest
X	O_2
	O_4

The information about the two groups' initial status is missing and must be assumed. Any assumption on the part of the researcher that the groups are equivalent is very tentative and may be incorrect. Patients from the same nursing care unit, clients of the same clinic, or infants from the same nursery may all differ on critical characteristics if not randomly selected and randomly assigned to treatment or control group. Without a pretest, there is virtually no information at all about their equivalence on variables of interest, especially the outcome variables.

Why, then, you might ask, is this design ever used? Often, a researcher encounters a situation calling for study where it is too late or not possible to collect pretest data. An example would be a comparison of the degree of posttraumatic stress disorder in hurricane victims who received crisis intervention counseling compared with those who did not. It is not possible in this case to test the prehurricane status of the people affected although it can be estimated through postdisaster interviewing.

The third quasi-experimental design is the one *group pretest-posttest* design in which there is only an experimental treatment group and no comparison or control at all (Cook & Campbell, 1979, p. 99).

Pretest	Treatment	Posttest
O_1	X	O_2

You can see that there is information about how much change occurred in the experimental group, but arguments for ascribing it to the experimental treatment have a very weak basis. In fact, the change, if there is one, could be due to an entirely different factor altogether. For example, a school nurse may be concerned about low immunization levels in incoming kindergartners. To remedy this, the school nurse sent a letter to all their parents about 6 weeks before the school term began in the fall. The rate of completed immunizations rose dramatically from 88% the previous year to 98% the new fall term. The school nurse was very pleased, of course, but was it possible to credit the letters sent home? In fact, the health department had received a small grant to place advertisements on local television and radio at the same time that the letters were sent out. Neither the school nurse nor the health department could differentiate between these two possible contributors to the improved immunization rates. In addition, neither was aware that the only pediatrician in town had, with the pediatric nurse practitioner in the practice, begun more actively urging parents to complete their children's immunizations as well, a potential third contributing factor.

Parenthetically, if there were several elementary schools in the same locality and only one school nurse sent letters, the response (immunization rate) could be compared across two schools. Of course, the schools themselves may not be comparable, and the parents and children in each school may differ on such important factors as income and confidence in the safety and efficacy of immunizations. For example, there are parents who fear that the mercury in some immunizations may be a cause of autism spectrum disorders and resist having their children immunized for this reason.

This one group design is often used when resources are limited or it is difficult or impossible to recruit a control group. At best, a positive outcome only *suggests* an effect for the experimental treatment.

The fourth and final quasi-experimental design to be discussed is the *one group posttest-only* design. This design lacks randomization, comparison with an equivalent group, even information on the experimental treatment group before treatment is given. The symbolic representation of this design is as follows (Cook & Campbell, 1979, p. 96):

Treatment	Posttest
X	O

Despite its limitations, there are times when this extremely simple design is appropriate. For example, it may be used in identifying the source of a contaminant in food that has sickened a large number of people. Or it may be used in evaluating the effects of a drug newly introduced to the public at large. In both cases, however, there exists prior information that can be used at "posttest": the manufacturer of the contaminated food, the manufacturing process and the ingredients included in the first instance, and the known actions of the drug ingredients and results of testing done prior to its introduction in the second. The path of the contaminant or drug from source to recipient can also be traced.

In most instances, however, this last and simplest design is inadequate if you want to study cause and effect related to a nursing intervention and patient outcomes.

CONCLUSION

Careful planning is essential to all research. The best time to do the work needed to ensure that you will have data of the type and quality needed to achieve your study objectives is before you begin the study (Piantadosi, 1997). Once the people are selected, the treatment provided, and the data are collected, it is very difficult to fill in the gaps, reduce preventable biases, or correct other mistakes that were made in planning the study. Experienced researchers appreciate the importance of careful planning before beginning a study. If you are planning a quantitative study, this includes consultation with a clinically oriented biostatistician to be certain that the data obtained will be sufficient to address the questions posed and conduct the desired analyses.

REFERENCES

Boring, E. G. (1954). The nature and history of experimental control. *American Journal of Psychology,* *67*(4), 573–589.

Campbell, D. T., & Stanley, J. C. (1963). *Experimental and quasi-experimental designs for research.* Boston: Houghton Mifflin.

Cook, T., & Campbell, D. T. (1979). *Quasi-experimentation: Design and analysis issues for field settings.* Boston: Houghton Mifflin.

Cook, T. D., & DeMets, D. (2008). *Introduction to statistical methods for clinical trials.* Boca Raton, FL: Chapman & Hall/CRC.

Davis, J. A. (1985). *The logic of causal order.* Newbury Park, CA: Sage.

DeMets, D., & Fisher, M. R. (2008). Introduction to clinical trials. In T. D. Cook & D. L. DeMets (Eds.), *Introduction to statistical methods for clinical trials* (pp. 1–28). Boca Raton, FL: Chapman & Hall/CRC.

Fleiss, J. L. (1999). *The design and analysis of clinical experiments.* New York: John Wiley & Sons.

Kerlinger, F. N. (1973). *Foundations of behavioral research.* New York: Holt, Rinehart & Winston.

Larson, E. L., Ferng, Y. H., McLoughlin, J. W., Wang, S., & Morse, S. S. (2009). Effect of intensive education on knowledge, attitudes and practices regarding upper respiratory infections among urban Latinos. *Nursing Research, 58*(3), 150–165.

Piantadosi, S. (1997). *Clinical trials: A methodological perspective*. New York: John Wiley & Sons.
    ✧ Probably the most readable of the many books on RCTs.

Robbins, L. B., Gretebeck, K. A., Kazanis, A. S., & Pender, N. J. (2006). Girls on the Move program to increase physical activity participation. *Nursing Research, 55*(3), 206–216.

Spector, P. E. (1981). *Research designs*. Beverly Hills, CA: Sage.

CHAPTER 6

Descriptive Research Designs, Mixed Methods, and Meta-Analysis

Just as a reminder, a research design is "the logical sequence that connects the empirical data to a study's initial research questions and, ultimately, to its conclusions" (Yin, 2003, p. 20). In less formal terms, it is our "plan for getting from here to there" (p. 20) in a research study.

In the previous chapter we considered a progression of experimental and quasi-experimental designs ranging from the true experiment epitomized by the randomized clinical trial to designs that lacked so many elements of the true experiment that they could almost be called descriptive. The more quantitatively oriented research designs, as you have seen with the experimental and quasi-experimental designs, are based upon well-defined principles and provide relatively clear guidelines. In contrast, research designs within the qualitative universe are much more ambiguous and far less predetermined. Denzin and Lincoln (1998) aptly compare the designs of quantitative studies to well-defined road maps while the qualitative designs more closely resemble paths of discovery (p. xii).

Perhaps the single most important difference between the experimental designs of the previous chapter and the mostly descriptive designs of this chapter is *manipulation*. In descriptive research, the investigator does not provide a treatment of any kind (in this case, the word *treatment* is used very broadly to include *any change* that is introduced by the researcher, whether it is new signage in a nursing home, a new vaccine for children, a physical aid, patient education, medication, meditation, psychotherapy, etc.).

Although there is no manipulation by the researcher in descriptive studies, many of these studies encompass what is informally called a *natural experiment* where comparisons can be made before and/or after something has happened. We can track the health outcomes of inactivity and overweight, for example, but cannot assign people to be inactive and overeat for a research study. Further, people who have been inactive and overeaters for a long time can be compared with people who have exercised regularly and maintained their weight within normal limits. After-the-fact comparisons can also be made: people who have had heart attacks or developed different type of cancers can be compared to those who live in their neighborhood, attend the same schools, and work in the same places but have not had a heart attack or developed cancer.

Descriptive designs are many and varied. They may involve collection of information on a single group or phenomenon in a very simple descriptive study, or they may be complex, multifaceted studies of the factors that contribute to the development of a major health problem. Their size varies as much as their complexity. The data collected may be quantitative, qualitative, or a combination of both.

We will begin with the simplest of descriptive designs and progress through some of the most common variations and elaborations of this design. We will also consider the use of mixed designs and meta-analyses in this chapter.

SIMPLE DESCRIPTIVE DESIGNS

These are the most basic of descriptive designs. A simple descriptive design focuses on a single group or population. Data are collected on the group's characteristics, attributes, and/or experiences and reported using descriptive statistics such as means, median, mode, percents, if quantitative, or a narrative, if qualitative. Case studies and surveys are two common types of simple descriptive designs.

Case Studies

Case studies typically focus on a single, unifying event or situation including both descriptive information and an analysis of the case, usually within a context that is also described. Stake (1998) adds that the case should be specific, unique, and bounded. Some cases are selected because they are intrinsically interesting, such as the deaf culture or the first cases of Kaposi's sarcoma noted in people with HIV. Other cases are selected because they provide insight into an issue or lend themselves to refining an existing concept or theory. A third reason for selecting certain cases is because they will lead to better understanding of people or events with similar circumstances (Stake, 1998). Sabat's (2009) case study of his aged father's conceptualization of a good life is an example:

> Sabat (2009) wrote a phenomenologically based case study of his father's last years as a caregiver for Sabat's mother who was wheelchair bound and suffering from advancing vascular dementia and then as a care recipient himself. His father lived with colon cancer (for which he did not want surgery) for 8 years after his wife's death. Both as caregiver and care recipient, his father defined a "good day" as one when no problems arose that he could not manage. He was happy to be at home even though he was alone most of the time because it meant that he could "do what I want," (p. 164). This included choosing what to eat and when; making phone calls at will; watching television or listening to the radio when he wanted to. Sabat then asks, "How can we understand this quality of life as being good?" (p. 164). Most of the professionals he encountered concluded that this man at 92 was "at risk" and should be in a facility. But this older man himself thought, based on his own experience and values, that his quality of life was actually quite good. "Good moments," writes Sabat, "are defined as such by each individual person," and our treatment of care recipients "must be deeply mindful of the lived experience of the person involved" (p. 166).

The qualitative approach to case study research has a dynamic behind it that differs from the epidemiologically oriented case studies described in the next chapter. Janesick (1998) likens this dynamic to an exercise or dance workout that begins with a warm-up phase, progresses to the total workout, and ends with a cool down as follows:

1. *Warm-up:* Begin the case study research project by framing the question for inquiry; define what is to be studied, and decide for how long, under what circumstances, and with whom the study will be done.

2. *Workout:* The researcher redefines and readjusts the design as data are collected and analyzed.

3. *Cool down:* This is the time to decide when to end data collection and how to withdraw from the situation in which the researcher has been immersed.

Qualitative case studies often include both descriptive and interpretive elements, both of which are evident in Sabat's (2009) case study. The analysis may be directed toward discovering meaning (phenomenology), thick description (ethnography), describing social processes (grounded theory), analyzing verbal interactions (discourse analysis and ethnomethodology), describing behavior (participant observation) or a mix of these (Morse, 1998).

Survey Research

Probably every reader of this book has been a participant in a survey at one time or another. Opinion polls are done by telephone, on the Internet, at shopping malls and by mail. People are asked who they would vote for, how often they have intimate relations, and what their favorite brand of peanut butter is. Most of these familiar polls are done for marketing purposes, but there are also health-related surveys that provide very useful information on people's attitudes and behavior.

We are interested in the most basic survey design here. Surveys are used primarily to obtain answers that can be tallied and reported numerically. Fowler (2002) uses the term *total survey design* to describe the elements of a survey plan. These elements include the type of sample to be used (probability or nonprobability), the design of the survey questions, and mode of data collection.

Most often survey research uses a sampling of the population of interest, not the total population unless that population is very small. The US Census count of everyone living in the United States that is done every 10 years is an exception: the intent of the Census is to collect information on every person in the population. Other well-known surveys provide us with unemployment rates, crime statistics, health conditions, health-related behaviors, and health service usage (Fowler, 2002).

Smaller surveys may tally patient satisfaction ratings, nurse retention rates, infection rates, and rates of adverse events. The following example about postvaccination syncope uses a combination of survey data from the VAERS reporting system and case studies:

The Centers for Disease Control and Prevention (CDC) published a report on syncope (fainting) after vaccination based on data from the Vaccine Adverse Event Reporting System (VAERS) (Sutherland et al., 2008). The rate of syncope after vaccination was calculated by dividing the number of reports by the total doses of vaccine given for the same time period. They compared the 2005–2007 rates of syncope with previously reported rates and found that the rates had increased primarily in females age 11–18. During the 2005–2007 time period, 463 syncope reports were received. Thirty-three (7%) were rated as serious. For the 23 patients on whom complete data were available, 52% of the episodes occurred within 5 minutes of vaccination, and 70% occurred within 15 minutes of vaccination. Ten reports indicated secondary injuries had occurred, 9 head injuries, and one motor vehicle accident. One fatality was documented: a 15-year-old suffered a fatal intracranial hemorrhage from head trauma received upon fainting. An editorial accompanying the report reiterates the importance of patient observation for 15 minutes after vaccination and notes the American Academy of Pediatrics 2006 report that recommends, in addition, that the recipient sit or lie down for 15 minutes after vaccination (Sutherland et al., 2008).

Note that this report presents simple descriptive statistics on a specific population—people receiving vaccinations. The only comparison made was with rates for previous years. Only raw numbers and percents are reported. No associations between types of patients and fainting or comparison of different types of vaccines or ways to administer them are made. The rates, however, are segmented by age group, and they are compared to historical rates. A simpler quantitative description without any segmentation or any comparison is less common, but many surveys and opinion polls have little or no statistical analysis beyond descriptive statistics or comparison of groups (Gliner & Morgan, 2000). In this example on syncope, several but not all of the cases in which a secondary injury occurred are described. A pure multiple case study report would describe all the cases encountered within a specific time frame, in a specific geographic area, or other commonality such as patients from the same hospital unit.

MORE COMPLEX DESCRIPTIVE DESIGNS

Descriptive study designs can be much more complex than the ones already discussed. The simplest ones involve a single observation on a single group. From this basic design, the number of groups may be increased, the number of observations may be increased, or both may be increased (see Figure 6-1).

Notice in Figure 6-1 that despite the increasing complexity, there still is no intervention or treatment (i.e., manipulation) and that the participants may be selected randomly or in a nonrandom manner, which is more often the case.

The first set of designs in Figure 6-1 becomes a *descriptive comparative* design when more than one group is observed. The second set becomes a *descriptive associational* design when several observations are made about one group and their interrelationships are analyzed. These may also be called correlational designs (Spector, 1981). The third set is simply a combination of the first two in which both comparisons and associations are made.

These designs are very common. What makes each study different are the purpose of the study, the choice of sample, and the variables that are measured and analyzed. The data collected may be quantitative, qualitative, or a mix of the two. Qualitative studies are more likely to use the simplest designs but are not limited to these.

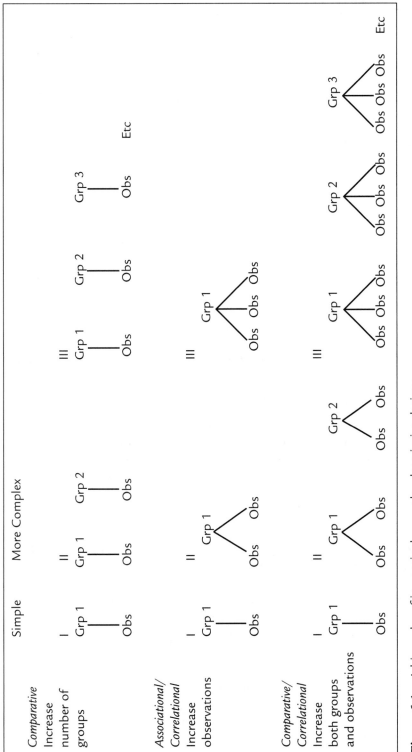

Figure 6-1 A hierarchy of increasingly complex descriptive designs.

Note: Grp = group; Obs = observation.
Source: Based on Clark-Carter, 1997 and Gliner and Morgan, 2000.

Comparative Descriptive Designs

These are the descriptive designs that resemble natural experiments. People cannot be deliberately exposed to such adverse events as violence, injury, prejudice, or to illness, but those who have had this experience can be compared to those who have not.

> Richmond and colleagues (2007) randomly selected 275 adults who presented to an urban emergency department (ED) with a physical injury that had not been self-inflicted. Those with major depression, psychosis, or physiologic abnormality were excluded. On the basis of a postdischarge interview and assessment, participants were classified as having past or current psychiatric history or no psychiatric history. The researchers found that 45% of the people injured also had a past or current psychiatric disorder. Those individuals with a current disorder were more likely to be unemployed and have a lower educational level, suggesting that they had fewer resources available to them post-ED discharge and that they may need more comprehensive assessment and intervention before leaving the ED. The researchers are careful to point out that their study results cannot be used to determine reasons why so many of the injured had an apparent psychiatric disorder. In other words, their study results could not provide an explanation for the link between injury and mental illness.
>
> Raymond and Lusk (2006) studied the use of hearing protection devices by 1245 workers in an automotive plant. Because this was a secondary analysis, the researchers had to use data from three measures to segment the sample by levels of hearing protection device use, from no use to 100% use in the past week, past month, and intention to use in the future. They compared stage of use to the Predictors of Use of Hearing Protection Model instrument variables including self-efficacy, barriers, and benefits. They found that self-efficacy (confidence in ability to use the devices correctly) scores differed significantly by level of use as did perceived barriers, which were lower in those who used the devices more often, and benefits, which were higher in the high users. The results support the influence of self-efficacy and other elements of the predictor measures used.

In the Raymond and Lusk (2006) study the five segments (subgroups) of the sample, from the subsample with lowest use to the subsample with high protective device use, were compared on their perceptions of self-efficacy, barriers, and benefits, a nice example of use of the comparative descriptive design. Note that it was the *existing* degree of use of the protective devices that was used in their analysis; the researchers had not taken any steps to change it before these data were collected.

Associational or Correlational Descriptive Designs

In studies using this type of design, a number of observations are made on the same group and the relationships (correlations) between them are calculated. The observations may be characteristics of members of the group or phenomena that affect the group. The following are two examples that illustrate use of the associational/correlational descriptive design:

Flanagan (2006) mailed questionnaires on job satisfaction and stress to 984 nurses working in state prison systems in the northeastern United States. Of these, 454 (56%) responded. The researcher used the Pearson product moment (bivariate) correlation statistic to identify what factors were related to job stress and satisfaction. Variables related to stress were unit specialty, presence of inpatient beds, supervisor status, and years in correctional nursing. Inpatient beds, years in correctional nursing, years at the current institution, race (scored as 0 = other and 1 = white), and stress were inversely related to satisfaction. The next step in the analysis involved multiple regression to calculate the extent to which the factors that were measured predicted job satisfaction. The top three sources of satisfaction were physician–nurse interaction, autonomy, and professional status. Job stress, which was moderate in this sample, was found to be a significant predictor of job satisfaction. It was expected that pay would also be a significant source of satisfaction, but it actually had the lowest amount of influence among the factors studied.

Zalon (2004) conducted a correlational/predictive study of recovery from major nonlaparoscopic abdominal surgery for adults age 60 and older. The researcher was particularly interested in the relation of pain, depression, and fatigue to patients' perception of recovery and functional status. Data were collected during hospitalization, 3–5 days after discharge, 1 month, and 3 months postdischarge. Pain and fatigue decreased over time but were significantly correlated with each other at each time interval as were fatigue and depression. Multiple regression analysis showed that pain, depression, and fatigue all contributed to self-reported functional recovery after discharge but not to perceived recovery during hospitalization. Their contribution decreased as time passed, accounting for 33% of the variation in perceived recovery at 1 month after discharge and 16.1% at 3 months postdischarge. The researcher concluded that interventions to reduce pain, fatigue, and depression after surgery need to be tested given their influence on recovery (Zalon, 2004).

Note that the results of these studies include *predictions* of relationships among measured factors (the independent variables).

Combined Comparative and Correlational Design

This next level of complexity in descriptive designs combines the comparison of multiple groups (or multiple segments of a single group) with analysis of multiple factors that might affect the groups in some way. For example, Youngblut and colleagues (2001) examined the effects of low-income single mothers' employment and infant prematurity on behavior problems and cognitive functioning of the children at preschool age in two groups: 60 children who were premature (preterm delivery) and 61 who were full-term infants. The abbreviated study aims reflect the combined comparative and correlational descriptive design:

1. Describe the effects of the mother's employment and preterm vs. full-term gestation on preschool child cognition and behavior.

2. Examine the relationships of the mother's employment, prematurity, child cognition, behavior, and related factors.

The researchers found that both premature and full-term children of employed mothers had higher cognitive scores than unemployed mothers, and, in those who had been premature, fewer behavior problems when compared to children of mothers who were not employed. Some relationships of interest:

- Higher income and higher education of the mothers and having fewer children related to higher cognitive function of the child.
- Mother–child attachment strain was related to behavior problems.

When characteristics of the mother, child, and family were controlled, however, the beneficial effect of employment was not significant (p. 353). Prematurity also had little effect. The researchers conclude that high levels of concern about employment of mothers of young children in low-income, single parent families may not be justified.

Prediction and Causation

A few words about the use of regression and related statistical techniques in relation to prediction and causation may be helpful here. Regression uses correlations between variables to test whether or not there is a relationship. If a relationship does exist, then knowing the score on one variable provides information to *predict* the score on the other variable. If the correlation was perfect, a -1.00 or $+1.00$, which is rare, then you could make a perfect prediction. A prediction equation can be created in which weights are assigned to each of the predictor variables based on their relationship to the outcome variable (Munro, 2005). Path analysis takes this a step further to create what is called a causal model. Such a model indicates both direct and indirect effects on the phenomenon of interest.

Descriptive, not experimental, data are used. There is also no manipulation of the independent variables (the predictor variables). Both independent and dependent (the outcome variable) variables are measured at the same time. Strictly speaking, causation cannot be tested in this manner. Instead, the *causal relationship* is supported by a theoretical argument that the independent variable preceded or led to the values of the dependent variable. For example, it is relatively persuasive to argue that a lifetime of parental abuse reported by an adolescent (the independent or predictor variable) contributed to the adolescent's current suicidal ideation (the dependent or outcome variable). The temporal (time) relationship is not always this clear, however. Because of these limitations of descriptive data, researchers are generally very careful about the terminology used in describing the relationships. The independent variables are called predictor variables, but their effect is referred to as an *influence* rather than a *cause* of the dependent variable (Norris, 2005).

SECONDARY ANALYSIS

The work required to obtain high-quality data on a large number of individuals, particularly if these individuals are difficult to find (examples would be depressed older adults who have isolated themselves as a result or individuals who consume excessive amounts of alcohol on the weekend but not during the work week) or to access (undocumented or illegal, immigrants would be an example) is reason enough to plan multiple analyses from one set of data. The study of self-efficacy and use of protective hearing devices by Raymond and Lusk (2006) is an example of a secondary analysis of data originally collected as a pretest before an intervention is introduced.

Another example of a secondary analysis is the addition of a new or relatively untested measure to the test battery. While not used to analyze the outcomes of the study, the data obtained on both the new instrument and more widely used instruments may be used in a separate analysis to evaluate the reliability and validity of the new instrument.

These examples are, in effect, studies within studies. They make efficient use of the expensive and time-consuming job of data collection without jeopardizing the quality of the parent study. The model used in the previous example of research by Raymond and Lusk (2006) is a combination of descriptive (the use of pretest data for descriptive analytical purposes) and experimental (the introduction of an intervention and collection of posttest data) factors.

MIXED DESIGNS AND MIXED METHODS

We turn now to *metadesigns* in which the basic designs discussed so far can be combined in various ways or in which the information that is obtained includes both qualitative and quantitative data. The epidemiological and longitudinal designs discussed in the next chapter also provide many examples of variations on the basic experimental and descriptive designs. Attention will be directed to the inclusion of both qualitative and quantitative approaches in a study, usually called mixed methods, as this raises many issues but also, if done well, may produce a more satisfactory result than one or the other can do alone.

Mixed Methods

The term *mixed methods* is usually used to refer to the combination of qualitative and quantitative research (Plano Clark et al., 2008). Several different goals may be met through the combination of qualitative and quantitative approaches (Greene, Caracelli, & Graham, 1989; Tashakkori & Teddlie, 1998, 2002):

- The researcher may be looking for convergence in the results from the two different approaches.
- The results from the two approaches may complement each other or better complete our understanding of a phenomenon. For example, the numbers of unemployed single parents who are the sole support for their families provide information about the scope of the problem, but qualitative data on the effect on both the parent and children (unable to afford health care, unable to pay the rent or the electric bill) fills in detail on the impact that numbers alone cannot do.

- Information from one approach may inform the design of the second approach. For example, the results of interviews of individuals with multiple sclerosis (MS) may be used to create a measure of coping with MS.

- Contradictions may be found between the two sources of data. If further studied and reconciled these may lead to greater insight and new directions for research. For example, nursing staff on a locked unit were very concerned about what they thought was an increased incidence of patient-to-staff violence. A count of the frequency of these incidences indicated they had not actually increased, suggesting that it was the *impact* and *severity* of the violence episodes that had affected staff, not the frequency alone. This new direction could then be explored through qualitative interviews.

Mixed Method Design Variations

There are a number of different ways to combine qualitative and quantitative approaches. Instead of listing each one (some are frequently used but others are relatively rare), we will first review the three parameters of the design that can be modified to answer a particular research question, and then we'll examine the levels or degrees of integration of the qualitative and quantitative data (Creswell, 2009):

1. *Timing:* Will you collect both types of data at the same time (simultaneously) or one before the other (sequentially)?

2. *Emphasis:* Will the study be primarily a quantitative study with the addition of some qualitative data, primarily a qualitative study with the addition of some quantitative data, or will the qualitative and quantitative portions be about equal?

3. *Data mixing:* Will you merge the quantitative and qualitative data into a single data set to be analyzed? Or will you keep them separate but link or compare the results? Or will you embed the qualitative results into the report of the quantitative (or vice versa)?

Creswell (2009) and Plano Clark and colleagues (2008) described four different mixed methods designs, which Happ (2009, p. 124) has ordered by the degree to which the qualitative and quantitative data are integrated. These four levels, beginning with the least integrated, are as follows:

1. *Separated:* The quantitative and qualitative data are collected, analyzed, and reported separately.

2. *Sequential:* Either qualitative or quantitative data are collected first, and the results are used to inform the design and collection of subsequent data.

3. *Comparative:* The data are collected and analyzed separately, but the results are then linked and compared.

4. *Integrated:* The qualitative and quantitative data are collected at (approximately) the same time, and the results are analyzed together. The data may be transformed, for example the qualitative data may be quantified and merged into a single quantitative dataset for analysis (this is discussed further in a later chapter).

Newlin (personal communication, 2010) conducted a mixed methods community-based participatory research design study of church-based diabetes education programs in the Atlantic Coast region of Nicaragua. This area is populated primarily by Miskitos and Creoles of African descent. The first phase of the study involved interviews with local nurses, church leaders, Nicaraguan Ministry of Health representatives and individuals with or at-risk for type II diabetes (T2D) who described diabetes as epidemic in this region of Nicaragua and identified factors contributing to this public health concern:

- Increasing rates of diabetes and related complications.
- Limited access to diabetes specialists
- Need for public education about diabetes and management of diabetes

The second phase of the study was a community survey of food availability, physical activity levels, availability of diabetes—related services and pharmaceuticals, and community residents' knowledge levels, attitudes and behaviors related to diabetes. Quantitative measures such as the SF-12, PAHO Nutrition and Exercise Survey, Diabetes Care Profile: Education, Attitudes and Barriers subscale, BMI (Body Mass Index) and HbA1c levels were obtained.

Results from the interviews were analyzed using content analysis (Krippendorf, 2004) and Atlas.ti software to create codes and identify themes that represent the views of the participants). Quantitative measures were analyzed using SAS 9.2.

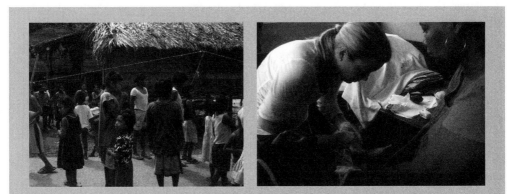

Dr. Kelley Newlin and research associate Yolanda McLean employed mixed methodology in her research on prevention and treatment of diabetes in the residents of several coastal towns in Nicaragua. These photos show a typical street scene in one of these towns (left) and Dr. Newlin providing foot care to a study participant (right).

Results supported the suspected high prevalence of type II diabetes and the need for education about diabetes. The sample ($N = 154$) was comprised largely of people who were of Creole (72.3%) or Miskito (23.2%) origin. Most were middle age adults (M = 54.9, SD ± 16.4) and women (77.8%). Most participants reported a diagnosis of T2D (62.5%), the remainder evidenced T2D risk (27.5%). In the quantitative component ($n = 112$), those with T2D had suboptimal glycemic control as measured by HbA1c (M = 10.6, SD ± 2.5) and elevated BMIs (M = 31.7, SD ± 8.1). A majority reported treatment (78%) to control their diabetes with medication only (43%) or medication and lifestyle factors (35%). In terms of medication accessibility, most indicated medications were generally available (78%) while a smaller percentage indicated medications were affordable (54%). Among those at-risk for T2D, most were obese BMI (M = 30.2, SD ± 6.0) with a majority reporting there is little they can do to prevent diabetes (58%) and feeling they had only modest control over their health (83%) (Newlin, Melkus, Mclean & Dekker, 2010). With respect to the qualitative component ($n = 54$), participants tended to perceive T2D as serious with complications to which they felt they were susceptible. Barriers to diabetes self-management included the belief that insulin causes blindness, that exercise is for the *young* not for older people, and medications may be taken on an as needed basis.

Community strengths included a strong commitment to volunteerism; local access to primary care; and local physicians, nurses, and physicians committed to raising diabetes awareness. Community action strategies included the development of "diabetes teams" with physicians, nurses, social workers, and community volunteers to deliver church-based diabetes education, offer diabetes support groups, and provide home visits for the home bound (Newlin, Melkus, Mclean, Mclean, Dekker et al., 2010). The community survey confirmed the need for more diabetes specialists and identified characteristics of the local food supply that reinforced a carbohydrate-rich diet. For example, a single piece of fruit cost $1 (converted to U.S. currency), the same as a one-pound bag of rice. Together, the quantitative and qualitative results presented a more comprehensive profile of type II diabetes as a public health concern in these communities.

Issues Related to Mixing Methods

Qualitative and quantitative research have different, often conflicting philosophies underlying them. Parse (2009) questions the soundness of using both in the same study, as do many others. They also ask if it is appropriate to merge data obtained in such different ways? Is this a problem of mixing "apples and oranges," to use a trite but relevant phase?

Another important issue is the expertise needed to use several different methods together. Many researchers have devoted entire careers to becoming expert ethnographers, phenomenologists, or a principal investigator on clinical trial studies. Can one person be expert in a multitude of methods? That certainly is unlikely and is one of the reasons that researchers work as teams, each contributing his or her expertise to the enterprise.

The Special Case of Participatory Action Research (PAR)

PAR (participatory action research) or CBPR (community-based participatory research) is both a philosophy and an approach to the design and conduct of research. It is a "participatory, democratic process concerned with developing practical knowledge," that "seeks to bring together action and reflection, theory and practice, in participation with others, in the pursuit of practical solutions to issues of pressing concern to people" (Reason & Bradbury, 2001, p. 1). Although the emphasis is usually on the kind of information best obtained through qualitative methods, quantitative methods may also be used in participatory action research.

Community-Based PAR

The key difference between participatory action research and most other types of research lies in the kind and amount of *participation* by the subjects of the study. Whyte writes that science is not about distancing oneself from the world but becoming engaged in it (1991, p. 21). In PAR the researcher engages the study participants in actual collaboration, ideally through every step in the research process, from deciding upon the purpose of the study to selecting the measures to be used or questions to be asked, to the final phase of interpreting the results. In effect, the study participants partner with the researcher to plan and implement the research study. This is in sharp contrast to the usual study in which the researchers are the experts and the subjects are willing but relatively passive participants (Whyte, 1991).

Clearly, the PAR approach requires some additional skills on the part of the researcher, including the ability to enter a community (broadly defined as the population of interest to the study), to engage community members in dialogue to design the study, to motivate and maintain interest and participation throughout what can be a lengthy process, and to be open to new ideas and new ways to conduct the study. In addition, the researcher must also respect the input of the participants in the study. They are, after all, expert on their needs and experiences and have much to offer. This process becomes one of colearning (Blair & Minkler, 2009), where the researcher shares his or her expertise in research and the problem to be studied, and community members contribute access to the people of the community and their experience. Without their input, there can be no PAR (van der Velde, Williamson, & Ogilvie, 2009, p. 1299):

> Van der Velde and colleagues (2009) describe the efforts involved in engaging members of immigrant and refugee populations in a mental health project in Canada. The experts were representatives of nonprofit human services and health and immigration services agencies. The community members represented five ethnic/cultural groups: Chinese, Somali, South Asian, Hispanic, and Vietnamese. One consequence of the project was that the communities learned much more about each other, particularly that other groups were also struggling to become integrated into Canadian society. They also found they could accomplish more by working together than in isolation.

Organization-Based Action Research

Participatory action research may be conducted within an organization as well as within a community at large. In fact, there is a long tradition of using action research to effect change within organizations. As with community-based PAR, action research aims not only to create knowledge but also to take action. Members of the organization take an active part in this collaborative process. It begins with planning, which is followed by taking action, evaluating the results, and, sometimes, returning to the planning stage to continue to improve the work environment (Coghlan & Brannick, 2001). The following is an example of action research within an organization:

> Vivian, Marais, McLaughlin, Falkenstein, & Argent (2009) describe the use of PAR with staff of a pediatric intensive care unit in South Africa. The study was undertaken in response to concerns about interpersonal relationship problems within the staff and about some of the caregiving practices on the unit. They used the PAR approach because they believed that "actively involving subjects in their own research process will produce knowledge that will empower them to change" (p. 1594). Ninety-seven percent of the staff agreed to participate. Two researchers conducted 12 focus groups, observed activity on the unit, and conducted eight semistructured interviews. Findings were presented to the staff who then rated their accuracy and relevancy.

A few of the findings:

- Relationships among nurses were seen as highly effective during critical incidents, but social disharmony among nurses otherwise was also noted.
- Medical staff were identified as the primary decision makers. Nurses were reluctant to challenge their decisions, often opting to remain silent.
- Conflict and dysfunction in management was noted.
- Inadequate training and staff shortages exacerbated these problems.

The researchers concluded that the unit was experiencing "problematic levels of dysfunction that potentially placed patients and staff at risk" (Vivian et al., p. 1595). Eighty-one percent of the staff agreed with this summary statement. The researchers commented that participation in the process empowered staff and that using PAR revealed the discord, increased their awareness of it, and prepared them for change.

The balance between qualitative and quantitative approaches was clearly weighted toward the qualitative side in the initial data gathering. Quantitative data were then used to summarize the feedback from staff on the researchers' findings.

META-ANALYSIS

Meta-analyses may be compared, somewhat tongue in cheek, to literature reviews on steroids. They are analyses of the results of multiple studies on a single topic. The analysis may be quantitative or qualitative.

Glass, one of the developers of meta-analysis, called it the "analysis of analyses" (1976, p. 3), but we could also call meta-analysis a study of studies or, more accurately, a study of study results. Quantitative meta-analysis is "the statistical analysis of a large collection of analysis results from individual studies for the purpose of integrating the findings" (p. 3).

Primary analyses, as Glass (1976) reminds us, are the original analyses of data collected in a research study. *Secondary analyses* are reanalyses of the data, either to refine the original analysis or to answer a new question using existing datasets. *Meta-analyses* are formal, structured analyses of the results of a number of studies on the same topic.

Traditional literature reviews, which are narrative reviews of existing research, have several limitations. Usually studies with similar findings are grouped together, but conflicting findings (e.g., in one study an intervention appears to be effective, in another it does not) are difficult to reconcile. It is also tempting to emphasize the results that agree with your hypothesis and to ignore those that do not. Furthermore, it is difficult to judge studies with samples that are too small to produce significant results (Rosenthal & DiMatteo, 2001).

There has been an increasingly urgent call for clearer direction upon which to base practice and healthcare policy. This will be addressed in detail in the chapter on evidence-based practice, but the usefulness of meta-analyses in reconciling or explaining conflicting results should be evident from its definition. Briefly, meta-analysis can be used to combine results from a number of completed studies. Results that appear to conflict can be examined statistically, and reasons for the disagreement may be found; for example, a particular drug may be more effective in a low dose than in a high dose or in women but not men, or an operative procedure may be more effective than conservative treatment in some instances but not in others. There are even efforts under way to provide *overviews* of groups of systematic reviews on health-related subjects (Ryan, Kaufman, & Hill, 2009).

Steps in Beginning a Meta-Analysis

Qualitative and quantitative meta-analysis begin in a similar way.

1. Most meta-analytic studies, qualitative or quantitative, begin by defining study aims and stating a research question or set of questions.

   For example, Conner, Pinquart, and Gamble (2009) had five aims for their meta-analysis of studies of the relationship between depression and alcohol use disorder. The primary aim was to test the association of depression, alcohol use, drug use, and involvement in treatment. Secondary aims were to look at associations of depression and socio-economic characteristics such as gender and describe changes in levels of depression over time.

   Similarly, de Bloom, Kompier, Geurts, de Weerth, Taris, and Sonnentag (2009) posed three research questions related to the health effects of taking a vacation: does it increase well-being? How long does the effect last? Does the type of vacation taken make a difference?

2. The next step in designing and conducting a meta-analysis is to clearly and specifically set boundaries on the search of the literature that will be done. This includes (a) the sources to be searched, (b) the time frame of the search, (c) the inclusion criteria, and (d) the exclusion criteria.

> For example, Conner and colleagues (2009) searched MEDLINE and PsycINFO plus the reference lists from related studies and review articles for their depression and alcohol use disorder study. They included only studies from peer-reviewed journals, studies related to adults, and studies that reported effect size or correlations. Excluded were reports that had not been peer reviewed, which included books, drug or therapy trials, and surveys that did not include data on all of the variables needed for the meta-analysis. Their time frame was 1986 to 2007.

> Yarcheski, Mahon, Yarcheski, Hanks, and Cannella (2009) conducted a meta-analytic study of the predictors of maternal-fetal attachment (MFA). For their literature search, CINAHL, PsycINFO, MEDLINE, Social Science Index, and dissertations and theses were used. The search terms included *maternal–fetal attachment* or *bonding, parental–fetal attachment*, and *prenatal attachment*. The time frame was 1980 to 2006. They also excluded books or studies that only reported results on sub-scales of MFA measures. The search yielded 115 studies and 68 dissertations and theses. Of these, 72 met their criteria and became the sample for their study. They found very low effect sizes for anxiety, self-esteem, and depression. Gestational age was the most powerful predictor of MFA.

> de Bloom and colleagues (2009) used a somewhat different approach, beginning with much broader boundaries for their search. They used almost a dozen separate search words including *vacation, holiday, well-being, health, stress, recovery*, and so forth, generating 829,536 hits. When they combined *vacation* or *holiday* with the other health- and well-being-related terms, the list was reduced to 125 possible studies. Elimination of non-English papers reduced this by another 22; elimination of non-peer-reviewed papers and dissertations (note the difference from Yarcheski et al., who retained the dissertations) eliminated another 38. This left 65 articles. Review of the 65 abstracts of these articles for relevant samples (working adults) and topics and for appropriate designs (they were looking for interrupted time series designs, which are described in the next chapter) left 11 articles of which 4 more were excluded because of overlaps in information (duplicate publications by the same authors) or irrelevancy, leaving 7 for their final sample. They used effect size to calcu-

late vacation effects and found that a vacation has a positive but weak effect on well-being that does not last long.

3. The results of the search are then analyzed. This is where quantitative and qualitative meta-analyses differ and must be discussed separately.

Quantitative Meta-Analyses

Probably the most frequently used statistic in quantitative meta-analysis is the *effect size*, which is explained further in the chapter on sampling. Correlations and odds ratios from epidemiological studies can also be transformed into effect sizes (Sutton & Higgins, 2008). These statistics are obtained from each of the selected studies or from their authors if not available in the published information, and combined for analysis. There are several different software programs available for use in these analyses.

The analyses may be further refined by weighting certain studies on the basis of their quality and analyzing the effects of certain characteristics for their potential influence. Quality may be rated on the basis of the design (experimental vs. nonexperimental, randomized vs. nonrandomized), the measures (standard instruments vs. investigator-created or subjective measures), and so forth. Potential influences on the outcomes are the effects of sample size and publication bias (when more studies that yielded significant results are published than are studies that did not).

> For example, Han, Lee, Kim, Hedlin, Song, and Kim (2009) used two raters to independently score the quality of the 23 studies of interventions to promote mammography in ethnic minority women the researchers had found. The two raters rated the studies on the basis of design, measures, clarity of outcome definition, and information on withdrawals from the study. They also calculated the impact of three of the most influential studies on the final results. Interestingly, they found small or negative effects (lower rates of mammography) in studies using *promotoras* (lay health advisors), but they suggested that weakness of the study designs may be a factor since all six studies using promotoras were nonrandomized community trials with low-quality ratings.

Metadata

An alternative approach to meta-analysis is the combination of the data itself on individuals from each of the studies to be analyzed. This can be a highly complex and challenging undertaking but is very valuable in some instances. For example, many studies of brain function have relatively small samples. Combined, however, they can be used to identify areas of the brain that are activated when different activities are undertaken such as solving a mathematical problem or areas affected when a disorder such as schizophrenia or autism is present (Van Essen, 2009; Laird, Lancaster, & Fox, 2009). These *metadata* banks can yield powerful results that are otherwise impossible or at least unrealistic for most research studies. In fact, Sutton and Higgins (2008) say that collecting and analyzing individual participant data from the original studies is the "gold standard" in quantitative meta-analysis (p. 636).

Meta-Analysis of Qualitative Data

Meta-analysis of qualitative data uses similar approaches to defining the aim of the analysis, stating research questions to focus the study and defining the boundaries of the literature search. The inclusion and exclusion criteria, of course, need to be suitable to the particular analysis and to the type of studies that will be analyzed.

The type of data that can be retrieved from a qualitative study will affect whether you conduct metasynthesis or a metasummary (Sandelowski & Barroso, 2003).

Metasynthesis

A *metasynthesis* may use grounded theory's constant comparison or a similar approach in the analysis after the findings of the selected studies have been reduced to a set of abstracted statements or into a taxonomy (Sandelowski & Barroso, 2007). This is appropriate for interpretive qualitative studies when models, metaphors, or concepts are generated in the original studies. Sandelowski and Barroso (2003) define qualitative metasynthesis as the:

> systematic review or integration of qualitative research findings . . . that are themselves interpretive syntheses of data including phenomenologies, ethnographies, grounded theories, and other integrated and coherent descriptions or explanations of phenomena, events, or cases. (p. 227)

A metasynthesis is "a complete study in itself" (Jensen & Allen, 1996, p. 554). It should be a rigorous procedure with as much attention paid to trustworthiness and credibility of the results as it is in other qualitative research (trustworthiness of qualitative research findings is discussed in detail in a later chapter). It should also be interpretive, reaching a higher level of abstraction than did the studies under analysis. The interpretive synthesis that is created may have two aspects: *hermeneutic*—portraying the individual constructions accurately; and *dialectic*—comparing and contrasting the individual constructions (Jensen & Allen, 1996, p. 555).

Jensen and Allen (1996) describe the steps in the analysis:

- Each study is read and reread.
- Key "metaphors" are identified in each study (*metaphor* in this usage means themes, perspectives, organizers, or concepts revealed by the qualitative studies) (Noblit & Hare, 1988).
- Study findings are "standardized" by using common codes (Jensen & Allen, 1996, p. 556).

- Relationships among study findings are identified by showing how the key metaphors from each study relate to each other (Paterson, Thorne, Canam, & Jillings, 2001).
- The studies' findings are then juxtaposed.
- Findings from the studies may be combined, set against each other, or organized into a line of argument.

This is an iterative process during which you will redefine the metaphors and revise decisions as you proceed with the metasynthesis (Sandelowski & Barroso, 2007). An example of a metasynthesis may make this clearer.

Xu (2007) conducted a metasynthesis of qualitative studies on the experiences of immigrant Asian nurses working in Ireland, the United Kingdom and the United States. CINAHL, MEDLINE, PsychINFO, Sociological Abstracts, ERIC, and Pro Quest Dissertations and Theses were searched using the terms *Asian nurses*, *foreign nurses*, and the like. The search was completed July 2006. Targeted journals were also searched by hand as were ancestral searches of references found in relevant papers. To be included, the papers had to address the experience of Asian nurses practicing in Western countries and they had to be qualitative studies or include qualitative data. The final sample of the papers included four doctoral dissertations, one thesis, and nine articles. The Asian nurses involved came from India, Korea, Pakistan, and the Philippines. Xu (2007) based the analytic approach on Noblit and Hare's (1988) work on meta-ethnography. Analysis began with reading and rereading the studies. Key metaphors (themes, concepts) from each study were listed and relationships among them identified. Then the key metaphors were translated so as to preserve the individual particulars yet bring them into a whole (synthesize them) that goes beyond the individual studies.

The researcher identified four themes, relating many examples and connecting them to Asian and Western culture. Communication challenges were the first theme identified. Although the nurses knew formal English, they did not understand such phrases as "you are a hell of a good nurse," or the frequent "uh-huhs," delivered in different tones signifying different meanings (Xu, 2007, p. 251). Not all of the problems were this benign, however. Instances of harassment and prejudicial bullying were also related under the marginalization, discrimination, and exploitation theme. Xu concluded that the experience of these immigrant Asian nurses needs to be viewed through the lenses of gender, race, and culture simultaneously to be fully understood.

Note that it is the findings (results) of the studies that are synthesized, not the raw data, in a metasynthesis. The goal in producing a new, more integrated interpretation may be to refine or better explain existing knowledge, build theory, or produce a clearer description of a phenomenon (Finfgeld, 2003). Metasyntheses generate theories, grand narratives, generalizations, or interpretive translations from the integration or comparison of the findings of qualitative studies (Sandelowski, Docherty, & Emden, 1997).

Questions About Metasynthesis

Qualitative research is "endangered by the failure to sum it up," note Sandelowski, Docherty, and Emden (1997, p. 366). Metasynthesis addresses this need to pull together disparate insights, theorizing, and explanations of phenomena. The results of the metasynthesis, if done well, make the findings from qualitative research more accessible and usable (Sandelowski, Docherty, & Emden, 1997).

There are questions about the conduct of a metasynthesis. Many are related to the great diversity of qualitative research methods and the different philosophical stances that underlie them. Can the findings of studies from such a diverse base be combined? Should they be clustered by the method used (ethnographies separate from phenomenological studies, for example)? If the levels of abstraction differ widely across studies, does this undermine the ability to synthesize the findings? Should only peer-reviewed articles be included? If yes, wouldn't some valuable work from dissertations and theses be lost (Jensen & Allen, 1996)?

Finally, the question of generalization needs to be addressed. It is said that qualitative studies are particularistic (i.e., they describe and interpret a given event, situation, experience, or phenomenon but are not designed to be generalized to other events, situations, or experiences). Sandelowski, Docherty, and Emden (1997) write that Glaser and Straus warned of this in 1971, that failure to link the studies' findings would leave them as "little islands" of knowledge remaining separate and unconnected (p. 367). Metasynthesis enhances the generalizability of qualitative research findings, producing a kind of "cross-case" generalization generated from a series of individual cases (Sandelowski, Docherty, & Emden, 1997, p. 367).

Metasummary

In contrast to the metasynthesis, a *metasummary* is more appropriately used when the data in the selected qualitative studies are summarized rather than synthesized. The data may be from a qualitative survey or other type of study that generates themes rather than concepts, models, or metaphors, which are generally at a higher level of abstraction. The results or findings of the studies selected are extracted from the articles and grouped by topic. Sandelowski and Barroso (2003) offer an example of a metasummary in which they extracted 800 statements or findings from 45 articles, books, and dissertations on mothers with HIV. These were reduced to 93 thematic statements (abstracted findings) organized into 10 topics such as stigma and disclosure or conceptualizations of motherhood. They then calculated the magnitude of treatment effect. Two effect sizes (which are not the same as the quantitative effect sizes), one based upon the *frequency* of the theme or number of articles and dissertations that contained this finding, and the other on the *intensity* of the findings (i.e., the concentration of findings in each report) (Sandelowski &

Barroso, 2003) were calculated. In this manner, qualitative results can also be characterized quantitatively.

CONCLUSION

The real test of the appropriateness of a research design selection is if it matches the purpose of the study and the research questions or hypotheses that are posed. The second question is whether or not the selected design suits the situation or context of the study. As mentioned earlier, you cannot assign people to be inactive or to overeat, although you can study the effects on people who have already done this. Likewise, you cannot impose an illness or disaster, but you can study what happens when they strike in order to intervene more effectively in the future. Descriptive designs often suit such situations.

Mixed method and meta-analysis studies are far from simple to plan or execute. However, they are designs that allow us to better answer some important questions. A mixed method design combines the richness of qualitative data with the precision of quantitative data, often producing a more comprehensive understanding than one or the other could do alone. Meta-analyses not only capitalize on research that has already been done, but they also enable us to answer questions in a more definitive way than most individual studies can do. Remember, however, that meta-analyses depend upon the original studies for the data that is to be analyzed.

REFERENCES

Atlas.ti Scientific Software Development. (2008). *Atlas.ti 5 multi educational license* [computer software]. Clevebridge AG: Cologne.

Blair, T., & Minkler, M. (2009). Participatory action research with older adults: Key principles in practice. *Gerontologist, 49*(5), 651–662.

Clark-Carter, D. (1997). *Doing quantitative psychological research: From design to report.* East Sussex, UK: Psychology Press.

Coghlan, D., & Brannick, T. (2001). *Doing action research in your own organization.* Thousand Oaks, CA: Sage.

Conner, K. R., Pinquart, M., & Gamble, S. A. (2009). Meta-analysis of depression and substance use among individuals with alcohol use disorders. *Journal of Substance Abuse Treatment, 37*, 127–137.

Creswell, J. W. (2009). *Research design: Qualitative, quantitative and mixed methods approach.* Los Angeles, CA: Sage.
   ✧ A basic textbook with a clear explanation of mixed methods.

de Bloom, J., Kompier, M., Geurts, S., de Weerth, C., Taris, T., & Sonnentag, S. (2009). Do we recover from vacation? Meta-analysis of vacation effects on health and well-being. *Journal of Occupational Health, 51*, 13–25.

Denzin, N. K., & Lincoln, Y. S. (1998). *Strategies of qualitative inquiry.* Thousand Oaks, CA: Sage.

Finfgeld, D. (2003). Metasynthesis: The state of the art-so far. *Qualitative Health Research, 13*(7), 893–904.

Flanagan, N. A. (2006). Testing the relationship between job stress and satisfaction in correctional nurses. *Nursing Research, 55*(5), 316–327.

Fowler, F. J. (2002). *Survey research methods.* Thousand Oaks, CA: Sage.

Glass, G. V. (1976). Primary, secondary, and meta-analysis of research. *Educational Researcher, 5*(3), 3–8.
  ◇ Another classic, this article explains the value of meta-analysis.
Gliner, J. A., & Morgan, G. A. (2000). *Research methods in applied settings.* Mahwah, NJ: Lawrence Erlbaum.
Greene, J. C., Caracelli, V. J., & Graham, W. F. (1989). Toward a conceptual framework for mixed-method evaluation designs. *Educational Evaluation and Policy Analysis, 11,* 255–274.
Han, H-R., Lee, J-E., Kim, J., Hedlin, H. K., Song, H., & Kim, M. T. (2009). A meta-analysis of interventions to promote mammography among ethnic minority women. *Nursing Research, 58*(4), 246–254.
Happ, M. B. (2009). Mixed methods in gerontological research. *Research in Gerontological Nursing, 2*(2), 122–127.
  ◇ Not just for those interested in gerontological research, this article provides a clear, basic explanation of mixed methods.
Janesick, V. J. (1998). The dance of qualitative research design: Metaphor, methodolatry and meaning. In N. K. Denzin & Y. S. Lincoln (Eds.), *Strategies of qualitative inquiry* (pp. 35–55), Thousand Oaks, CA: Sage.
Jensen, L. A., & Allen, M. N. (1996). Meta-synthesis of qualitative findings. *Qualitative Health Research, 6*(4), 553–560.
  ◇ Useful explanation of meta-synthesis.
Krippendorf, K. (2004). *Content analysis: An introduction to its methodology.* Thousand Oaks, CA: Sage.
Laird, A. R., Lancaster, J. L., & Fox, P. T. (2009). Lost in localization? The focus is meta-analysis. *NeuroImage, 48,* 18–20.
Morse, J. M. (1998). Designing funded research. In N. K. Denzin & Y. S. Lincoln (Eds.), *Strategies of qualitative inquiry* (pp. 56–85). Thousand Oaks, CA: Sage.
Munro, B. H. (2005). Regression. In B. H. Munro (Ed.), *Statistical methods for health care research* (pp. 259–286). Philadelphia: Lippincott, Williams & Wilkins.
  ◇ A basic and unusually readable introduction to statistics with examples from health-related fields of study.
Newlin, K., Melkus, G. D., Mclean, Y., & Dekker, R. (2010). Exploration of diabetes-related factors in Nicaraguan adults with or at-risk for diabetes. *Clinical and Translational Science, 3*(2) 1:S48.
Newlin, K., Melkus, G. D., Mclean, Y., Mclean, E., Dekker, T., & Chyun, D. (2010). *Participatory action research: Exploring Diabetes-related factors & community action strategies in Nicaragua.* Poster presentation, Eastern Nursing Research Society 22nd annual scientific sessions, Providence, Rhode Island.
Noblit, G. W., & Hare, R. D. (1988). *Meta-ethnography: Synthesizing qualitative studies.* Newbury Park, CA: Sage.
  ◇ This is the classic work on meta-synthesis.
Norris, A. E. (2005). Path analysis. In B. H. Munro (Ed.), *Statistical methods for health care research* (pp. 377–403). Philadelphia: Lippincott, Williams & Wilkins.
Parse, R. R. (2009). Mixed methods or mixed meanings in research? *Nursing Science Quarterly, 22*(2), 101.
Paterson, B. L., Thorne, S. E., Canam, C., & Jillings, C. (2001). *Meta-study of qualitative health research.* Thousand Oaks, CA: Sage.
Plano Clark, V. L., Huddleston-Casas, C. A., Churchill, S. L., Green, D. O., & Garrett, A. L. (2008). Mixed methods approaches in family science research. *Journal of Family Issues, 29*(11), 1544–1566.
Raymond, D. M., & Lusk, S. L. (2006). Testing decisional balance and self-efficacy applied to workers' use of hearing protection. *Nursing Research, 55*(5), 328–335.

Reason, P., & Bradbury, H. (2001). *Handbook of action research: Participatory inquiry and practice.* Thousand Oaks, CA: Sage.

Richmond, T. S., Hollander, J. E., Ackerson, T. H., Robinson, K., Gracias, V., Shults, J., et al. (2007). Psychiatric disorders in patients presenting to the emergency department for minor injury. *Nursing Research, 56*(4), 275–282.

Rosenthal, R., & DiMatteo, M. R. (2001). Meta-analysis: Recent developments in quantitative methods for literature reviews. *Annual Review Psychology, 52,* 59–82.
  ◇ An excellent overview of quantitative meta-analysis, from its value to the data analysis that is performed.

Ryan, R. E., Kaufman, C. A., & Hill, S. J. (2009). Building blocks for meta-synthesis: Data integration tables for summarizing, mapping, and synthesizing evidence on interventions for communicating with health consumers. *BMC Medical Research Methodology,* 9:10 doi:10.1186/1471-2288-9-16.

Sabat, S. R. (2009). Existential phenomenology and the quality of life of carers and care recipients: A case study. *Dementia, 8*(2), 163–166.

Sandelowski, M., Docherty, S., & Emden, D. (1997). Qualitative metasynthesis: Issues and techniques. *Research in Nursing and Health, 20,* 365–371.
  ◇ Also helpful, this article is a good introduction to meta-synthesis.

Sandelowski, M., & Barroso, J. (2003). Creating metasummaries of qualitative findings. *Nursing Research, 52*(4), 226–233.
  ◇ A helpful description of the conduct of a metasummary of certain types of qualitative data. There is also additional information available on the Editor's website.

Sandelowski, M., & Barroso, J. (2007). *Handbook for synthesizing qualitative research.* New York: Springer.
  ◇ The authors call their book a "methodological toolbox" and "stimulus to thinking and creativity" for doing metasynthesis.

SAS/STAT (2007). Software, Version [9.2] of the SAS System for [Windows], © SAS Institute Inc., Cary, N.C.

Schlotzhauer, S. D., & Littell, R. C. (1997). *SAS system for elementary statistics.* SAS Institute Inc., Cary, N.C.

Spector, P. E. (1981). *Research designs.* Beverly Hills, CA: Sage.

Stake, R. E. (1998). Case studies. In N. K. Denzin & Y. S. Lincoln (Eds.), *Strategies of qualitative inquiry* (pp. 86–109). Thousand Oaks, CA: Sage.

Sutherland, A., Izurieta, H., Ball, R., Braun, M. M., Miller, E. R., Broder, K. R., et al. (2008). Syncope after vaccination—United States, January 2006-July 2007. *Morbidity and Mortality Weekly Report, 57*(17), 457–460.

Sutton, A. J., & Higgins, J. P. T. (2008). Recent developments in meta-analysis. *Statistics in Medicine, 27*(5), 625–650.

Tashakkori, A., & Teddlie, C. B. (1998). *Mixed methodology: Combining qualitative and quantitative approaches.* Thousand Oaks, CA: Sage.

Tashakkori, A., & Teddlie, C. B. (2002). *Handbook of mixed methods social and behavioral research.* Thousand Oaks, CA: Sage.
  ◇ An excellent resource on mixed methods.

Van der Velde, J., Williamson, D. L., & Ogilvie, L. D. (2009). Participatory action research: Practical strategies for actively engaging and maintaining participation in immigrant and refugee communities. *Qualitative Health Research, 19*(9), 1293–1302.

Van Essen, D. C. (2009). Lost in localization—but found with foci?! *NeuroImage, 48,* 14–17.

Vivian, L., Marais, A., McLaughlin, S., Falkenstein, S., & Argent, A. (2009). Relationships, trust, decision-making and quality of care in a paediatric intensive care unit. *Intensive Care Medicine, 35,* 1593–1598.

Whyte, W. F. (1991). *Participatory action research.* Newbury Park, CA: Sage.

Xu, Y. (2007). Strangers in strange lands: A metasynthesis of lived experiences of immigrant Asian nurses working in western countries. *Advances in Nursing Science, 30*(3), 246–265.
   ✧ A good example of meta-synthesis done in a textbook-like and organized fashion. It is also quite interesting to read.

Yarcheski, A., Mahon, N. E., Yarcheski, T. J., Hanks, M. M., & Cannella, B. L. (2009). A meta-analytic study of predictors of maternal–fetal attachment. *International Journal of Nursing Studies, 46,* 708–795.

Yin, R. K. (2003). *Case study research: Design and methods.* Thousand Oaks, CA: Sage.

Youngblut, J. M., Broota, D., Singer, L. T., Standing, T., Lee, H., & Rodgers, W. L. (2001). Effects of maternal employment and prematurity on child outcomes in single parent families. *Nursing Research, 50*(6), 346–355.

Zalon, M. L. (2004). Correlates of recovery among older adults after major abdominal surgery. *Nursing Research 53*(2), 99–106.

CHAPTER 7

Epidemiological and Longitudinal Designs

We turn our attention now to the design of "big picture" studies, particularly to the epidemiological and longitudinal studies that have contributed significantly to our understanding of health and health-related concerns. The majority are descriptive in design. Several, like the case study, will already be familiar from the previous two chapters on research designs.

EPIDEMIOLOGICAL DESIGNS

Epidemiology is the study of the distribution and determinants of health-related states and events in human populations. The emphasis is on populations (Rothman, Greenland, & Lash, 2008, p. 32) rather than on individual clients.

In epidemiological studies, incidence and prevalence are often of interest. *Incidence* is the frequency (count of new cases) of *new* occurrences of the disease, illness, or injury being studied within a given population. *Prevalence,* on the other hand, is the count of all existing cases at a given time in a specified population (Bhopal, 2002). These numbers are different but related since prevalence includes the new as well as the continuing cases. Disease registries, reporting systems such as VAERS for adverse events related to immunizations, and surveys conducted for the specific purpose of the study are typical sources of data. The following is an example of a survey study of the prevalence of pressure ulcers (decubiti) in healthcare facilities in the Netherlands:

> Bours, Halfens, Abu-Saad, and Grol (2002) conducted a survey of hospitals, long-term care facilities, and home care organizations in the Netherlands for the prevalence of pressure ulcers in their patients. They invited all facilities in their country to participate, which would have been a study of the entire population rather than a probability sample of the population. Partially because they had to pay to participate but also because some were not particularly concerned about pressure ulcers given their client population, some facilities declined the invitation. None of the psychiatric hospitals participated. Altogether, 89 facilities did participate, and data were obtained in each of these facilities.
>
> A study coordinator was appointed in each facility. The researchers trained them in staging of pressure ulcers and assessing risk for pressure ulcers. The coordinators, in turn, trained staff to collect the data on the date that was set for the survey. Two nurses conducted independent assessments of each consenting patient: one nurse

was from the unit, and one nurse was unfamiliar with the patient. The data collected also included characteristics of the facility, staff, and patients; assessment of risk using the well-known Braden Scale, plus presence of malnutrition and incontinence, staging of existing decubiti, and use of preventive treatments such as positioning. The prevalence rates, which they reported by type of institution, were higher than have been reported in the literature. For example, the overall prevalence rates ranged from 13.2% in the university hospitals to 34.8% in an institution for the physically handicapped. Heels and the sacral area were the most common sites. When researchers compared the use of preventive treatment to existing Dutch guidelines for prevention, they found that only 27% of those at risk received the recommended nutritional support, and only 31% who should have been repositioned periodically actually were.

The researchers also discussed some of the limitations of this study, particularly the potential for bias that arises when a nonprobability sample is used. It is possible, for example, that data from hands-on assessments might produce a higher rate than asking staff how many patients had pressure ulcers. The facilities that were willing to participate are also likely to have been interested in improving their prevalence rates. On the other hand, units such as maternity or psychiatry were excluded by many facilities because pressure ulcers are rare occurrences there. More specific guidelines for selection of the units to survey would have been helpful in this case, and the researchers recommended that guidelines be developed so rates from various prevalence surveys can be compared. They also concluded that the rates they found were too high (Bours et al., 2002).

Case Studies

In an epidemiological case study or case study series, clinical case notes are compiled and then analyzed to better understand the event or health problem (Bhopal, 2002). Such case studies often provide new insights into existing problems or raise new concerns that are further explored in more complex studies.

Case study research may involve one case, called the *single case study* design, or several cases, the *multiple case study* or *case study series* design. The case or cases selected are those that are critical, sentinel, unique, representative, or typical. The researcher investigates each case, recording the information pertinent to the research question as well as contextual information that may explain the situation, and then the researcher writes up each case description. When multiple cases are used, the researcher then draws cross-case conclusions and concludes with implications for practice. Yin (2003) suggests that a series of cases often presents a more compelling picture, not just because of the increased number but because of seeing each additional case as a replication of the previous case study. The following is a case study of a single event:

An elementary school nurse informed the Ravalli County, Montana, Public Health Department of an incident of human exposure to a dead bat (Dickerson et al., 2009). The day before, a family cat brought a dead bat into the house of one of the students. The bat was put in a jar and brought to school the next day and to soccer practice later that same day. Many teachers, students, and school staff touched the bat. School officials sent letters home the next day with students in five classes informing the parents of the incident. When the bat was found to be rabid, they called each household that had a potentially exposed child. One hundred seven students and staff were interviewed: one had had contact with the bat's teeth and was recommended for rabies postexposure prophylaxis (PEP) treatment. Seventy-four of the students and staff actually elected to receive PEP at the cost of $75,000. No serious reactions occurred, and no case of human rabies was reported after the incident. The family cat was given a rabies booster shot and remained healthy at the time this report was made.

The editorial note at the end of this case study suggests that more communication between medical and public health officials would have reduced the number who received PEP to those who met Advisory Committee on Immunization Practices (ACIP) criteria for PEP.

Epidemiological research employs a wide range of designs. You will note that the next two are actually quasi-experimental designs, which allow the researchers to test specific interventions (Cwikel, 2006); the others have a variety of descriptive designs.

Field Trials and Community Trials

Field trials typically are designed to test an intervention to prevent a health-related problem. Examples would be trials of protective sports equipment, reduction of emergency response time, or a new vaccination for chicken pox. Gerstman (2003) compares field trials with the already familiar clinical trial: clinical trials are designed to evaluate an intervention for individuals who already have a problem, whereas a field trial is usually designed to test a preventive measure, although the lines between the two are sometimes blurred. A *community trial* is even broader than the field trial; it is usually a test of a community-wide intervention such as fluoridation of the public water supply (which is very common today but was quite controversial when originally introduced). Typically, the number of people affected by a field or community trial is quite large. Data may be collected at the aggregate level rather than at the individual level, particularly in community trials. When data is analyzed at the aggregate or the population level, descriptive epidemiological studies are often called ecological studies (Gerstman, 2003). For example, birth rates in underdeveloped countries may be compared with the rates in industrialized countries or rates in rural areas may be compared to those in urban areas.

Cohort Studies

A *cohort* is a group of people who have a characteristic, problem, or experience in common. This characteristic may be age, gender, residence in a single neighborhood, employment in a certain type of workplace (a chemical plant) or occupation (migrant worker), or having developed a particular disease (multiple sclerosis, for example). Cohort studies may be *retrospective* or *prospective*. In *retrospective* cohort studies, individuals are interviewed to identify past exposures or events that might have increased their risk. For example, residents of a neighborhood that has a high rate of childhood leukemia may be asked about their children's use of a local playground that was built over a former hazardous waste site or attendance at a poorly constructed school. In *prospective* studies, individuals are tested or interviewed about present characteristics or behavior. They may then be followed to determine what happens to them in the future.

> For example, Gerstman (2003) described a study of 40,564 British physicians who were asked if they smoked and how much they smoked. They were then followed prospectively. Forty years after the study began, the researchers Hill and Doll (in Gerstman, 2003) found that 50% of the heavy smokers died before reaching the age of 70 compared with only 20% of the nonsmokers. Only 8% of the heavy smokers survived to the age of 85, while 33% of the nonsmokers did survive this long (p. 206). This British study, as are many prospective studies, is very similar in design to the longitudinal studies to be described in the next section of this chapter.

Case-Control Design

To compare the characteristics and experiences of people who have a particular problem with those who do not, the cohort design can be extended to add what is called a control group. This control group differs from the control groups of an experimental study. It is a sample of people without the problem who are drawn from the same population. The people with the problem are the *cases*.

> For example, Gilbert and colleagues (2009) used the case-control design in a study of the possible effects of sun exposure over a lifetime on development of prostate cancer in British men. Men age 50 to 69 were offered prostate specific antigen (PSA) tests at 400 general medical offices. Those with elevated PSA results ≥ 3 ng/ml were offered a diagnostic biopsy. Altogether 55,172 men had the PSA test; 5873 had raised PSA levels, and 1933 had prostate cancer. Of those with prostate cancer, 1374 completed the study questionnaire and became the cases. Six other men in the sample who were from the same age group and geographic area were selected per case; these became the controls. The researchers found significantly more case subjects had a family history of prostate cancer than did the controls (7.8% vs. 5.4%), but fewer were or had been smokers. Sun exposure was collected retrospectively back to childhood years. The researchers had hypothesized that low sun exposure was related to low vitamin D levels, which raised the risk for prostate cancer. Their results provided only weak evidence to support their hypothesis.

LONGITUDINAL STUDIES

Most of the descriptive designs discussed so far are *cross-sectional* in nature. There are a few exceptions; the prospective design is one. Also, in most experimental and some quasi-experimental studies, data are collected at more than one time interval). In a cross-sectional study, data are collected at one point in time. In retrospective designs, data are collected about several past time points but all at the same time, even if it is done in multiple interviews. In contrast, data are collected over at least two time periods, often called *waves*, for longitudinal studies.

The following sections cover the several variations of the longitudinal study design described by Menard (2002, 2008).

Longitudinal Panel Design

This is the basic longitudinal study design in which participants are enrolled at the beginning of the study and followed through a planned number of successive *waves* of data collection.

A prospective cohort (longitudinal) study of 1880 older individuals living in upper Manhattan (New York City) enrolled in 1992 and 1999 was assessed every 1.5 years from 1992 to 2006. Information on their cognitive status, physical activity levels, and food consumption was obtained. The data enabled researchers to classify participants as having developed dementia or not and to calculate a physical activity score as well as a Mediterranean-type diet score (beneficial components were fruits, vegetables, legumes, cereals and fish; detrimental components included meat and dairy). Both higher Mediterranean-type diet scores and higher physical activity levels were associated with a lower risk of development of Alzheimer's disease (Scarmeas et al., 2009).

Total Population Design

In this design, an attempt is made to interview or obtain needed information about every individual in the population of interest. The US Census is a well-known example of a total population design.

Repeated Cross-Sectional Design

The name of this design is a little confusing since it is a longitudinal design, not a cross-sectional design. It is a series of cross-sectional samples drawn from the same population at planned time intervals. Although the samples should be equivalent if drawn appropriately, each sample is composed of different people. Election studies and opinion polls such as the consumer confidence survey reported periodically in the media are examples.

Revolving Panels

The term *panel* is often used for the people who constitute the sample of a longitudinal study. In the revolving panel design, segments of the panel may be added and/or dropped at different time intervals. In the Framingham study, for example, younger generations have been added to the original panel.

In the Framingham study, the initial cohort of 5209 individuals age 28 to 62 was enrolled in 1948. A new segment, the offspring of the original cohort, was added in 1971. It included 5124 individuals age 5 to 70 (Eaker, Sullivan, Kelly-Hayes, D'Agostino, & Benjamin, 2007). In the offspring cohort, data were collected on marital and work strain as well as heart disease and stroke. Results were reported on 1769 men and 1913 women average age 48 ± 10 years, range 18 to 77 at baseline. This is a relatively well-educated sample. The generally beneficial effect for men of being married that was found in this sample has also been found in other studies. However, men with working wives who reported work strain that spilled over into home life were more likely to develop coronary heart disease within a 10-year period. Women who self-silenced (usually or always kept their feelings to themselves) had four times the risk of dying during those 10 years than those who did not (Eaker et al., 2007). Self-silencing had no effect on these outcomes in men. Marital satisfaction and marital disagreement were not significantly related to development of coronary heart disease or mortality.

In another Framingham offspring study, those offspring whose parents lived to 85 or more were found to have "advantageous" cardiovascular risk profiles in middle age when compared to those whose parents died at an earlier age (Terry et al., 2007).

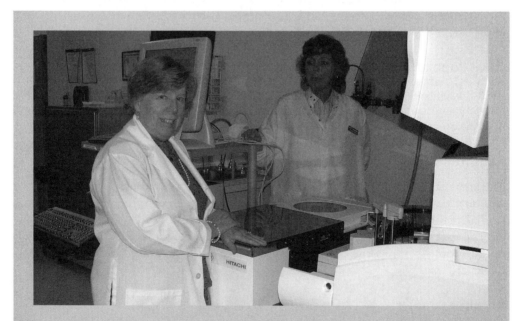

Dr. Margaret Kelly-Hayes, an expert on the epidemiology of stroke, is seen here with a colleague in their lab. Dr. Kelly-Hayes has been a member of the well-known Framingham, Massachusetts longitudinal studies investigative team for many years.

The first Framingham study illustrates the advantage of following people over an extended period of time and of being able to add variables of interest during succeeding waves of assessment and testing. The second one illustrates the advantage of adding new segments, in this case the offspring, to the original panel to allow additional comparisons.

Interrupted Time Series

A time series design involves a collection of data on the same variables at multiple time points. A simple interrupted time series study has just one group (Shadish, Cook, & Campbell, 2002). This group might be all licensed drivers in a state on whom data regarding use of seat belts or child safety seats are collected at regular intervals before and after the seat belts or safety seats became required by law. The passage of the law is the treatment or "interruption" that occurs during the study. Often two or more groups are compared, one affected by the treatment/interruption, the other not. An example would be to compare the use of safety seats in a state that passes a strict law to use in a state that does not have a strict law. Using the notation introduced in Chapter 5, this may be diagrammed as follows (Shadish, Cook & Campbell, 2002; Abraham & Neuendorff, 1990):

X = treatment
O = observation or testing
    O O O O X O O O
    O O O O   O O O

Advantages of the Longitudinal Design

A limitation of cross-sectional designs is that they often ignore what has preceded or will follow the time point at which the data are collected (Abraham & Neuendorff, 1990). Of course, some of this can be accomplished retrospectively as was done in the case control study of sun exposure and prostate cancer. However, the accuracy of these reports of events that occurred 5, 10, or more years ago is difficult to assess: people often forget, misplace an event in time, telescope events—making them come closer together than actually happened, or simply misremember details (Lynn, 2009). Interviewing people at frequent intervals or asking them to keep calendars or diaries generally provides more accurate information.

The order of events, which is so important in establishing a causal relationship, is better identified through longitudinal research than in cross-sectional studies. How often a problem arises, how long it persists, and what else is happening to the person at the same time are also better captured in longitudinal studies. The following is drawn from a discussion of the advantages of the longitudinal design in the study of drug abuse:

> Recent evidence emphasizes the chronic nature of substance abuse and the long-term nature of the treatment needed. However, the typical research study of substance

abuse treatment is only 6 or 12 months in length. Hilton, Chandler, and Compton (2008) call these studies "snapshots in time" (p. 3). In contrast, the average treatment and relapse cycle in people with substance abuse problems, from admission to treatment, relapse and back to readmission to treatment takes 9 years.

For these and other reasons, Hser and colleagues (2007) argue for a life course perspective when studying substance abuse to better understand what leads people to become substance abusers and the factors that contribute to persistence of substance abuse, to successful treatment and to relapses or cessation. Understanding the natural course of substance abuse and recovery and the interactions with multiple service systems that may occur over time (mental health, social services, criminal justice, and so forth) is best captured in longitudinal studies. It is hoped this improved understanding will eventually lead to development of more effective long-term interventions (Hser, Longshore, & Anglin, 2007; Hser & Teruya, 2007).

Disadvantages of Longitudinal Designs

Longitudinal studies are complex and challenging for even the most experienced researcher. Samples are often large. Recruitment and testing of participants is costly in terms of both time and money. Keeping track of participants for follow-up testing and managing missing data when participants cannot be found or decline to continue are also difficult tasks (Laurie, 2008; Lynn, 2009).

A different challenge is the effect of *conditioning*, which is a change in response due to having been asked a question before. Asking questions may lead to raising participants' awareness, cementing attitudes by asking people to express or explain them, increased honesty of the responses after trust has been established, and the effects of practice (Cantor, 2008). Although of particular concern in longitudinal studies, these threats to the reliability of the data may arise whenever participants who are tested are interviewed more than once.

CONCLUSION

Most of the research designs described in this chapter are complex and challenging to implement. A new researcher is more likely to be a member of an investigative team rather than the leader of the team on these very large studies. However, if you have a chance to become part of such a team, you are likely to find it an excellent learning opportunity.

REFERENCES

Abraham, I., & Neuendorff, M. M. (1990). The design and analysis of time-series studies. In L. E. Moody (Ed.), *Advancing nursing science through research* (pp. 550–553). Thousand Oaks, CA: Sage.
  ✧ Readable introduction to designs employing multiple time points.
Bhopal, R. (2002). *Concepts of epidemiology: An integrated introduction to the ideas, theories, principles and methods of epidemiology.* Oxford, UK: Oxford University Press.

Bours, G. J. J. W., Halfens, R. J. G., Abu-Saad, H. H., & Grol, R. T. P. M. (2002). Prevalence, prevention, and treatment of pressure ulcers: Descriptive study in 89 institutions in the Netherlands. *Research in Nursing and Health, 25,* 99–110.
    ◇ This article has some interesting details about the conduct of a descriptive study.

Cantor, D. (2008). A review and summary of studies on panel conditioning. In S. Menard (ed.), *Handbook of longitudinal research: Design, measurement and analysis* (pp. 123–138). Burlington, MA: Academic Press.

Cwikel, J. G. (2006). *Social epidemiology: Strategies for public health activism.* New York: Columbia University Press.
    ◇ A fresh approach to epidemiology. See especially the chapter on research design and Figure 7.1, which is a guide to selecting the appropriate research design.

Dickerson, S., Park, N., Hamilton, S., Parmenter, D., Squires, K., McKillip, K., et al. (2009). Human exposures to a rabid bat-Montana 2008. *Morbidity and Mortality Weekly Report, 58*(20), 557–561.

Eaker, E. D., Sullivan, L. M., Kelly-Hayes, M., D'Agostino, R. B., & Benjamin, E. J. (2007). Marital status, marital strain, and risk of coronary heart disease or total mortality: The Framingham Offspring Study. *Psychosomatic Medicine, 69,* 509–513.

Gerstman, B. B. (2003). *Epidemiology kept simple.* Hoboken, NJ: Wiley-Liss.

Gilbert, R., Metcalfe, C., Oliver, S. E., Whiteman, D. C., Bain, C., Ness, A., et al. (2009). Life course sun exposure and risk of prostate cancer: Population-based nested case-control study and meta-analysis. *International Journal of Cancer, 125,* 1414–1423.

Hilton, T. F., Chandler, R. K., & Compton, W. M. (2008). Longitudinal research that can inform dynamic models for the treatment of addiction as a disease. *Evaluation Review, 32*(1), 3–6.

Hser, Y-I., & Teruya, C. (2007). Introduction to the special issues on longitudinal research on substance abuse and health services: Current knowledge and future directions. *Evaluation Review, 31*(6), 511–518.

Hser, Y. I., Longshore, D., & Anglin, M. D. (2007). The life course perspective on drug use. *Evaluation Review, 31*(6), 515–547.

Laurie, H. (2008). Minimizing panel attrition. In S. Menard, *Handbook of longitudinal research: Design, measurement and analysis* (pp. 167–184*)*. Burlington, MA: Academic Press.

Lynn, P. (2009). *Methodology of longitudinal surveys.* Chichester, UK: John Wiley & Sons.
    ◇ An excellent, although advanced, text on longitudinal research.

Menard, S. (2008). *Handbook of longitudinal research: Design, measurement and analysis.* Burlington, MA: Academic Press.
    ◇ Another excellent text on longitudinal research.

Menard, S. (2002). *Longitudinal research.* Thousand Oaks, CA: Sage.

Rothman, K. J., Greenland, S., & Lash, T. L. (2008). *Modern epidemiology* (3rd ed.). Philadelphia: Walters Kluwer.

Scarmeas, N., Luchsinger, J. A., Schupf, N., Brickman, A. M., Cosentino, S., Tang, M. X., et al. (2009). Physical activity, diet, and risk of Alzheimer disease. *Journal of the American Medical Association, 302*(6), 627–637.

Shadish, W. R., Cook, T. D., & Campbell, D. T. (2002). *Experimental and quasi-experimental designs for generalized causal inference.* Boston: Houghton Mifflin.

Terry, D. F., Evans, J. C., Pencina, M. J., Murabito, J. M., Vasan, R. S., Wolf, P. A., et al. (2007). Characteristics of Framingham offspring participants with long-lived parents. *Archives of Internal Medicine, 167*(5), 438–444.

Yin, R. K. (2003). *Case study research: Design and methods.* Thousand Oaks, CA: Sage.

CHAPTER 8

Sampling

Imagine conducting a study in which you interview your family, friends, neighbors, and colleagues—no one else. Is this acceptable? Is it sound research? That depends on the purpose of the interviews. If you want to generalize to other people, then this sampling frame is inappropriate. If you are writing an autobiographical case study, then it may not be inappropriate.

Sampling involves decisions about who or what will be tested, observed, or interviewed in your study (Morse, 2007). Two primary questions need to be addressed:

1. *Composition:* There are two questions related to composition: (a.) Who should be included in the study? (these are the *inclusion* criteria), and (b.) Who should not be included in the study? (these are the *exclusion* criteria). Together, the inclusion criteria and the exclusion criteria define the sample.

2. *Size:* Size addresses this deceptively simple question: How many should be included in the study?

The answers to these questions are very different in quantitative research and qualitative research, reflecting their different objectives. In fact, Patton (2002) suggests that "nothing better captures the difference between quantitative and qualitative methods than the different logics that undergird sampling approaches" (p. 230). For example, in quantitative research, decisions about sample size can be based upon existing formulas for calculating the power of a study. In qualitative research, the decision is based primarily upon thoughtful, informed judgment about how best to achieve the purpose of the study.

PROBABILITY SAMPLING

Probability

The concept of probability is fundamental to much of the decision making in sampling for a quantitative study as well in analysis of study outcomes. In many of these studies, we want to be able to conclude that the result was due to a real difference, not to chance or to a bias that has been inadvertently introduced. Probability theory provides a basis for drawing one conclusion or the other (Runyon, Coleman, & Pittenger, 1999).

Probability is the likelihood that an event or condition will occur. It is reported numerically in terms of the *relative frequency* of the occurrence (Henkel, 1976). For example, people say "I have about as much chance of getting that promotion as I have of winning the lottery," or "You are no more likely to see that happen as you are to be struck by lightning." If the lottery is fair and you know (a) how many lottery tickets were sold and (b) how many tickets you bought, then you can calculate your chances (i.e., the probability) of winning the lottery. Let's say this is a small lottery: 10,000 tickets were sold, and you bought 10 of those tickets. In the case of the lottery, you can precisely and accurately calculate your probability of winning once you know how many tickets were sold and how many of those were sold to you. Your chance of winning is 1 out of 1000:

$$\text{Probability} \quad = \quad \frac{10}{10,000} \quad = \quad \frac{1}{1000}$$

In the case of a lightning strike, however, the probability of being struck by lightning is not as easy to calculate. If you are on the beach and a thunderstorm is approaching, the probability of being struck by lightning is much higher than if you are inside working at your computer. In neither case is the probability zero. In both cases, the probability is very small.

In the first case, the lottery tickets, you had information about the entire population of interest (all lottery tickets). In the second, at best you could only obtain an estimate based on reported lightning strikes under various conditions. This second situation more closely resembles probability in many research studies because it is affected by the conditions under which the event may occur.

There are several different ways to express probability. You can, as in the above lottery ticket example, describe it in terms of the chance that the event will occur, which was 1 out of 1000. Or you can express it in percentages, which would be .001 or less than 1% chance, actually one tenth of 1% or 0.1%. Your chances of winning can also be described in terms of odds. The odds against your winning the lottery were a discouraging 999 to 1. Expressed again in more positive terms, your odds were 1 in a 1000 of winning.

Levels of Significance

Significance levels are set by the researcher at the outset of a study. In behavioral studies this level is usually $P \leq .05$, which means that there is a 5% likelihood, or probability, that what appears to be a real difference (between treatment groups, for example) is actually due to chance. A stricter level of significance $P \leq .01$ reduces this chance to 1%, and a looser criterion of $P \leq .10$ allows a 10% likelihood.[1]

These levels are conventions adopted by researchers. They indicate the difference that will be accepted as too large to be attributed to chance (Henkel, 1976) and are usually set before a study is done. As you can see, they are expressed in terms of probability.

---

[1]P is the symbol for probability; $\leq$ is the symbol for less than or equal to.

Probability Samples

Probability samples are samples formed to assure that each subject, whether person, animal, object, or event, has an equal chance (probability) of being included. In other words, given a specified population from which the sample is drawn, being chosen to be in the research study is by chance. Another way to say this is that every possible combination of potential subjects has an equal chance of occurring (Henkel, 1976). The goal of probability sampling is an unbiased sample although most recognize that a perfectly representative, absolutely unbiased sample is unlikely to be attained. More formally, the purpose of probability sampling is "to allow one to make statements about a population of interest without actually obtaining data on all people in that population" (Pedulla & Airasian, 1980, p. 807).

A *sampling frame* is the set of people (subjects) you will draw your sample from. It includes everyone who has a chance of being selected. Technically, a sample is representative only of those who are part of this sampling frame, although generalization is usually extended to others with the same or similar characteristics who constitute the *theoretical* or *target* population (Fowler, 2002, p. 6):

> Turner-Henson, Holaday, and O'Sullivan (1992) describe an effort to develop a sampling frame for a relatively rare pediatric population: chronically ill children age 10 to 12 in Alabama and California. They defined their sampling frames as the SMSA (Standard Metropolitan Statistical Areas) of San Francisco, California, and Birmingham, Alabama. Within these areas, they identified potential clusters where these children could be found: university medical centers, community hospitals, children's hospitals, other agencies serving this population, and private pediatrician offices (those not being served would not be identified using this approach).
>
> In some instances, records were computerized, facilitating their search. Many duplications were found and deleted. Researchers also found that many Alabama families had relocated owing to loss of a major employer in the locale. They reviewed thousands of medical records and interviewed many healthcare providers. This work took 1 year to complete and resulted in a sampling frame of 936 participants with characteristics similar to previously published estimates. Children with asthma were the largest diagnostic group within this sampling frame.

A *sampling design* describes the process used to choose subjects for the sample (Gliner & Morgan, 2000). It should include details about the size of the sample (number of subjects); how they will be accessed, screened, and selected; and the inclusion and exclusion criteria that will guide the screening and selection process. The following is an example of specific inclusion and exclusion criteria used in a clinical trial of a testosterone replacement therapy:

> In a report of a randomized double-blind, placebo-controlled clinical trial of a testosterone gel compared with a placebo gel in men 50 years of age and older who had androgen deficiency, the researchers specified several inclusion and exclusion criteria:

Inclusion Criteria	Exclusion Criteria
Age $\geq$ 50	History of prostate, breast, or testicular cancer
Serum total testosterone level on screening of $\leq$ 280 ng/dl (the lower limit of the normal range)	Hospitalization within the last month
	Prostate-specific antigen (PSA) level of $\geq$ 3.0
Meet DSM-IV criteria for dysthymia or mild depression	Abnormal digital rectal exam
	Psychiatric instability or suicidality
Did not meet criteria for major depression disorder	

Men who were treated with antidepressants were eligible if they had been receiving a stable dose for at least 3 months (Shores, Kivlahan, Sadak, Li, & Matsumoto, 2009). You can see that these criteria are very specific and clearly define individuals who would be eligible for the study.

The *selected sample* is the smaller group who are actually chosen to participate. Not all will actually participate, however. Some will decline, others will not exactly meet the inclusion or exclusion criteria, and others will not want to or be able to complete the study for some reason. Those who do enroll in the study and complete it constitute the *actual sample*. If the selected sample includes 100 people, but only 80 finish the study, the *response rate* will be only 80%. Too low a response rate is a threat to study quality and may even invalidate the results (Gliner & Morgan, 2000).

Random selection may be accomplished in several ways. First you need to have a list of all subjects that are within the sampling frame. Manual (by hand) random selection is done by putting all the names in a container, mixing them up well and drawing the number you need, one by one. Alternatively, you can number each potential subject and select the sample using either a table of random numbers or a computer-generated list of random numbers. You can also randomize the list and then select them by beginning at a random starting point and then selecting every 4th, 10th or 100th person, depending upon how many you need (Fowler, 2002).

The goal in each of these methods is to achieve randomness and avoid any systematic procedure that might introduce bias. For example, if the list of potential subjects for an acute care study is in order by patient room number and you take the first 25 out of 50, you may be selecting those that are placed nearest to the nurses' station, often those that need the most monitoring. Or if you use a list of students provided by the school system, they might be in order by age or grade achieved, either of which might introduce a bias.

There are several possible variations of the simple random sampling just described. There may be an important theoretical rationale for needing an equal number of males and females, of certain age groupings, ethnic group membership, type of diagnosis, or type of procedure (e.g., repair of hip fracture vs. hip replacement). To do this, the subjects in the sampling frame are separated into strata and randomly selected from each stratum. This is called *stratified random sampling*. A more complex, *multistage* method may be needed in some instances. For example, if you want to do a survey of pediatric intensive care units

(PICUs) across the country, you probably would decide that there are too many to survey the entire population of PICUs. Instead, you may divide the hospitals that have PICUs into clusters such as for-profit, private not-for-profit, and municipal hospitals. Or you might divide the hospitals by size, such as under 100 beds, 100–500 beds, and over 500 beds. You can then sample randomly from each of the nine clusters (three types of hospitals in each of the three sizes) that were created.

McCall (1982) differentiated strata and clusters this way: In *stratified* sampling the sampling units are the *elements* or individuals that make up the population; in *cluster* sampling the sampling units are groups of individuals. Which is preferable? That depends on the design of your study, but the following example may also be helpful:

> Pedulla and Airasian (1980) conducted an interesting study using existing data collected from 1481 teachers in the Republic of Ireland. The teachers had been selected using stratified random sampling. The strata used were gender of the student body of their schools, location of the school (city, town, rural) and primary or postprimary type of school. The teachers had been asked questions on their attitudes toward standardized testing. The investigators wondered if they could draw subsamples from the larger sample that would still be representative. They drew 21 10%, 25%, and 50% subsamples (e.g., a 10% sample would include 148 teachers, a 50% sample would be 740 teachers) by simple random sampling, cluster sampling using individual schools as the clusters, stratification by gender, and stratification by school size. The cluster sampling was found to be least effective: 19 of the 21 25% sample results differed significantly from the total sample compared with 1 out of the 21 for simple random sampling, none for stratification by gender, and 2 for stratification by school size. They concluded that, in this case, at least, simple random sampling was as good as the stratified random samples, and the cluster sample was clearly inferior.

Nonprobability Sampling

If any type of choice, discretion, or preference enters into the selection process, the sample becomes a nonprobability sample. There are many reasons why researchers use nonprobability samples despite the advantages of probability sampling. The following are just a few of the possible reasons:

- Limitations on resources: You may not have the time or funds available to develop an accurate sampling frame or purchase what are often expensive lists of potential subjects.

- Accessibility: The information needed to identify all the potential subjects may not be available to you or may not exist in an accessible form.

- Limited number of subjects: If you are studying an infrequent event or health problem such as a rare form of anemia or the occurrence of spina bifida, you may recruit *all* known cases within your target area instead of sampling them.

- Subject availability: Some groups of potential interest, such as high-risk youth, victims of domestic violence, or substance abusers, are not only difficult to find but may also be difficult to persuade to participate in a research study.

- Nonresponse: Subjects may simply not return questionnaires or answer the telephone. Others decline to participate for personal reasons, lack of interest, or desire for privacy (Fowler, 2002).

- Experimental mortality: Sometimes involvement in a study requires more time, more attention, or is more unpleasant than anticipated leading to high subject "mortality" (loss) from an intervention group (Gliner & Morgan, 2000). Other times, individuals desire treatment and do not want to risk being placed in a no-treatment or placebo group.

The following example illustrates some of these challenges, even in a large multistate study:

Kim and colleagues (2009) point out that most research studies on caregivers of individuals with cancer have relied on small, geographically restricted (local) samples that lack power and may not be generalizable. They may also be limited to a particular type of cancer, which may or may not affect outcomes. One option, which is to develop and maintain multisite collaborations, is time consuming and expensive.

An alternative strategy, to reach cancer survivors through state cancer registries and ask them to name their caregiver, was tested by Kim et al. (2009). About 30% of the 19,294 survivors identified through this means completed the survey. Of these, 42% named a caregiver. Middle-aged (45–54), female, non-black survivors and those with breast or ovarian cancer were more likely to complete the survey. Those with advanced cancer or bladder or lung cancer were less likely to complete the survey. Given these findings, they suggest oversampling of groups less willing to participate to ensure sufficient numbers and using incentives to encourage participation. Formulas for estimating the probability of participation for various subgroups within this large sample were provided. For example, to recruit 200 caregivers of survivors who are 75 years old or more with colorectal cancer would require a selected sample of 1170 survivors from registries of this type.

While these efforts do help to identify hard-to-find caregivers and produce a more representative sample, the fact that only 30% of those contacted responded suggests that the resulting sample is not a probability sample.

Many pilot studies and exploratory work are done with nonprobability samples. You also can see that even if a probability sampling design is attempted, a very low response rate can lead to unintended creation of a nonprobability sample.

There are several different types of nonprobability samples:

- Quota sampling: When a theoretical basis is used to select people with certain characteristics, a quota sample is created. For example, a study of ethnic group differences in activity levels of preschool children might use a sample of 50 European Americans, 50 Hispanic Americans, 50 African Americans and 50 Asian Americans.

- Convenience sampling: This very common approach to sampling uses people available to the researcher. For example, a study of adherence to dietary recommendations in people with end-stage renal disease might be conducted in several dialysis centers that have agreed to participate in the study.

- Snowball network or referral sampling: When there are no easily accessed means for identifying individuals who have had a particular experience (urinary incontinence, for example) or a health problem (multiple sclerosis, for example) researchers may advertise their study, which is often very expensive, or begin with known individuals and ask them to refer others who have the same concern.

It is important that the limitations of nonprobability sampling need to be recognized when analyzing data and reporting the results.

Tracking and Reporting Sample Development

Created to improve reporting of randomized controlled trials (RCTs), the CONSORT (Consolidated Standards of Reporting Trials) statement includes a checklist for authors reporting on RCTs and a flow diagram (Figure 8-1) that illustrates the flow of participants through the study (Altman et al., 2001), beginning with the selection of participants and proceeding to randomization to treatment or no-treatment group, how many were lost to follow-up, and so forth. The flow chart can be adapted for multigroup studies as well.

Although not emphasized by its creators, the flow diagram represents a very useful guide for tracking sample development as it occurs rather than only after the fact (similar to the audit trail in qualitative research described in a later chapter). It is often difficult to go back and recreate this information, but it is not difficult to track and record it as sample development occurs. Also valuable is recording reasons for loss of subjects, whether it is due to ineligibility, refusal to participate, illness, or discontinued intervention. An example from an article by Buchbinder and colleagues (2009) illustrates the many and various reasons why potential subjects are lost to the study.

As you can see in Figure 8-2, the researchers initially assessed 468 potential participants of whom 78 were enrolled and randomized to treatment and placebo intervention. The placebo in this case was a sham intervention in which the needle for injection of the treatment under study (polymethylmethacrylate or PMMA) was actually inserted but nothing was injected. Notice that, once enrolled, few participants failed to complete the study. The researchers found no beneficial effect of the PMMA in these individuals, all of whom had unhealed, painful osteoporotic vertebral fractures of less than 12 months duration.

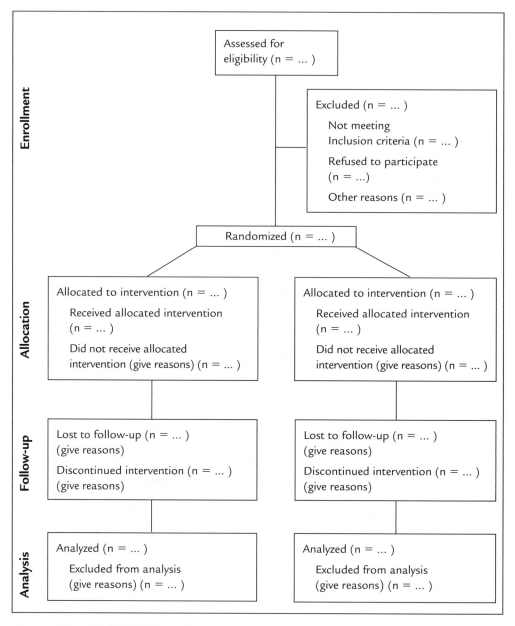

Figure 8-1 CONSORT flow diagram.

Source: Altman et al., 2001.

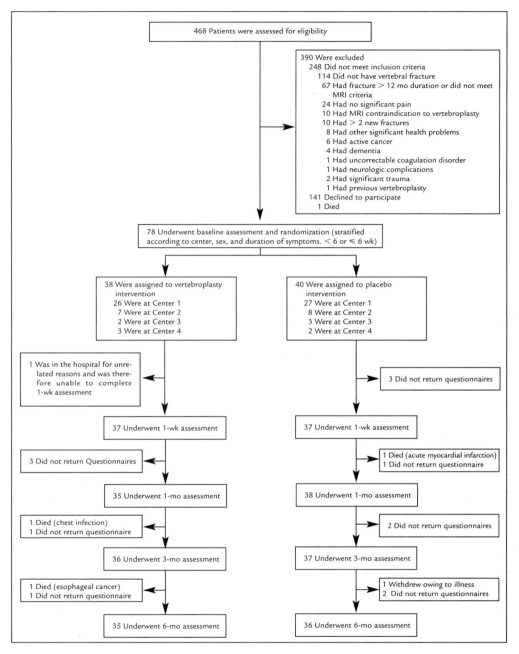

Figure 8-2 Example of CONSORT flow diagram.

Source: Buchbinder et al., 2009.

In 1990, Selby and colleagues reviewed 30 research reports randomly selected from five clinical nursing journals, *Public Health Nursing, Heart & Lung, Journal of Gerontological Nursing, Journal of Obstetric, Gynecological and Neonatal Nursing,* and *Oncology Nursing Forum.* Most first authors were nurses. The sampling method was found to be unclear in 4 (13%) of the articles. In 21 (70%), there was an unclear or missing report of the sampling frame, sample size, number of refusals, withdrawals, or cases lost. Forty-three percent of the authors did not report the limitations of the sample, and in 53% generalizations were inappropriate given the sampling method used. Such findings support the need for better reporting of sampling procedures and for use of guides such as the CONSORT flow diagram.

Sample Size in Quantitative Research

In quantitative studies sample size is estimated numerically, based upon either the desired significance level or confidence intervals. Before explaining this, several fundamental concepts will be reviewed.

Type I error occurs when a null hypothesis that is actually true is rejected (Cohen, 1988; Newman, 2001). The null hypothesis predicts that no difference between groups will be found. If the significance level is set too high, at $P = .10$, for example, there is a risk of concluding that a true difference exists when the difference only occurred by chance (type I error).

Type II error is the opposite. It occurs when we accept (fail to reject) a false null hypothesis. In other words, there is a true difference between the groups, but it was not detected. If the significance level is set too strictly, for example, we risk missing a real difference.

Power Analysis Using Effect Size

The *power* of a statistical test is the probability that it will yield a statistical significant result (Cohen, 1988, p. 1). In other words, it is a calculation of the chances that, if a true difference exists, this difference can be detected given the study design that is proposed. An *underpowered* study typically has too few subjects or an insensitive measure of change, or both, leading to increased risk of type II error. An *overpowered* study is too large, not only wasting resources but also risking a variation of type I error, finding effects that are too small to be of importance clinically (Cook & DeMets, 2008).

The *effect size* is another important parameter in the estimation of power. Effect size is the estimated magnitude of the phenomenon under study. In other words, it is the answer to the researcher's question, "How large an effect do I expect?" (Cohen, 1988, p. 12).

If the null hypothesis is true, the effect size will be zero; however, most researchers anticipate a real effect in most of their studies. The size of this effect may be calculated from prior research or it may be based on existing theory. The calculated effect size is generally preferred because it is based upon data; the theory-based one usually is less solidly grounded.

The way in which an effect size is calculated depends upon the study design and the plan for analysis of the outcomes as well as the estimated effect size and significance level selected. An effect size calculation indicates the strength of the relationship between the independent and dependent (outcome) variables. It can be calculated by subtracting the mean of the control group ($\overline{X}_c$) from the mean of the intervention group ($\overline{X}_I$) and then dividing the result by the pooled standard deviation from both groups. The effect size index for t tests is represented by d (Cohen, 1988; Gliner & Morgan, 2000):

$$ d \quad = \quad \frac{\overline{X}_I \quad - \quad \overline{X}_c}{S \text{ pooled}} $$

Cohen (1988, p. 82) has also provided correlation coefficient (r) equivalents to effect size d as follows and suggested conventions for considering them to be small, medium, or large effects:

	d	r
Small	.20	.10
Medium	.50	.30
Large	.80	.50

A good statistical textbook and the tables found in Cohen's 1988 book may be sufficient guides for very simple designs, especially those using correlations that are readily interpreted. There are also useful software packages that can calculate power for you, but they are frequently limited in the number of designs they can be applied to and may require input of estimates you find hard to calculate. For a complicated design and resultant complicated calculations, statistical consultation is recommended.

Another, less preferable, approach to estimating effect size is to predict the size of an effect (small, medium, or large) on the basis of the literature and experience.

Another important convention is the level of power thought to be acceptable. Most researchers generally accept a power of .80 although a higher power level (.85 or .90 or more) is certainly desirable. (Remember, this figure estimates the chances of achieving a significant result.) Once you have calculated the effect size and set the significance level and the desired power for a study, you can calculate the number of people needed in your sample.

The following are some helpful generalizations about the relationship of effect size, sample size, and the power of a proposed study:

- If the null hypothesis is not true, then the effect size will be greater than zero (> 0).

- The larger the effect size, the greater degree to which the phenomenon (e.g., the outcome of an intervention study) is manifested.

- The larger the effect size is, the greater the power will be; so a smaller sample will be needed to detect the phenomenon and reject the null hypothesis (Cohen, 1988).

There is a second use of power analysis that arises after a study has been completed. If results of a study are equivocal or nonsignificant, a power analysis can be done to determine if the study was underpowered. This is useful information for the researcher as well as the reader of the research report.

Confidence interval calculations provide valuable information that a *P* value alone cannot (Hennekens, 1987). Significance levels or *P* values do not provide information about the magnitude or size of the outcome. The way in which the *P* value is interpreted also presents some problems. Usually it is presented as an all-or-none conclusion—significant or not significant. Yet a significance level of .06 clearly differs from a significance level of .60 (Gliner & Morgan, 2000). Instead the significance level really indicates the *probability* that a result is significant, usually at the .05 or .01 level. The use of confidence intervals is helpful here. A confidence interval (CI) indicates the estimated range within which the true difference between the means lies. Of course, we are never absolutely sure of this unless the entire population of interest is measured, which is usually not possible (Newman, 2001). You are probably familiar with the idea of a *margin of error* typically reported by pollsters. This margin of error rate is actually one half of the confidence interval (Clark-Carter, 1997).

The confidence interval may also be used to estimate sample size. Although, like the effect size, an estimate of the margin of error can be based on theory, it is far better to use previous data as a guide. From this data, you can enter the actual margin of error into a formula to estimate needed sample size. A larger sample size is needed when a narrow margin of error is desired. Conversely, a smaller sample can be used if a wider confidence interval or margin of error is acceptable (Clark-Carter, 1997).

A 95% confidence interval is the most commonly reported. The following is an example of its use in a large national survey of breastfeeding practices:

> Data from the 2004 National Immunization Survey (NIS) were used to evaluate differences in breastfeeding. NIS data is obtained through random digit dialing of households with children age 19–35 months. It is designed to obtain nationally representative data. US Census Bureau definitions were used to classify households. The comparison reported was between white, non-Hispanic ($N = 16,977$) and black, non-Hispanic households ($N = 4,112$) only. The researchers reported that 71.5% of white, non-Hispanic children (95% confidence interval [CI] 69.1–73.0) and 50.1% of black non-Hispanic children (95% CI 44.4–55.8) were ever breastfed. The greatest difference between people of the two races were found in children living in rural areas. The smallest were found in those living in the Northeastern part of the United States. In the editorial note, the researchers note that racial and economic disparities in breastfeeding have decreased but have not been eliminated. They also urge continuation of public health education efforts to promote breastfeeding, especially to black mothers in rural areas or aged 20 years or under. (Grummer-Strawn, Scanlon, Darling, & Conrey, 2006)

PURPOSEFUL SAMPLING

The sampling done for qualitative studies is called *purposeful* because it is directed by the purpose of the study, not by statistical calculations. It may also be called *purposive* sampling, *judgmental* sampling, or *theoretical* sampling. There are a variety of strategies that can be used to make the decisions about who should be included. Some of these are generic; others are specific to the research design.

Composition of the Sample

Creswell (1998) provides a helpful overview of the different types of sampling used in different qualitative designs.

Case Study Research

The case or cases selected are often unusual in some way, such as a rare form of skin cancer or new infectious disease. There are times when the case is selected because it is judged to be typical of a certain set of circumstances such as the "usual" progression of untreated glaucoma or of a chronic progressive dementia.

Ethnography

Sampling begins with the selection of a culture, subculture, or ethnic group of interest and the site or sites in which they will be studied. This site could be a rural health clinic in Appalachia or a tertiary care hospital in a major city. Unless the focus is already defined, Fetterman (1998) suggests beginning with the "big net" approach of mixing with as many people as possible and then narrowing the focus (and sampling) as the topic of interest becomes more defined. Fetterman uses the term *judgmental sampling*, as this approach relies on the judgment of the researcher to guide selection of the most appropriate people, events, and artifacts to study.

Phenomenology

The primary criterion for selecting subjects for a phenomenological study is that they have experienced the phenomenon under study. Often the first participant is the researcher who writes a personal lived-experience description before asking others about their experiences. Additional sources of data include close observation, anecdotes, literature, poetry, biographies, diaries, journals, art, and the phenomenological literature (van Manen, 1990).

Grounded Theory

Theoretical sampling is used in grounded theory. Selection of subjects and sources of data are based upon ability to contribute to the evolving theory (i.e., whether or not their inclusion has theoretical purpose and relevance). The initial selection is based upon a general idea of the topic of interest. When first selecting subjects and other sources of data, Glaser and Strauss (1967) suggest that differences between people and groups of people studied should be minimized. After the basic framework has emerged, differences should be maximized for purposes of comparison and extension of the theory. In other words, the boundaries of the sample evolve and expand as theory develops, beginning with a homogeneous sample and extending outward to a more heterogeneous sample.

Biography
Like case studies, historical biographies may focus on typical people from a selected time and place or on individuals who are politically important, marginalized, or insightful, depending on the purpose of the biography.

We turn now to a list of generic strategies for developing a sample in a qualitative study from Patton (2002). They are not all appropriate for every type of qualitative study or for every group that may be studied. In some studies a combination may be used.

1. *Extreme cases:* These are the people, groups, or organizations that stand out in some way. They may be the sickest, the most abused, or the poorest. On the positive side, they may have achieved excellence (magnet hospitals, for example), been the most effective, or recovered the fastest. For example, a lot of attention has been directed toward individuals who survived HIV infection before the more recent, more effective treatments were available. They were the outliers whose survival provided insights for AIDS researchers. Extreme cases are often the ones from whom we can learn a lot—they are likely to be information-rich cases.

2. *Intense experiences:* In some instances, extreme cases may be too unusual or may distort the phenomenon too much (Patton, 2002). On the other hand, mild, low-key experiences are not likely to be as information-rich as intense experiences. The goal in sampling is to study examples of sufficient intensity, although not necessarily extreme intensity, to be rich in information. For example, it could be helpful to study people who manage their diabetes well, to identify the coping strategies they use that could be used by others as well.

3. *Maximum variation sampling:* Variability or differences in important characteristics or dimensions may be deliberately sought in the people included in a sample (Miles & Huberman, 1994). For example, it might be important to be sure to include men as well as women or to include individuals from different ethnic groups when studying beliefs about end-of-life treatment and advance directives.

4. *Negative instances or confirming and disconfirming cases:* As will be discussed in the chapter on trustworthiness of qualitative research, it is particularly important to consider both examples that support a tentative conclusion and those that do not.

5. *Homogeneous sampling:* In some ways, this is the opposite of the maximum variation sampling. Intensive, in-depth study of individuals with important characteristics in common may be valuable. For example, children of parents who are substance abusers may be at risk for substance abuse themselves and may have in common some important emotional needs.

6. *Criterion sampling:* Similar to some of the other sampling strategies, criterion sampling is done on the basis of one or more criteria for selection. For example, you may want to interview school age children and their parents to understand the reasons for high levels of absenteeism. To do this, you may decide to sample those who were absent 15 days or more in the last year. You might also exclude those who were absent this long owing to suspension rather than illness if your focus is health-related issues.

7. *Stratified purposeful sampling:* Similar to stratified random sampling described earlier, this approach also divides the sample into strata or subsamples on the basis of important characteristics such as low, moderate, and high income; degrees of depression; or levels of impairment; selecting participants from each stratum.

Evolving or Iterative Sampling

Another characteristic of sampling for qualitative research that differs substantially from quantitative research sampling procedures is the willingness, sometimes the necessity, to change the sampling strategy during the course of the research.

Morse (2007) lists several reasons why the sampling strategy is altered during the study:

- *Saturation:* Saturation occurs when new information is no longer appearing. This may occur in some areas while others may need continued work, necessitating a larger sample.

- *Scope:* As others have also noted, it is important to identify the boundaries of the phenomenon under study. A more narrowly focused study will saturate faster, but in other cases it may become necessary to push the boundaries out, expanding the focus.

- *Variation:* Like maximum variation, increasing awareness of the structure of the phenomenon under study may lead to examination of extreme cases, disconfirming cases, and so forth.

- *Verification:* New data may be needed not only to confirm conclusions but also to explore new issues that have emerged.

Bias in Qualitative Sampling

The name *purposeful* or *purposive* given to qualitative sampling emphasizes the deliberate selection of individuals, groups, organizations, or communities to study. This is in contrast to *random* selection where the researcher sets the criteria for inclusion and exclusion but does not exercise discretion in selection of the particular individuals or cases. In a sense, this means that qualitative samples are deliberately biased but in a deliberate, thoughtful manner. Morse (2006) distinguishes between this purposeful bias and an unintended bias that may weaken the conclusions. A few examples of problematic unintended bias include the following:

- Overreliance on one or two key informants (often people with whom the researcher has become comfortable)

- Too much attention to dramatic events, thereby missing the usual but important events and routines of everyday life

- Presence, sometimes active participation, of the researcher in activities under observation. In some forms of action research, researcher involvement is expected, but it is important to recognize and record the effects of this participation.

Purposive Sample Size

There are some qualitative designs for which it is possible to specify an expected number of subjects in a study. For most, however, the number to include is difficult to specify when the study begins, and the ultimate decision is based upon what is learned as the study progresses.

Some very influential qualitative research has been done with small samples. Piaget, for example, closely observed the cognitive development of his own two children to develop his theory. Freud also based his theory on in-depth analysis from his clinical experience with only 10 patients. Patton (2002, p. 245) also mentions the work of Clair Claiborne Park who, with her husband, systematically observed and recorded data on 40 years of their daughter's experience with autism: her development, emotions, obsessions, and challenges. These are examples of the incredibly rich data that may be gained from some small samples.

As you can see from these examples, case study research often uses a sample of $N = 1$ (N stands for the number in the sample) although multiple cases are also used in case study research (Yin, 1993).

Contrasting the sampling done in qualitative and quantitative research, Miles and Huberman (1994) describe qualitative sampling as "taking a smaller chunk of a larger universe" (p. 31). Obviously, you cannot conduct in-depth interviews with everyone of interest, so you need some principles to guide your decision to stop collecting data.

Rules of Thumb

The rule of thumb for the size of focus groups is 8 to 12 participants per group. However, some believe this is too many people, and that having only 5 to 6 participants allows each one enough time to speak. Some even suggest only 3 people per group. The subject under discussion and the nature of the group (all strangers vs. an established support group where members know each other) should be considered in finding the optimal group size. You may also need to experiment with different group sizes to find the best one for your participants and your topic (Kitzinger & Barbour, 1999).

Miles and Huberman (1994) emphasize that most qualitative samples involve a small number of cases. These cases may be a group, class, or whole organization. Each setting (a school, for example) has subsettings (individual classrooms). Because in-depth information is obtained about each case, a study that involved 15 or more cases would become unwieldy. If you are considering including as many as 20 or 30 cases, they ask, why not just do a survey instead? (p. 30).

Number-Free Guidelines
Although these rules of thumb do not use statistical formulas, they do employ numbers. There are number-free means for deciding how large a qualitative sample should be as well. Lincoln and Guba (1985) suggest continuing sampling to the point of redundancy (i.e., repetition of what has already been seen or heard). This is similar to Glaser and Strauss' (1967) use of *theoretical saturation* as the determinant for ending data collection. Saturation is achieved when the researcher sees and hears "similar instances over and over again" (p. 61). It is not achieved with an *N* of 1. Instead, comparisons are made across groups and across the various properties and categories of the developing theory. Once this is achieved, they say it is a waste of the researcher's time to collect more data from the same group on the same subject.

COMPLEX SAMPLING STRATEGIES

The following is an example of the type of work that may be done to better understand and learn how to access a group of interest before sampling is done:

> As part of a longitudinal study, Auerswald and colleagues (2004) conducted an ethnographic study to obtain the information needed for development of the sampling frame for the parent study. They did not want to use traditional sampling techniques for fear of missing significant segments of their difficult-to-reach population: at-risk Latino youth age 14 to 19 living in San Francisco's Mission District. For example, if the researchers recruited their participants from clinics, they would only be able to study those who were "service exposed." Household counts are inaccurate in this case because many of these youth are missed when the census is conducted. In particular, those who are undocumented, not in school or not living at home, would be missed altogether if census data were used to create the sampling frame. To overcome these limitations and learn how to access their populations, the researchers took walks and drives through the Mission District, met with selected youth in focus groups of 7 to 12 participants, and conducted a series of interviews on the streets, in cafes, in fast food restaurants, and in clinic waiting areas. They asked participants to draw maps of the places where at-risk Latino youth could be found. Altogether, 62 participants were interviewed, 44 from street sites, and 18 from the clinics. From the participants, they learned of 94 venues: gang venues, street corners, commercial centers, recreation centers, parks, nearby schools, and day laborer sites. With this information in hand, the researchers could design a more effective approach to accessing this hard-to-reach population for future research.

In some large, complex studies both probability and purposive sample strategies may be used in a multilevel sampling design:

Wilson, Huttly, and Fern (2006) described the complex sampling design created for a multinational study of children growing up in poverty in Peru, Vietnam, Ethiopia, and India. This cohort of children aged 6 to 17 months at the beginning of the study would be followed from 2002 until 2015. At the same time, they would be tracking changes at other levels so that they would have information at the individual, community, regional, and national levels over this time and would be able, for example, to see the effect of a national policy or economic change on the lives of these children. Their decision to enroll 2000 children from each country was primarily made on a theoretical basis. They estimated a 95% confidence interval for change of approximately 2% within each country and allowed for detection of moderate size differences between subgroups that were at least 20% of the total sample in size (p. 354). They made clear that the sample size of 2000 would limit their ability to capture relatively rare events such as mortality but pointed out that this data is obtained through national health surveys and was not the goal of their study.

The sites within each country were chosen on a purposive basis. They selected 20 sentinel sites in each country with equal numbers at each site. They specified that each sentinel site meet the definition of a poor area with a ratio of 3 to 1 poor to nonpoor in that area using the purposive sampling of typical instances described by Shadish, Cook, and Campbell (2001). Within these sites, households were selected randomly. Here is how they described their sampling design:

A sampling method designed to represent *equally* the whole national population of children born in the qualifying period was not appropriate [but] a method which over-samples the poor but enables comparison of the poor with the non-poor, where necessary, is more suitable. (p. 356)

CONCLUSION

Whether your sample is an *N* of 1 or an *N* of 1000, the choice of subjects determines the information you will obtain. Matching the criteria for selection to the objectives and design of the study helps to ensure that you have the desired data at the conclusion of the study.

REFERENCES

Altman, D. G., Schulz, K. F., Moher, D., Egger, M., Davidoff, F., Elbourne, D., et al. (2001). The revised CONSORT statement for reporting randomized trials: Explanation and elaboration. *Annuals of Internal Medicine, 134*(8), 663–694.

◇ The Altman et al. (2001) article and other useful information about CONSORT are available on this website (www.consort-statement.org/consort-statement/flow-diagram), including the flowchart and checklist for authors reporting results of RCTs. The information is updated periodically so you may find it useful to refer back to it when you are ready to use the flowchart or checklist.

Auerswald, C. L., Greene, K., Minnis, A., Doherty, I., Ellen, J., & Padian, N. (2004). Qualitative assessment of venues for purposive sampling of hard-to-reach youth: An illustration in a Latino community. *Sexually Transmitted Disease, 31*(2), 133–138.

Buchbinder, R., Osborne, R. H., Ebeling, P. R., Wark, J. D., Mitchell, P. M., Wriedt, C., et al. (2009). A randomized trial of vertebroplasty for painful osteoporotic vertebral factures. *New England Journal of Medicine, 361*(6), 557–568.

Clark-Carter, D. (1997). *Doing quantitative psychological research.* Hove, UK: Psychology Press.
   ◇ Appendix II has an explanation of estimating required sample size using confidence intervals.

Cohen, J. (1988). *Statistical power analysis for the behavioral sciences.* Hillsdale, NY: Lawrence Erlbaum Associates.
   ◇ This book contains all the formulas and tables needed to conduct a power analysis but it is a relatively complex presentation.

Cook, T. D., & DeMets, D. L. (2008). *Introduction to statistical methods for clinical trials.* Boca Raton, FL: Chapman & Hall/CRC.

Creswell, J. W. (1998). *Qualitative inquiry and research design: Choosing among five traditions.* Thousand Oaks, CA: Sage.

Fetterman, D. M. (1998). *Ethnography: Step by step.* Thousand Oaks, CA: Sage.

Fowler, F. J. (2002). *Survey research methods.* Thousand Oaks, CA: Sage.

Glaser, B. G., & Strauss, A. L. (1967). *The discovery of grounded theory: Strategies for qualitative research.* New York: Aldine de Gruyter.

Gliner, J. A., & Morgan, G. A. (2000). *Research methods in applied settings.* Mahwah, NJ: Lawrence Erlbaum.

Grummer-Strawn, L., Scanlon, K. S., Darling, N., & Conrey, E. J. (2006). Racial and socioeconomic disparities in breastfeeding—United States, 2004. *Morbidity and Mortality Weekly Report, 55*(12), 335–339.

Henkel, R. E. (1976). *Tests of significance.* Beverly Hills, CA: Sage.

Hennekens, C. H., & Buring, J. E. (1987). *Epidemiology in medicine.* Boston: Little, Brown.

Kim, Y., Kashy, D. A., Kaw, C. K., Smith, T., & Spillers, R. L. (2009). Sampling in population-based cancer caregivers research. *Quality of Life Research.* DOI 10.007/s22236-009-9518-7.

Kitzinger, J., & Barbour, R. S. (1999). Introduction: The challenge and promise of focus groups. In R. S. Barbour & J. Kitzinger (Eds.), *Developing focus group research* (pp. 1–20). Thousand Oaks, CA: Sage.

Lincoln, Y. S., & Guba, E. G. (1985). *Naturalistic inquiry.* Newbury Park, CA: Sage.

McCall, C. H. (1982). *Sampling and statistics handbook for research.* Ames, IA: University of Iowa Press.
   ◇ This handbook offers very clear explanations of fundamental sampling and statistical concepts. Descriptions of different types of samples and combinations of different sampling designs are helpful.

Miles, M. B., & Huberman, A. M. (1994). *Qualitative data analysis* (2nd ed.). Thousand Oaks, CA: Sage.

Morse, J. M. (2007). Strategies of intraproject sampling. In P. Munhall (Ed.), *Nursing research: A qualitative perspective.* Sudbury, MA: Jones and Bartlett.

Morse, J. M. (2006). Six biased reflections. Principles of sampling and analysis in qualitative inquiry. In J. Popay, *Moving beyond effectiveness in evidence synthesis: Methodological issues in the synthesis of diverse sources of evidence* (pp. 53–60). London: NICE.
   ◇ An interesting, readable article about purposive sampling.

Newman, S. C. (2001). *Biostatistical methods in epidemiology.* New York: John Wiley & Sons.

Patton, M. Q. (2002). *Qualitative research and evaluation methods.* Thousand Oaks, CA: Sage.

Pedulla, J. J., & Airasian, P. D. (1980). Sampling from samples: A comparison of strategies in longitudinal research. *Educational and Psychological Measurement, 40*, 807–813.

Runyon, R. P., Coleman, K., & Pittenger, D. (1999). *Fundamentals of behavioral statistics*. New York: McGraw-Hill.

Selby, M. L., Gentry, N. O., Reporteller-Muller, R., Legault, C., & Monahan, K. M. (1990). Evaluation of sampling methods in research reported in selected clinical nursing journals: Implications for nursing practice. *Journal of Professional Nursing, 6*(2), 76–85.

Shadish, W. R., Cook, T. D., & Campbell, D. T. (2001). *Experimental and quasi-experimental designs for generalized causal inference*. Boston: Houghton Mifflin.

Shores, M. M., Kivlahan, D. R., Sadak, T. I., Li, E. J., & Matsumoto, A. M. (2009). A randomized, double-blinded, placebo-controlled study of testosterone treatment in hypogonadal older men with subthreshold depression (dysthymia or minor depression). *Journal of Clinical Psychiatry, 70*(7), 1009–1016.

Turner-Henson, A., Holaday, B., & O'Sullivan, P. (1992). Sampling rare pediatric populations. *Journal of Pediatric Nursing, 7*(5), 329–334.

◇ A detailed description of the development of a sampling frame in this article provides the reader with a good idea of how it is done and how much effort is involved.

Van Manen, M. (1990). *Researching lived experience: Human science for an active pedagogy* (2nd ed.). Albany, NY: State University of New York Press.

Wilson, I., Huttly, S. R. A., & Fern, B. (2006). A case study of sample design for longitudinal research: Young lives. *International Journal of Social Research Methodology, 9*(5), 351–365.

◇ A very rich description of complex sampling in a multinational longitudinal research study called Young Lives.

Yin, R. K. (1993). *Applications of case study research*. Newbury Park, CA: Sage.

CHAPTER 9

Reliability

It is important to achieve the highest quality of measurement possible in your research. Reliability and validity are the two primary aspects of the quality of quantitative research measures. This chapter addresses issues of reliability in quantitative studies. The following chapter addresses validity in quantitative studies. Then we will turn our attention to the quality of the data collected in qualitative studies.

WHAT IS RELIABILITY?

Evaluation of the reliability of research measures is concerned with questions of *consistency*. Other terms for reliability are *repeatability* (Nunnally & Bernstein, 1996), *reproducibility, stability, consistency, predictability* (Engstrom, 1988), *agreement*, and *homogeneity*. If two people use this measure in the same situation, will they get the same result? If they use it on two different occasions, will the results be the same? Are all the items within the measure measuring the same phenomenon in the same way? Will two different versions of the measure produce the same result? All of these are questions of reliability. If the answers to any of these questions is no, then the measure or the way the measure is being used is not reliable.

WHEN IS RELIABILITY A CONCERN?

Reliability is always a concern in quantitative research. When a new measure is being developed, it is a primary focus, along with validity. When a standard, well-tested measure is being used, your main concern is whether or not it continues to evidence reliability in your study. In this instance, you will want to know if your raters are consistent and if the measure provides consistent results when used with your sample.

The importance of reliability is emphasized by Lynn (1984):

> No study, no matter how sophisticated the design, analyses, theoretical background, or other components, can rise above the threat of nonreliability of the measures used in the study. (1984, p. 255)

Ways to improve reliability will be discussed along with the several types of reliability that can be estimated in quantitative studies. First, however, we will briefly consider some fundamental ideas related to the use of measurement in quantitative research.

MEASUREMENT

Definition

The classic, often repeated, definition of *measurement* in quantitative research is the assignment of numbers to objects or events according to certain rules. Carmines and Zeller (1979), however, point out that many times what we are interested in measuring is a far more abstract phenomenon than an object or event. Often it is something we cannot see or touch. Pain, anxiety, self-esteem, and comfort are common examples of abstract phenomena of interest in nursing.

Nunnally and Bernstein (1994) offer a better definition of measurement: rules for assigning numbers to objects so that they represent quantities of attributes of these objects. However, we still need to address the often abstract nature of what we want to measure and so will consider one more definition: linking empirical indicants (numbers) to a phenomenon of interest (Carmines & Zeller, 1979). This last definition is well suited to quantitative nursing research.

Uses

Why is measurement so important in quantitative research? The following are several reasons:

- Quantification (assigning numbers) allows us to perform powerful analyses that would not otherwise be possible to do.

- Numbers are often more clearly communicated. For example, which is clearer, "She had a huge baby," or "Her baby weighed 14 lb"?

- Subjectivity is reduced; objectivity is increased. Here is an example from Tryon (2005): "In one study, teachers rated certain children as hyperactive who, when their activity was measured quantitatively, were found to be no more active than other children in the class."

- Efficiency is sometimes increased by use of brief measures as opposed to long hours of observation or interview.

Levels of Measurement

Numbers may be assigned to each subject as a label, sometimes to replace identifiable names. This is the lowest level of measurement, called the nominal level, which provides a means of identification but nothing more. The next level of measurement is categorical in which numbers are assigned to people by group (Nunnally & Bernstein, 1994). For example, all males could be grouped as 1s and all females as 2s. These numbers specify the category in which a subject belongs but provide no other information. In fact, you could just as easily group the males as 2s and the females as 1s or males and females as 3s and 4s.

Ordinal level measurement provides for some type of ordering of subjects on a characteristic. For example, you could rank subjects from the earliest arrival at the clinic to the latest arrival. Or you could order students in a study according to their rank in their class, from highest grade point average to the lowest or from A to F. The order implies a sequence from most to least or vice versa but *not how far apart* the first is from the second and so forth.

The next two levels are important because many types of statistical analyses depend upon interval or ratio levels of measurement. Interval measurement is also ordered but there is, at least in the abstract, an estimation of the distance between one score and the next. Many well-developed scales such as those for depression and anxiety are considered to be interval level measures. IQ scores and professional licensure testing are also considered interval level scores. The highest level of measurement, ratio measurement, not only has a defined distance between the values assigned but also a zero point. Height, weight, and age are all ratio measures.

Measurement Error

Our measurements are never perfect. Even ratio level measures such as height and weight are subject to several possible sources of error. For example, let's say you are working with two other researchers to monitor the weight of school age children. Each of you is assigned three elementary schools and expected to obtain the weight of every 3rd-grade child every 6 weeks. The following are some potential sources of error:

- One of the three scales is not accurate; it adds 1.5 lb to everyone's weight (this is a source of systematic error).
- The scale readout is difficult to see so the wrong results are being recorded.
- One of the researchers has poor eyesight and is unable to read the weights accurately.
- One of the scheduled weigh-ins is the Monday after Thanksgiving.
- The children are having trouble standing still long enough for the scale to register their real weight.
- Some of the children are wearing heavy winter clothes and boots that add to their weight.

The sources of error causing unreliability may be one or more of the following:

- The measure itself is inconsistent or inaccurate. For example, a self-esteem scale may include items about depression, making the scale results inconsistent.
- The raters or testers are inconsistent or inaccurate. For example, the raters may not have been well trained or they may be subjective as in the previously mentioned example of teachers rating hyperactivity in children.
- The phenomenon being measured varies from one measurement time to the next. For example, pain may vary from one test point to the next. Likewise, state anxiety may fluctuate in response to anxiety-producing situations such as a test or public speaking event.

- The situation (environment) in which measuring is being done is confounding (interfering with) the measurement. For example, there may be many distractions—other people talking within earshot or a thunderstorm occurring outside.

All of these sources of error are potentially important. Any one or all may reduce the reliability of a measure. In classical measurement theory, each of these sources is tested separately. Generalizability theory, a newer approach, makes it possible to evaluate them altogether (Burns, 1998).

The observed score that is obtained whenever something is measured is thought to contain both the true score and error. The equation for this is:

$$X = t + e$$

| Observed score | True score | Random error |

Because our measurements are never perfect, there is always some error in the scores we obtain in research (Carmines & Zeller, 1979). The more error that enters into a measurement, the less reliable our results will be. Our goal is to reduce the error as much as possible so that our observed scores are as close as possible to the true score.

Several types of reliability need to be considered in designing a research study and evaluating the measures you might use. These are the *consistency* of results between and within the people (raters or examiners) or instrument used to collect the data, *stability* from one testing time to the next, and *homogeneity* of items within a measure. The basic references upon which much of the following is based are Carmines and Zeller (1979), Nunnally and Bernstein (1996), and Waltz, Strickland, and Lenz (2005).

CONSISTENCY

It is essential that the people and instruments employed in a research study are consistent in the way data is obtained and recorded from one subject to the next, one data collector to the next, and one data collection point to the next. Imagine having a research assistant who rates an infant as calm and easily quieted one day but rates the same infant as irritable and difficult to quiet the next day despite no change in the infant. Or having a sphygmomanometer that reports a blood pressure of 135/72 on a person one day and 175/105 the next day without any change in the person's actual (true) blood pressure. These discrepancies are obviously unacceptable. Referring back to the $X = t + e$ equation, you could say that the observed score (X) had too much error (e) in addition to the true (t) score, making these measures very unreliable.

These examples, by the way, refer to intrarater reliability (i.e., reliability within the same rater). The other important type is consistency between or across raters and instruments where more than one is used in a study. The simplest type of interrater reliability evaluation is a comparison of the ratings produced by two examiners done at the same time with the same subjects. A hypothetical example:

A new observational form to detect breaks in infection control during wound care has been developed. To determine interrater reliability of the new form, two research nurses are trained in its use and then assigned to observe and rate adherence to infection control procedures during wound care together on one surgical unit on two randomly selected days. The two examiners complete the form without discussion or sharing of observations. On a busy surgical unit, they were able to complete 30 dual observations over the 2 assigned days. To evaluate the interrater reliability, their observations are entered into a statistical database and a Pearson correlation coefficient is calculated.

Percent agreement between two examiners can also be calculated in some instances. This is discussed further under intercoder reliability, as well as calculation of Cohen's kappa, which corrects for chance agreement.

INTRARATER RELIABILITY

It is also important that a single rater be consistent from one subject to another and from one time to another, such as from pretest to posttest. This is tested and evaluated in much the same way as interrater reliability. A particular concern with intrarater reliability, however, is that the situation be the same in both instances, and that the rater does not remember what was recorded at the first time point. This is difficult to achieve. One useful approach is to use videotaped encounters. Another is to test a relatively large number of people on consecutive days if the phenomenon being measured can be assumed to be sufficiently stable from one day to the next in a given group of subjects.

INTERCODER RELIABILITY

Intercoder reliability is similar to interrater reliability in that a comparison is made of the results produced by more than one rater. However, in the case of intercoder reliability, it is the coding or classification of data that is compared. The degree of agreement between coders is the result of interest when calculating intercoder reliability (Burla et al., 2008). A hypothetical example:

> One hundred twenty middle school children with type I diabetes were asked to describe what made it difficult for them to adhere to their prescribed diets. The interviews were tape recorded, transcribed, and uploaded into Atlas.ti (Atlas.ti, 2008). The research team created a coding scheme for the various reasons given by the children: peer pressure, desire to "be like others," eating away from home, desire for sweet and satisfying foods, unavailability of appropriate foods, unacceptability of appropriate foods, and difficulty estimating types and amounts of various foods allowed.
>
> The transcribed data was coded by a pediatric diabetes clinic nurse who checked each of the categories mentioned by each of the children. A second clinic nurse independently coded 30 randomly selected interviews as well. The percent agreement was calculated on this subset of 30 interviews.

If you have just two coders, you can calculate the percent agreement between them by hand. In the hypothetical example above, if the second nurse's coding of each child's response was the same for 24 of the 30 interviews this yields an 80% agreement. This calculation does not account for chance agreement, however. In fact, Cohen (1960) called this approach "primitive" and suggests using the coefficient K (Cohen's kappa), which corrects for change agreement. Cohen's kappa uses both the proportion in which the coders (or judges) agreed and the proportion of agreement that would be expected by change. K is calculated by subtracting the frequency of agreement (fo) by the frequency of agreement expected by chance (fc) and dividing this by the number evaluated (N) minus the frequency expected by chance (fc):

$$K = \frac{fo - fc}{N - fc}$$

In the hypothetical example, the two nurse coders agreed on the coding of 24 of the responses to be the question on adherence to the prescribed diabetic diet. Assuming (this can be calculated; see Cohen [1960] or Waltz, Strickland, and Lenz [2005] for details) that 50% agreement or 15 out of 30 would occur by chance, this can be entered in the formula for K as follows:

$$K = \frac{24 - 15}{30 - 15} = \frac{9}{15} = .60$$

There are other kappas that can be calculated when more than two coders are used (see Burla et al., 2008).

When high levels of disagreement or inconsistency between coders are found, it is important to find out why this has occurred. The first step is to identify the codes on which disagreement has occurred. Next, evaluate why disagreement occurred: Was it due to a poor coding scheme or inadequate explanations given to the coders? If the coders did not understand the codes, then retraining and recoding can be done. If the coding scheme itself is poorly done, then it may be necessary to revise it. When a small amount of disagreement occurs, it is sometimes possible to bring the coders together to discuss and reconcile disagreements.

STABILITY

Test-Retest Reliability

Test-retest reliability is evaluated by administering the same test to the same people or taking the same measurement on the same people after a specified period of time. The results of the two testing times are then compared statistically.

For example, Rossen and Gruber (2007) evaluated the stability of their Self-Efficacy Relocation Scale (a measure of older adults' perceived self-efficacy to relocate to a congregate living facility) by testing the measure on a subsample of 30 participants a second time 2 weeks following the first test. They compared the results using the Pearson correlation coefficient which yielded an *r* of .69 (*P* = .001). They concluded that this result indicated adequate stability of the measure over time.

On the other hand, Tluczek, Henriques, and Brown (2009) found differences in parent anxiety across three time points in the first year of their infant's life (at 2 months, 6 months, and 12 months). They found higher state anxiety in parents of infants with medical conditions at the first time point (age 2 months) than at the 6 month or 12 month time points. The researchers suggest that by 6 months the parents had adjusted and developed some confidence in their parenting. Does this difference indicate instability of the measure? State anxiety is a transient type of arousal, while trait anxiety is conceptualized as an enduring characteristic. Therefore, the measure is expected to change over time and is not expected to be stable over months. This is an example where test-retest stability is not expected or especially desirable.

Factors Affecting Test-Retest Reliability

Test-retest reliability is a relatively simple, straightforward idea but its application in real life research can become more complicated. The use of test-retest reliability *assumes stability* in the phenomenon being measured. Many phenomena of interest in nursing cannot be assumed to be stable over time: fever, pain, nausea, hypoxia, hormone levels, and so forth may all change from day to day, even from hour to hour. For these phenomena, test-retest reliability is not useful.

Another important issue is *reactivity*. Carmines and Zeller (1979) note that "sometimes the very process of measuring a phenomenon can induce change in the phenomenon itself" (p. 39). Asking questions about a person's attitude toward people with disabilities, for example, may increase their sensitivity to the needs of people with disabilities. In the same way, asking questions about diet or consumption of alcohol may increase a person's awareness of some very unhealthy behaviors and could lead to a change in behavior.

The *practice effect* is another issue. A test of cognition or physical ability may be easier to do the second time. In some instances, people practice what they have been asked to do (standing on one foot with eyes closed, for example, to test balance) and so will perform better on the second testing.

Calculating Test-Retest Reliability

There are several ways to calculate test-retest reliability. The most common is the Pearson product moment correlation, which is easy to calculate and has a straightforward interpretation. There are limitations to using the correlation coefficient that are addressed by using intraclass correlations (ICCs). Intraclass correlation coefficients control for systematic bias that is not controlled by using Pearson correlation coefficients alone by combining correlation with testing the difference between means (Leidy, 1999). There are a number of different forms of the ICC (Shrout & Fleiss, 1979). Choice of the appropriate form depends upon three factors:

- Whether one-way or two-way analysis of variance is most appropriate
- If the differences between mean ratings are relevant
- Whether an individual rating or the mean of several ratings is the unit of analysis

For most beginning nurse researchers, consultation with a statistician to select the right form of the ICC is likely to be necessary.

Limitations of Correlation Coefficients

Pearson correlation coefficients test for an association or relationship between sets of results; they actually do not test for agreement. In other words, you can have what appears to be a perfect correlation (1.00) but considerable disagreement between raters. How is this possible? Engstrom (1988) provided a very simple hypothetical example. If the second (comparison) rater consistently scored people 1, 5, or 10 points higher than did the first rater, the ratings would not agree but the correlation would be 1.00. Yet the difference of 1, 5, or 10 points can be clinically very significant (Engstrom uses an example of differences in measuring the fundal height but this applies to virtually any clinical measurement). Correlation coefficients are also affected by the range of scores obtained. If, for example, the possible range is 1 to 10 on one scale and 1 to 50 on another, comparison of ratings on the scale with the larger range of scores would produce a higher correlation coefficient, all other things being equal.

HOMOGENEITY

Many educational tests, such as the national tests for college admission and professional licensing exams, have alternate forms. This means that if you take the test a second time, you will encounter items of similar difficulty, but you will not be asked the same questions as you were asked on the first test. The effort behind creating these parallel forms of the tests is massive and beyond the resources of many nurse researchers.

Most research measures do not have these alternate forms to prevent practice effects or remembering items from the last test administration, issues that were mentioned earlier. It may also be difficult to persuade research subjects to return to take a test the second time. For these reasons, researchers often resorted to use of the split-half technique for assessing reliability: comparing the first half of the measure to the second half or odd-numbered items to even-numbered items. For a number of reasons, including the questionable comparability of various items, this technique was far from satisfactory. However, the idea of comparing items within the measure was potentially useful and led to a test of the homogeneity of items within a measure called Cronbach's alpha. This widely used test of reliability is the equivalent of all possible combinations of items into two halves. It may also be thought of as an estimate of the correlation of the existing measure with a hypothetical alternative form of the measure (Carmines & Zeller, 1979; Nunnally & Bernstein, 1996). A practical advantage of this statistic is that the measure only has to be administered one time. It also produces the correlations of individual items within a measure to the total score and estimates of the effect of removing an item (removal of a troublesome item may increase the alpha). Cronbach's alpha is also affected by the number of items in a measure. Generally, adding items will raise the alpha unless the added items are inappropriate, irrelevant, or poorly written.

Values of Alpha

Judging the strength of Cronbach's alpha and interpreting its value are additional steps in its use. Nunnally and Bernstein (1996) suggest that a Cronbach's alpha of .70 is acceptable for new measures, indicating that this level represents a modest degree of homogeneity. An alpha of at least .80 is expected for established measures used in research. However, if a measure is to be used in clinical evaluation of a particular individual, at least .90 or better .95 or higher is desirable.

Interpreting Cronbach's Alpha

Cronbach's alpha is an indicator of the internal consistency or homogeneity of a scale. Fundamentally, and perhaps a little simplistically, Cronbach's alpha tells you the extent to which all of the items on the test are "behaving" similarly. A low alpha suggests that there are errors in the selection of items to be included in the measure. If a measure has several subscales, alphas are calculated and reported for each of the individual subscales. It may or may not make sense to report an alpha for the scale as a whole as well, depending upon the degree to which the scale as a whole is measuring the same phenomenon. The following is an example of the use and interpretation of Cronbach's alpha from research on the Mini AQLQ, a measure of health-related quality of life for people with asthma reported by Baghi and Atherton (2004).

> The Mini AQLQ was completed online by 307 individuals participating in a Web-based intervention study. Cronbach's alpha was calculated for the four factors (dimensions) of the scale (activities, symptoms, emotions, and environment) and for the scale as a whole. At pretest the alphas were .92, .82, .78, .65, and .91, respectively. As the researchers point out in their report, all but the fourth factor (environment) and the scale as a whole have satisfactory alphas, demonstrating "that the items of the instrument are homogeneous within each [sub] scale" (p. 28) and that they exceed Nunnally and Bernstein's threshold of .70 for a new scale (Baghi & Atherton, 2004).
>
> The researchers do not discuss any changes that might be made to raise the alpha of the environment subscale, but it is noted that it is one of the shorter ones, containing only three items. Addition of another item of a homogeneous nature might bring this subscale alpha into the .70 or above range.

RELIABILITY OF PHYSICAL MEASURES

There is a wide range of physical measures that are used in nursing research, from laboratory analyses to pulse oximetry, actigraphy, and polysomnography. Each has its individual characteristics and, therefore, individual reliability issues. A review of some common issues follows, but use of any particular physical measure requires in-depth knowledge of that measure and expertise in its use and interpretation.

Systematic and Random Error

Both systematic and random types of error are of concern in evaluating reliability. A scale that consistently adds 2 lb to everyone's weight is producing a result that contains systematic error. A data collector who is easily distracted by conversation with study participants and occasionally records the wrong weight is introducing random error. Physical measures are more likely to introduce systematic error (as well as random error) into the observed score than are psychological and behavioral measures.

Detecting Error in Physical Measures

Engstrom (1988) offers an interesting example of the way in which random errors can cancel each other out unless the researcher knows how to detect them:

> Three examiners obtained fundal height measures on 30 subjects using four different techniques for obtaining this measurement. An error within 1 cm of the true value (true fundal height) would be considered clinically acceptable because that is the approximate change expected over a week in a pregnant woman. Although there were differences on the fundal heights obtained, since the erroneous results were both too high and too low, they cancelled each other out leaving a mean error of close to zero. However, if the errors were treated as absolute values (no negative or positive sign), the mean error rate was found to be 1.08 cm instead of .013 cm, higher than the maximum considered clinically acceptable.
>
> The technical error of measurement (TEM) can be obtained with a hand calculator: square the sum of the differences between a pair of examiners and divide this by 2 times the number of paired scores being evaluated. Then calculate the square root of this result.

$$\sqrt{\frac{\sum d^2}{2N}}$$

d = the difference between scores of paired examiners

N = number of pairs of scores

> The TEM for the fundal height measures was .97 cm, very close to the clinically accepted limit of 1.00 (Engstrom, 1988).

Often employed in nursing research, actigraphs are devices that use a microcontroller to measure and store data on movement. Tryon (2005) compared the means, standard deviations, and correlations produced by four Motion Logger and four Buzz Bee actigraphs in a laboratory test using a precision pendulum to provide the motion (activity) to be measured. Ten trials were conducted for each actigraph. The results were interesting, especially if you've believed that most of these mechanical measuring devices can be assumed to be relatively accurate. The lowest mean activity units produced by a Motion Logger was 204, the highest was 297. Compare this to the Buzz Bees which produced a low mean of 245 and a high mean of 269. The unit difference in the first case was 93, in the second it was 24. The Motion Logger means differed by approximately 8% on repeated testing, the standard deviations by about 7%. The Buzz Bee means and standard deviations differed about 3%, considerably better. The test-retest correlation coefficients exceeded .98 for both, again demonstrating the limitations of this popular statistic. Tryon (2005) noted that there would likely be even more variability in these measures when used outside the laboratory. People move in various ways, affecting the measurement. Positioning of the actigraphs may also affect results. Recalibration of the devices can reduce any systematic error produced by a particular device. Consistent application of the devices can help to reduce random error.

Measurement of peak expiratory flow rate was an example used by Bland and Altman (1986). They tested the Wright peak flow meter and the mini Wright meter on volunteers. The correlation coefficient of their results was $r = .94$. However, as many others have done, they point out that the correlation is a measure of the strength of the relationship but not of agreement. They found that the correlation actually concealed considerable lack of agreement between the two sources of measurement finding discrepancies as high as 80 liters per minute between the two types of meters.

We will consider one more example of the reliability of physical measure factors that may affect the values reported after laboratory analysis of specimens submitted, in this case, a blood sample:

> Seventeen-year-old Bonnie G. is a participant in a study of adolescents with diabetes who are hospitalized because of problems related to glucose control. To track progress in improving control, participants' blood glucose levels are measured every 4 hours during waking hours. The fasting blood sugar was drawn at 7:30 a.m. by the IV team. The tech on the team picked up the correct order, checked the patient's name on her ID bracelet, and chose a plain tube for the specimen. If analysis of the sample was expected to be delayed, then a tube with preservative would have been needed because unpreserved glucose can fall 10 to 15 mg/dl an hour in a plain tube. The blood was drawn correctly, but no one asked if Bonnie had eaten before the blood was collected. Bonnie has a drawer full of snacks brought by her friends, but the staff did not know this yet. Bonnie also has an IV—was the sample drawn from the IV line? If so, was the line cleared sufficiently to prevent IV fluid from getting into the sample?

The runner delivered the sample to the lab within 15 minutes, and it was bar coded and centrifuged quickly. But the main chemistry analyzer was backed up. Maintenance had been done early that morning, and it was not operating well. Lab personnel ran quality controls after maintenance was done and found the glucose tests were running too low. The control test read 131, but the target value was 151. Lab personnel had to check several things: was the reagent fresh or expired? Was it stored at the right temperature? Was it matched with the correct value? All these items checked out so the machine was recalibrated using additional quality control samples with known values.

Bonnie's results are high despite strict dietary management and insulin administration. The research nurse is sent in to talk with the IV team about their blood draw technique, with the medication nurse about the time and amount of insulin administered, and with Bonnie about her diet and activity. Everything seems to check out, and no reason was found for the high fasting glucose. But was this really a fasting glucose? Did anyone ask Bonnie about her snack stash?

This example illustrates the potential number of factors that can affect a physical measurement. It also illustrates the importance of correct interpretation of the results. Bonnie eventually revealed her snack stash to the research nurse, her treatment plan was modified accordingly, and she was discharged with her diabetes well controlled.

There are a number of considerations in obtaining reliable physical measures. The most important is to know what factors may affect the accuracy and consistency of the measure and how these may be controlled. Correct interpretation of the result is also important. Each measure and each device used to produce data is different. To ensure reliability of the data, the researcher needs to know the specifications and sensitivities of the measure used.

IMPROVING RELIABILITY

There are a number of actions you can take to improve the reliability of the measures used in your study. Some are very specific, others quite general. Those that refer to changes in the measure itself are more difficult to use because they require a reevaluation of the measure. The following are ways in which reliability (consistency, stability, and homogeneity) may be enhanced:

- Be sure the people collecting the data (called raters, examiners, or judges) are responsible, competent, and thoroughly trained in the use of each specific measure used.

- Supervise the people collecting the data, and periodically check interrater, intrarater, and intercoder reliability. As time passes, people develop their own "favorite" ways to ask a question or "shortcuts" to save time that may unwittingly threaten reliability. Fatigue and the effect of repetition may also contribute to rater drift.

- Periodically retest and recalibrate instruments used. Ensure regular equipment maintenance and quality control testing as specified by the manufacturer.

- Add appropriate items (lengthening a test), and delete those that lower the alpha coefficient to increase homogeneity.

- Standardize the conditions under which testing is done, and minimize any distractions. The manual for a computerized driver test (DriveABLE, n.d.) is an excellent example of how standardized conditions and reduced distractions are achieved. The following are a sample of the specifications for the conditions under which the test should be administered:

  ○ Use a windowless room to administer the test in.

  ○ Remove pictures, posters, other distractions from walls and doors.

  ○ Close the door to reduce outside noise; no interruption by phones.

  ○ Maintain a moderate level of lighting; overhead lights may need to be dimmed.

  ○ Place the touch screen at eye level.

  ○ Use an adjustable height chair in front of the screen.

  ○ Use an *L*-shaped testing table.

- Ensure that instructions and wording of items are not subject to interpretation. Pilot test them if necessary to ascertain their clarity.

- Standardize the instructions for data collection. In large studies, a manual or testing protocol is usually created for data collection and thoroughly reviewed with data collectors before testing is done. These manuals provide very specific instructions for introducing the measure, administering, scoring, and recording the results. Reliability is improved when administration is consistent. For example, if a person cannot name an object, a stimulus cue may be allowed in some tests. In other tests, they are not allowed. The person administering the test needs to know if cues or words of encouragement are allowed. The following is an example of instructions provided for administering a very simple cognitive test called category fluency, which tests a person's ability to generate words within a given category:

  1. "I'm going to name a category. I want you to name as many things that belong to the category as you can. The category is *animals*. You will have 1 minute. Tell me all the animals you can think of as quickly as you can, starting now."

  2. Start timing and recording the answers. Plurals and repetitions are not counted.

  3. After 60 seconds, say "Stop."

  4. You may prompt the person once if he or she makes no response or pauses for 15 seconds, saying "Tell me all the animals you can think of."

  5. You may repeat the instructions or category if the person requests it, but do not extend the time limit (Potter & Schinka, 2008).

As people who are committed to caring for others, nurses often find it difficult at first to avoid coaching research study participants, "helping" them to do well on the tests administered. Once they've learned more about the importance of the accuracy of the measurements, they usually find it easier to withhold their help on test questions while still being supportive of the individual and sensitive to their tolerance of the testing being done.

CONCLUSION

It is often noted that the reliability of measures used in research is specific to the situation in which they are applied. This means that reliability should be established in every study in which a measure is employed. The choice of reliability test depends on the study and the measures being used.

Reliability of the measures used in a quantitative study is a necessary component of the quality of measures. Validity is the second, equally essential component. Nunnally and Bernstein (1996) advise never switching to a less valid measure because it is more reliable. Instead, improve the reliability of the more valid measure as much as possible.

REFERENCES

Atlas.ti Scientific Software Development. (2008). *Atlas.ti 5 multi educational license* [computer software]. Cologne, France: Levebridge AG.

Baghi, H., & Atherton, M. (2004). Construct validity and reliability of scores on scales to measure the impairment of health-related quality of life in persons with asthma. *Journal of Nursing Measurement, 12*(1), 21–31.

Bland, J. M., & Altman, D. G. (1986). Statistical methods for assessing agreement between two methods of clinical measurement. *Lancet, I,* 307–310.

Burla, L., Knierim, B., Barth, J., Liewald, K., Duetz, M., & Abel, T. (2008). From text to codings: Intercoder reliability in qualitative content analysis. *Nursing Research, 57*(2), 113–117.
   ◇ Definitely worth reading if you plan to code and quantify qualitative data.

Burns, R. J. (1998). Beyond classical reliability: Using generalizability theory to assess dependability. *Research in Nursing and Health, 21,* 83–90.

Carmines, E. G., & Zeller, R. A. (1979). Reliability and validity assessment. Newbury Park, CA: Sage.
   ◇ Some sections may be difficult to read but this is a classic resource on reliability.

Cohen, J. (1960). A coefficient of agreement for nominal scales. *Educational and Psychological Measurement, XX*(1), 37–46.

DriveABLE. (n.d.). DriveABLE assessment centre's site license requirements. Edmonton, Canada: Author.

Engstrom, J. L. (1988). Assessment of the reliability of physical measures. *Research in Nursing & Health, 11,* 383–389.

Leidy, N. K. (1999). Psychometric properties of the functional performance inventory in patients with chronic obstructive pulmonary disease. *Nursing Research, 48*(1), 20–28.

Lynn, M. R. (1984). Reliability estimates: use and disuse. *Nursing Research, 34*(4), 254–256.

Nunnally, J. C., & Bernstein, I. H. (1994). *Psychometric theory.* New York: McGraw-Hill.

Potter, H., & Schinka, J. (2008). *Memory screening studies to detect progression of mild cognitive impairment in patients* [#CSG2007-08, research study]. Tampa, FL: Johnnie B. Byrd Alzheimer Center and Research Institute.

Rossen, E. K., & Gruber, K. J. (2007). Development and psychometric testing of the relocation self-efficacy scale. *Nursing Research, 56*(4), 244–251.

Shrout, P. E., & Fleiss, J. L. (1979). Intraclass correlations: Uses in assessing rater reliability. *Psychological Bulletin, 86*(2), 420–428.

Tluczak, A., Henriques, J. B., & Brown, R. L. (2009). Support for the reliability and validity of a six-item state anxiety scale derived from the State-Trait Anxiety Inventory. *Journal of Nursing Measurement, 17*(1), 19–28.

Tryon, W. W. (2005). The reliability and validity of two ambulatory monitoring actigraphs. *Behavior Research Methods, 37*(3), 492–497.

Waltz, C. F., Strickland, O. L., & Lenz, E. R. (2005). Measurement in nursing and health research. New York: Springer.
  ◇ Excellent textbook on measurement and instrument development in nursing and health research.

CHAPTER 10

Validity

Validity is the extent to which the measure you use is *true to its intended purpose.* In other words, an anxiety scale should measure either state (short-term) or trait (long-term) anxiety, not stress or depression. A pediatric behavior scale should measure what children do, that is, their activities, not their mood or health status. Further, the measure needs to be *accurate*, especially when it is used to diagnose a problem such as developmental delay, hypertension, or risk for such problems as pressure sores or heart attack.

The validity of a measure is always important. Sometimes, it is critical. Point of care testing, for instance, has become widespread for several reasons: the results are immediately available and the specimen does not have to be passed through different hands, saving time and money. The accuracy of point of care testing, however, is not always as high as testing done in the central laboratory. This difference was made clear in an unfortunate incident that nearly cost a life:

> Walt Gibson was on glucose checks at bedside four times a day. When the afternoon shift arrived, he said that he was not feeling well so they checked his blood glucose a little early with their handheld glucometer. The reading was very high, and they notified the resident. A blood glucose assay with blood gases done by respiratory at about the same time had produced a very low blood glucose reading of 20. To clarify the discrepancy a laboratory glucose was ordered. That test indicated his blood glucose was 35. The resident asked the staff to repeat the handheld glucometer test. The reading was very high again so she ordered insulin to be given immediately. An hour later she ordered additional insulin because the glucometer result remained stubbornly high. Soon after, Walt was found unresponsive and transferred to intensive care. Intensive care staff found his blood glucose to be very low and began to treat him for severe hypoglycemia. He survived but has some residual effects from this episode.
>
> What happened? A thorough investigation of this event was launched by an interdisciplinary team with medicine, nursing, respiratory, and the laboratory represented. They eventually found that the vial of reagent sticks used on the unit had been left open. This causes the reagent to rapidly deteriorate (the vial contains desiccant to prevent this when it is closed). The result can be falsely high or low glucose readings. In Walt Gibson's case, the results were falsely high. Neither the resident nor the nursing staff could explain why they trusted the handheld glucometer reading and ignored the respiratory department and main lab results. From a validity perspective, they had trusted the least accurate measurement available to them (L. Marchand, personal communication, April 14, 2010).

The goals of being as accurate as possible and as true to the intended purpose as possible are straightforward. Assuring that this actually happens, however, can be quite challenging because of the following reasons:

1. Many phenomena that we try to measure, especially psychosocial ones, are not precisely defined and often overlap with other phenomena. *Function*, for example, is a term that is used many different ways: from kidney function (e.g., ability to concentrate urine) to cognitive function (e.g., ability to balance a checkbook).

2. The measures or instruments themselves are often less accurate than they appear to be. Blood test results, for example, can vary a little from one testing time to another. Interpretation of the results, especially of changes from one testing time to another, needs to take this into account. Questionnaire and survey results usually have even more measurement error in them.

In this chapter, we will consider the three types of validity—content, construct, and criterion validity—as well as the two faces of accuracy in diagnostic tests—sensitivity and specificity.

CONTENT VALIDITY

Content validity refers to the extent to which a measure includes all of the dimensions of the phenomenon to be measured but does not include any extraneous dimensions. In other words, does the instrument address the domain it is meant to measure? For example, if you were considering use of a measure of readiness for kindergarten, you would look for items related to independence in putting on shoes and jackets but also a number of other dimensions such as social skills and prereading skills but not height, weight, or hair color. Knowledge of the phenomenon, its boundaries, dimensions, and indicators (explained further in the theory chapter) is essential to judging content validity.

There are several ways to judge content validity. One of these, face validity, is not recommended, as you will see.

Face Validity

Face validity means that the measure looks appropriate. In other words, a sleep measure would contain questions about how long you sleep, and a pain measure would contain questions about how much something hurts. Most researchers consider face validity to be virtually worthless, but it does have one or two useful aspects. When the items look relevant, people responding to them generally feel that the questions are reasonable and appropriate. This usually makes it easier to persuade them to use the measure or to answer the questions. Other than that, just because a measure looks appropriate, this does not establish its validity. The next three types of content validity better address this question, but before we consider them, let's look at an approach that has almost no face validity.

The implicit measurement approach, often used to ferret out prejudice and biases, has virtually no face validity! Here is an example:

> When you go to the Project Implicit (n.d.) website, you are asked to consent to participate, provide some information about yourself, and answer one or two sets of questions that might be about an upcoming election, the amount of risk you are willing to take, how you feel about older people, or how you feel about people of a different gender or race. If you do this, however, you will see that the questions do not directly address the issue of interest. Instead, the *response latency* or time it takes for a person to respond to the various items is used to measure how much easier it is to associate the concept of interest, "female," for example, with the attributes presented, such as *pleasant* or *unpleasant*.
>
> In another experiment using the implicit approach, 30 undergraduate students were asked to select "good" or "bad" when presented with an onscreen trait such as "friendly" or "selfish." They were not told that a word, either *young* or *old*, would be randomly flashed on the screen for 55 milliseconds (almost too fast to detect even if told it would happen ahead of time) before the traits appeared. The researchers found that there was a quicker response to negative traits when the word *old* was flashed on the screen than if the word *young* was flashed on the screen before the trait appeared. Positive traits received a faster response if *young* was flashed on the screen beforehand (Perdue & Gurtman, 1990).
>
> Not everyone agrees, by the way, that people are really unaware of these attitudes. They say, instead, that it is the measure itself that is implicit, not the attitude (Fazio & Olson, 2003). The indirect or implicit approach may be capturing attitudes people are unwilling to report rather than unaware they have.

Is this measurement approach valid? Does it really detect biases that people are unwilling to report or are entirely unconscious of having? There is some evidence that people's behaviors are congruent with the biases detected through implicit approaches. Validity of the results from indirect or implicit measures has been demonstrated by comparing implicit study results with direct observation of behavior. Examples are finding that responses to photos of overweight and normal weight women predicted how far away from an overweight woman the participant placed his or her own chair and finding a relationship between older persons' association of the "elderly" with "forgetfulness" and their own memory limitations (Fazio & Olson, 2003).

Expert Review and the Content Validity Index

To evaluate how well a measure encompasses the phenomenon of interest, you need either a map of its dimensions and indicators or a very clear definition in the case of a simpler concept. For many phenomena, you can turn to the literature for guidance. In cases where the literature is not sufficient, you will need to develop a concept tree as described in the theory chapter.

Once you have mapped the elements of the phenomenon, you may either do your own comparison between the measure and the map you created, or you may ask several experts to do this. For new measures, especially if it is one you have created, a review by a panel of experts is recommended.

The experts may be asked to provide general comments or to specifically rate the extent to which each dimension is represented. Waltz, Strickland, and Lenz (2005) explain how to calculate a Content Validity Index (CVI) from judges' ratings. Judges are first asked to rate the relevance or appropriateness of each item as 1 = not relevant; 2 = somewhat relevant; 3 = quite relevant; or 4 = very relevant. Scores of 1 or 2 are combined as a low rating and 3 and 4 are combined as a high rating. The scores are then totaled for each expert judge. If you have just one judge, you simply divide the number of items rated as highly relevant by the total number of items. For example, if your measure has 20 items and 10 are rated as 3 or 4, the CVI is .50.

If you have several judges, you calculate each judge's ratings the same way and average them. More complex calculations of interjudge agreement that adjust for chance agreement are described by Cohen (1960) and by Wynd, Schmidt, and Schaefer (2003).

Empirical Data

A powerful way to provide evidence of content validity is through the collection of data. This is often done during the development of a new measure. The following is an example:

> What kinds of moods do people with advanced Alzheimer's disease experience? The literature on moods in people with Alzheimer's disease is sparse, so a qualitative study was done to find out what moods were observed by family and formal caregivers of people with Alzheimer's disease. The moods described by the caregivers became the basis for individual items in the ADRD (Alzheimer's Disease and Related Dementias) Mood Scale (Tappen, & Williams, 1998).

Factor Analysis

Factor analysis is an analytic strategy for looking at the way individual items in a measure cluster together. A *factor* is a cluster of interrelated items or variables (Carmines & Zeller, 1979) produced statistically but interpreted theoretically. The strength of the relationship is indicated by the *factor loadings* that are produced. The further from zero (higher) this value is, the more salient the item is to the factor (Gorsuch, 1983). An example will make this clearer:

> The Cross Cultural Measure of Acculturation (CCMA) (Tappen & Williams, 2009) was designed to measure the degree of acculturation to mainstream American culture in various ethnic groups. Literature on the process of acculturation and how acculturation is evidenced, existing measures, and expert consultants were the primary sources for items. The CCMA has 19 items related to orientation to a person's culture of origin (heritage) and 19 parallel items related to orientation

to mainstream American culture. We will look at the results of a factor analysis for the first subscale, orientation to one's culture/ethnic group of origin (see Table 10-1).

To conduct a factor analysis, individual items from a measure are entered into a statistical program that runs the factor analysis and produces the result. (There are a number of choices to be made in performing this analysis. For further information about them see Hatcher [1994] or talk with a statistician.) The basic sample size requirement for factor analysis is 5–10 cases per item to be factored. The data must be continuous in nature, not categorical.

In the acculturation measure example, the responses of almost 300 university students, primarily nursing and psychology students of African American, Afro-Caribbean, European American, and Hispanic American origin, who were asked to provide consent and fill out this questionnaire were analyzed. The results of a factor analysis of the 19 items are pictured in Tables 10-1 and 10-2 and Figure 10-1. Table 10-1 shows the factor loadings. Any item with a factor of loading of .40 or higher is starred. This is the first decision you need to make in interpreting results of a factor analysis, the level at which you will consider a factor loading to be of some significance. In this case .40 was selected, but you can make it higher. The second decision is how many factors should be generated. You can specify this, or let the default option be used. The default option is usually based on what is called an eigenvalue. Eigenvalues of 1.00 or above are considered evidence of a meaningful factor (Table 10-2). In this illustration, the eigenvalues suggest five meaningful factors. Another criterion you can use is a visual one called a scree plot (see Figure 10-1). You look for a break in the slope of the scree plot to determine the cutoff point. In the case illustrated, the scree plot is not as clear as the eigenvalue table, but it does support a five-factor solution.

Going back to Table 10-1, you can see the items that loaded at the .40 level on each of the five factors. You are looking for clean loadings (little or no overlap of items loading on the different factors) and that are strong (higher factor loading values) (Youngblut, 1993). The factor loadings illustrated in Table 10-1 are exceptionally clear and strong and easy to interpret. Look down the list; you will see that none of the items load on more than one factor. The factor loadings are also relatively high (strong). The next step is to list all of the items that load on each factor in order of the strength of the factor loading (Table 10-3). For example, the degree that childhood friends of the respondent identified themselves with the respondent's culture of origin is the highest loading factor, but the respondent's mother's degree of identification is a strong second. The factor may be named for the strongest item or the theme across the items that loaded on the factor in contrast to those that did not (Gorsuch, 1983). In this case, *identification* seems to be the theme of the first factor and a reasonable name for it. Identification, by the way, is theoretically an important aspect of acculturation. The second factor could be named *traditions* or *celebrations*, the third could be named *language*, and so forth.

TABLE 10-1   Factor Loading for the Cross-Cultural Measure of Acculturation: Orientation to Culture/Ethnic Group of Origin

	Factor 1	Factor 2	Factor 3	Factor 4	Factor 5
1. Father identifies as _____ **	.87*	.15	.01	.00	.00
2. Mother identifies as _____	.97*	.11	.01	.00	.00
3. Respondent identifies as _____	.76*	.09	.02	.04	.00
4. Friends growing up identified as _____	1.00*	.01	.01	.02	.04
5. Current friends identify as _____	.95*	.01	.01	.04	.03
6. Socialize with _____ people	.63*	.07	.06	.05	.01
7. Eat _____ food	.22	.66*	.02	.00	.01
8. Wedding celebrations	.08	.87*	.02	.01	.01
9. Birthday celebrations	.06	.84*	.03	.01	.02
10. Holiday celebrations	.04	1.00*	.01	.01	.00
11. Listen to _____ musicians	.18	.04	.01	.08	.60*
12. Listen to _____ radio	.02	.01	.02	.09	1.00*
13. Television about _____ characters	.02	.01	.02	.78*	.04
14. Movies about _____ characters	.02	.00	.00	1.00*	.00
15. Books, magazines	.02	.01	.01	.82*	.03
16. Speak _____ dialect/ language every day	.10	.05	.71*	.00	.01
17. Speak to younger people in _____ language	.04	.02	.89*	.00	.01
18. Think in _____ language	.05	.01	.87*	.02	.00
19. Write in _____ language	.00	.01	1.00*	.03	.00

Notes: * Values on factor loadings greater than .40 are starred.
** Respondents are asked to identify their family's ancestry, country, or culture of origin, which might be Nigerian, Mexican, Irish, Japanese, Spanish, or Native American, to name just a few possibilities, before answering each question. For each item, respondents rate from "not at all" to "very much" the extent to which they agree with each item.

TABLE 10-2 Eigenvalues Indicating Five Factor Solutions of CCMA Subscales

Factor	Eigenvalue
1	29.85
2	5.53
3	4.47
4	2.43
5	1.58
6	.86
7	.58
8	.20

If the factors generated are congruent with the original theoretical mapping of the domain (see the Concept Tree in the theory chapter), they support the validity of the measure. If not, they raise questions about the validity of the measure. An observant reader may have noticed that factors 4 and 5 have fewer items and very closely related themes. Additional analysis may support combining them into one *media* factor.

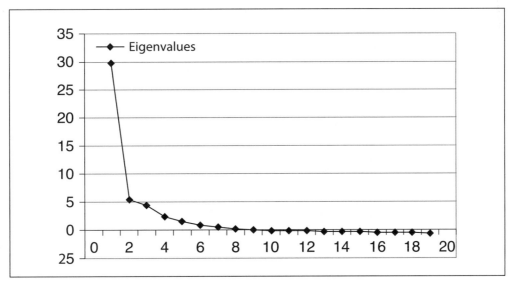

Figure 10-1 Scree plot for factor analysis.

TABLE 10-3 Items Loading on Individual Factors

Factor 1 Identification		Factor 2 Traditions		Factor 3 Language		Factor 4 Other Media		Factor 5 Music	
Childhood friends	1.00	Holiday celebrations	1.00	Written	1.00	Movies	1.00	Favorite musicians	.60
Mother	.97	Birthdays	.84	Speaking with younger people	.89	Print	.82	Radio	1.00
Current friends	.90	Weddings	.87	Thinking	.87	TV	.78		
Father	.87	Food choices	.66	Everyday use	.71				
Self	.76								
Social acquaintances	.63								

CONSTRUCT VALIDITY

Construct validity is concerned with how a measure relates to other measures. It focuses upon the extent to which the measure of interest produces results consistent with other measures of the same phenomenon. For example, you might be interested in using a new measure of depression. To evaluate its construct validity, you could compare it with existing measures that have well-established reliability and validity such as the Beck Depression Inventory-II (BDI-II) (Beck, Steer, & Brown, 1996) and the Center for Epidemiological Studies Depression Scale (CES-D) (Radloff, 1977). To evaluate construct validity, the following need to be done:

1. Specify the theoretical relationship between the concepts measured by the instrument of interest and the comparison instruments.

2. Examine the relationship between these instruments' results. Often this is done by looking at the correlation between the two instruments, although there are other statistics that can also be used.

3. Interpret the results of the comparison (Carmines & Zeller, 1979).

One of the reasons to carefully evaluate the theoretical relationship between the instruments being compared is that different instruments frequently measure different aspects of a phenomenon. The differences between state and trait anxiety is an example of this.

Correlations

Before proceeding to a more complex form of construct validity testing, let's take a minute to consider what a correlation coefficient means. Represented by a lowercase r, a simple correlation can range in value from -1.00 to 0 to $+1.00$ (-1.00 and $+1.00$ actually do not occur too often) (Schlotzhauer & Littell, 1997). Correlations of the same amount but different valences such as $-.40$ and $+.40$ are the same strength but indicate different directions for the relationships under study. If the correlation between a measure of anxiety and a test of attention is $-.40$ for example, it means that as anxiety goes up, attention goes down and vice versa. If the correlation were .40 instead (the plus sign is often omitted), it would mean that attention increases when anxiety increases.

It is also helpful to consider the strength of the relationship: does attention decrease a great deal if anxiety goes up? If the correlation is $-.40$, it means that anxiety explains 16% of the variability in the attention measure. This figure is obtained by squaring the correlation r and producing an R^2, a statistic that is relatively easy to interpret:

$$r \times r = R^2$$
$$-.40 \times -.40 = .16$$

The R^2 tells you the percent of the variability in the first variable (attention) that is associated with the second variable (anxiety) (Girden, 2001).

Multitrait-multimethod (MTMM) is an extension of the simple test of construct validity already discussed. It sounds complex at first, but it is just a set of comparisons of measures and data collection methods that are either *like* the one being tested (mono) or *unlike* (hetero) the one being tested (Nunnally & Bernstein, 1994; Ferketich, Figueredo, & Knapp, 1991). The correlations generated by these comparisons are put into a matrix, which is a table that displays the results in an orderly fashion.

To illustrate MTMM, we will use a set of fictional data. Imagine you want to evaluate a new observational measure of fatigue. Using MTMM, you plan to compare it to a self-report measure of fatigue (monotrait, heteromethod) and two measures of depression, one observational (heterotrait, monomethod) and one that is self-report (heterotrait, heteromethod). Good comparison measures are not always easy to find. The different methods need to be really different, not just a long questionnaire versus a short questionnaire but two substantially different ways to collect data. On the other hand, the concepts to be measured need to be relatively closely associated, so close that one is sometimes confused for the other. Fatigue and pain, for example, are close, but fatigue and depression would be closer and are a better choice for the comparison. It is important to specify the theoretical relationship between the two concepts and to predict the strength of the relationships that should be found if all the measures are valid:

- The observational and self-report measures of fatigue should have the strongest relationship (correlation).

- The observational measures of fatigue and depression should have a weak relationship.

- The observational measure of fatigue should have an even weaker relationship with self-report of depression.

The results of the comparisons are illustrated in Table 10-4. As you can see, the correlation between the new observational fatigue scale and the self-report fatigue scale is quite high, and the correlations with the depression scales are much lower. Similarly, the two depression scales have strong correlations. The relationships between the depression and fatigue scales are much lower, which supports the idea that they are not measuring the same concept ($.30 \times .30 = .09$ or 9% of the variability in the observational fatigue scale is accounted for by the results of the self-report depression scale). You can see also that results on the two fatigue scales *converge*, while comparisons of fatigue and depression measures show considerable *divergence*. You can use the terms *convergent* and *divergent validity* to describe this difference (Nunnally & Bernstein, 1994).

A serious disadvantage to MTMM, even in its simplest form, is the number of tests that have to be administered, which increases respondent burden. Further, the correlation comparisons are often far from perfect, suggesting not only some potential overlap between the fatigue and depression measures but also some other problems including accuracy, reliability, and other sources of measurement error.

TABLE 10-4   Simple Multitrait Multimethod (MTMM) Table (Fictional Data)

	Method 1 Observation		Method 2 Self-Rating	
	Fatigue	Depression	Fatigue	Depression
Observation				
Fatigue (new)	1.00			
Depression	.40	1.00		
Self-report				
Fatigue	.82	.28	1.00	
Depression	.30	.81	.36	1.00

Source: Based on Nunnally and Bernstein, 1994, and Ferketich, Figueredo, and Knapp, 1991.

CRITERION VALIDITY

Criterion validity is concerned with the ability of the measure to predict an outcome of interest that occurs either at the same time (concurrent) or in the future (predictive), even in the past in some cases. What might be predicted? Success in preschool, occurrence of pressure ulcers, wound healing, falls, SIDS, suicide, and so forth could be predicted.

For example, Metheny, Smith, and Stewart (2000) developed a new scale to evaluate the colors on test strips used to determine whether nasogastric and nasointestinal tubes are correctly placed. The criterion measure against which they tested their color scale results was a quantitative assay for bilirubin done by a research laboratory. Since it was done on samples taken at the same time, this was a measure of concurrent validity.

The research laboratory test results are also an example of what is commonly called a "gold standard" measure, a measure in which there is a high degree of confidence based on well-established reliability and validity.

Another example of criterion validity was reported by Bergstrom and Braden in 2002. They used the National Pressure Ulcer Advisory Panel (NPUAP) criteria to identify the occurrence of pressure ulcers on 843 subjects who had not had a pressure ulcer upon admission. These results were used to examine the predictive validity of the Braden Scale for Predicting Pressure Sores (often called the Braden Scale).

You can see that the choice of the criterion to be used for comparison should be based upon in-depth knowledge of the specialty area as well as of the quality of the measure chosen.

SENSITIVITY AND SPECIFICITY

Sensitivity and specificity are two aspects of a single question: how accurately does this measure characterize or diagnose individual people? Sensitivity and specificity calculations help us answer important clinical questions such as: Can lung cancer be found on physical examination or an x-ray? Does an MRI diagnose Alzheimer's disease? Is the Beck Depression Inventory accurate enough to diagnose depression?

Sensitivity is the proportion of positive results obtained on the measure of interest in people who are known to have the disease or problem that the measure is designed to identify. It refers to the true-positives. *Specificity* is the proportion of negative results obtained on the measure of interest in people who are known not to have the disease or problem. It refers to the true negatives (Agresti, 2002; Stokes, Davis, & Koch, 2000).

Sensitivity and specificity are easy to calculate. Let's say that a new screening test for colon cancer has been found to identify 40 out of 50 people who were found on biopsy to have colon cancer (note that biopsy is the gold standard here). Sensitivity is calculated by dividing 40 by 50:

$$40 \div 50 = .80$$

Specificity is calculated the same way. Let's say this same new test was found to produce negative results for 90 out of 100 people who did not have colon cancer. Specificity is calculated as:

$$90 \div 100 = .90$$

The specificity in this case is better than the sensitivity.

Receiver operator characteristic (ROC) curves can also be constructed by plotting the true positives against the false positives at different cutoff points on the test of interest (Fletcher, Fletcher, & Wagner, 1996). For example, Beck and Gable (2001) compared the sensitivity and specificity of their Postpartum Depression Screening Scale (PDSS), the Edinburg Postnatal Depression Scale (EPDS), and the more general Beck Depression Inventory-II to a structured clinical interview based on the DSM-IV. They found a 94% sensitivity and 98% specificity on their PDSS. The PDSS identified 94% of the women diagnosed with major postpartum depression, the EPDS identified 78%, and the BDI-II identified only 56%. Clearly, these results suggest that a specific measure for postpartum depression is superior to the more general measure for this purpose. The researchers also plotted ROC curves for these depression measures (Figure 10-2) which clearly shows a larger area under the curve of the PDSS than the others.

When you consider the importance of correctly identifying people with such serious problems as colon cancer or postpartum depression, you can see why calculation of sensitivity and specificity of a screening measure and plotting the ROC curves are essential to the evaluation of the measure. Selection of the appropriate criterion measure (the gold standard) is equally important.

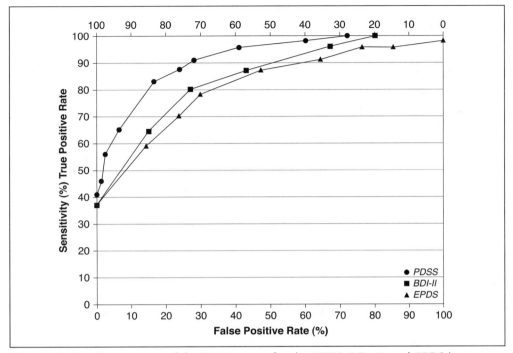

Figure 10-2 Comparison of the ROC curves for the PDSS, BDI-II, and EPDS in screening for major and minor postpartum depression.

Source: Beck and Gable, 2001. Used with permission.

CONCLUSION

We have come a long way in this chapter from the almost-useless face validity to examining the sensitivity and specificity of screening and diagnostic measures. When you select a measure to use in your research study, be sure that its validity has been thoroughly evaluated.

REFERENCES

Agresti, A. (2002). *Categorical data analysis*. Hoboken, NJ: John Wiley & Sons.

Beck, A. T., Steer, R. A., & Brown, G. R. (1996). *BDI-II manual*. San Antonio: The Psychological Corporation.

Beck, C. T., & Gable, R. K. (2001). Comparative analysis of the Performance of the Postpartum Depression Screening Scale with two other depression instruments. *Nursing Research, 50*(4), 242.
   ✧ This article is an excellent example of a thorough evaluation of a new instrument.

Bergstrom, N., & Braden, B. J. (2002). Predictive validity of the Braden Scale among black and white subjects. *Nursing Research, 51*(6), 398–403.

Carmines, E. G., & Zeller, R. A. (1979). *Reliability and validity assessment*. Newbury Park, CA: Sage Publications.
   ✧ Probably the best introduction to the basics of reliability and validity. Relatively easy to read as well.

Cohen, J. (1960). A coefficient of agreement for nominal scales. *Educational and Psychological Measurement, 20*(1), 37–46.

DeVon, H. A., Black, M. E., Moyle-Wright, P., Ernst, D. M., Hayden, S. J., Lazzara, D. J., et al. (2001). A psychometric toolbox for testing validity and reliability. *Journal of Nursing Scholarship, 39*(2), 155–164.
    ◆ An excellent, readable review of validity and reliability in nursing research. Includes some quotes from the editors of the leading research journals in nursing.

Fazio, R. H., & Olson, M. A. (2003). Implicit measures in social cognition research: Their meaning and use. *Annual Review of Psychology, 54*, 297–327.

Ferketich, S. L., Figueredo, A. J., & Knapp, T. R. (1991). The multitrait-multimethod approach to construct validity. *Research in Nursing and Health, 14*, 315–320.

Fletcher, R. H., Fletcher, S. W., & Wagner, E. H. (1996). *Clinical epidemiology: The essentials.* Baltimore, MD: Williams & Wilkins.

Girden, E. R. (2001). *Evaluating research articles from start to finish.* Thousand Oaks, CA: Sage Publications.

Gorsuch, R. L. (1983). *Factor analysis.* Hillsdale, NJ: Laurence Erlbaum.

Hatcher, L. (1994). *A step-by-step approach to using SAS for factor analysis and structural equation modeling.* Cary, NC: SAS Institute.
    ◆ Much practical information on conducting a factor analysis, even some guidance on reporting the results (see p. 107).

Kim, J-B., & Mueller, C. W. (1978). *Factor analysis: Statistical methods and practical issues.* Newbury Park, CA: Sage Publications.
    ◆ More advanced, more detailed than Carmines and Zeller, but still quite readable.

Metheny, N. A., Smith, L., & Stewart, B. (2000). Development of a reliable and valid bedside test for bilirubin and its utility for improving prediction of feeding tube location (2000). *Nursing Research, 49*(6), 302–309.

Nunnally, J. C., & Bernstein, I. (1994). *Psychometric theory.* New York: McGraw-Hill.
    ◆ Difficult to read but this is an authoritative source of information on reliability and validity.

Perdue, C. W., & Gurtman, M. B. (1990). Evidence for automaticity of ageism. *Journal of Experimental Social Psychology, 26*, 199–216.

Project Implicit. Retrieved March 14, 2010, from https://implicit.harvard.edu/implicit
    ◆ If you would like to read more about this project and/or try out one of their questionnaires, you might like to go to this website. Remember though, that you are agreeing to be a research subject if you take the test.

Radloff, L. S. (1977). The CES-D Scale: A self-report depression scale for research in the general population. *Applied Psychological Measurement, 1*(3), 385–401.

Schlotzhauer, S. D., & Littell, R. C. (1997). *SAS system for elementary statistics.* Cary, NC: SAS Institute.

Stokes, M. E., Davis, C. S., & Koch, G. G. (2002). *Categorical data analysis using the SAS system.* Cary, NC: SAS Institute.

Tappen, R. M., & Williams, C. (1998). Attribution of emotion in advanced Alzheimer's disease: Family and caregiver perspectives. *American Journal of Alzheimer's Disease and Other Dementias, 13*(5), 257–264.

Tappen, R. M., & Williams, C. L. (2009). Development and testing of a measure of acculturation that is useful across cultural groups. Paper presented: Southern Nursing Research Society Annual Conference, Baltimore, MD.

Waltz, C. F., Strickland, O. L., & Lenz, E. R. (2005). *Measurement in nursing and health research.* New York: Springer Publishing.
    ◆ An excellent textbook for any nurse researcher, a must-have if you want to do instrument development.

Wynd, C. A., Schmidt, B., & Schaefer, M. A. (2003). Two quantitative approaches for estimating content validity. *Western Journal of Nursing Research, 25*(5), 508–518.

Youngblut, J. M. (1993). Comparison of factor analysis options using the Home/Employment Orientation Scale. *Nursing Research, 42*(2), 122–124.

Trustworthiness of Qualitative Research

Quality is as essential to qualitative research as it is to quantitative research. The term often used to describe the desirable characteristics of both the process and the product of qualitative research is *rigor,* which refers to adherence to high standards in the conduct of research (Davies & Dodd, 2002). Morse (2003) defines rigor as the (1) adequacy and appropriateness of the method to address the questions proposed, and (2) solidity of the research design (p. 837). Morse and colleagues have argued that without rigor, the research is worthless (2002).

Some scholars use the terms *reliability* and *validity* to define rigor in qualitative research, but others protest that the underlying philosophy is different and the criteria are different, so different terms should be used. Best known of these alternative terms are those Lincoln and Guba (1985) proposed to describe *trustworthiness* in qualitative research:

Credibility: Equivalent to internal validity

Transferability: Equivalent to external validity

Dependability: Equivalent to reliability

Confirmability: Equivalent to objectivity (p. 300)

They note that trustworthiness is a particular concern to the consumer of research, the person who reads the research report and is considering whether or not to use the results. The rigor of a study or its trustworthiness is what persuades others that the findings reported are worth paying attention to, that they are credible, dependable, confirmable, and transferable to other situations.

Meyrick (2006) tried to pull together these disparate views, dividing them into two principles, *transparent* and *systematic.* Transparency refers to clear disclosure of the research processes employed. Systematicity refers to use of a consistent approach to data collection and analysis:

- *Transparency* includes criteria such as a clear description of the sampling procedures used or a clear explanation of the reason for a change in the way questions are asked. An audit trail also contributes to transparency.

- *Systematicity* includes use of an articulated analytic framework, analysis of all cases, and a logical connection between the purpose of the study and the methods employed (Meyrick, 2006).

These two terms, *transparency* and *systematicity,* are a helpful way to think about quality in qualitative research when planning a study and reporting your findings. Most of the criteria discussed in the following section fall under one or the other of these two principles.

EXAMPLE: COMING OF AGE IN SAMOA

A classic example of the challenges in establishing the trustworthiness of qualitative research results is the controversy over anthropologist Margaret Mead's characterization of adolescence in the Pacific islands of Samoa (Lincoln & Guba, 1985). During her 9 months in Samoa, Mead concentrated her attention on 50 adolescent girls in three small villages. In her writings, she addressed an important theoretical question: are the conflicts and stresses of adolescence due to the physical changes of adolescence (i.e., biology) or to the society in which the adolescents are raised (i.e., culture)? She found that, while the girls experienced the same physical changes as girls in the United States, adolescence seemed to be emotionally "painless" in Samoa. She also noted a lack of neuroses among Samoans. She attributed these characteristics to the slower pace and more casual attitude toward life in Samoa as compared to Western countries such as the United States, describing Samoa as a "complacent, peaceful society," (Mead, 1949, p. 147).

Her book was a sensation. It was praised as an outstanding example of ethnographic research and an affirmation of the greater effect of nurture (culture) as opposed to nature (biology). More popularly, her book was considered a portrayal of Polynesian free love, an example for the uptight Western society of the time.

Not so, countered Derek Freeman (1983) who conducted additional ethnographic research in Samoa 15 years after Mead. He lived there for 2 years with a Samoan family and was welcomed into their chiefly [sic] assemblies. Freeman reports that Samoan leaders asked him to help them correct Mead's characterization of life in Samoa. They made court and police records of juvenile delinquency available to him, which painted a very different picture of life in Samoa. Freeman found as much adolescent delinquency in Samoa as in Western societies, concluding that adolescence in Samoa was not at all untroubled. This was the darker side of life in Samoa that Mead had missed.

What happened? Whose description of life in Samoa was correct? Freeman points out that Mead lived with an American family and had not mastered the nuances of the Samoan language during her time there. Other ethnographers' work in Samoa generally supported the idea of a more complex Samoan society with its share of conflicts and troubles. Even Mead reported conflicts she had observed there but these were lost in the excitement and romance of the idea of free love on a peaceful tropical island. Freeman attributes the difference to Mead's "deeply [held] belief in the doctrine of extreme cultural determinism" (p. 292), in other words, to her conviction that culture trumps biology. Others have pointed out that Freeman's sources of information were primarily adult males while Mead's sources were young girls. Further, Samoans are likely to be insulted by any suggestion that their adolescents are sexually active (Kirk & Miller, 1986). Would adult American males and adolescent American girls describe their life in the United States the same way? Could it be that Mead and Freeman saw different aspects of the same society? Or did Mead not stay long enough to develop a deeper understanding of Samoan society and the way young girls tell their stories (Lincoln & Guba, 1985)? If Mead had been aware of the other ethnographies of Samoa, would she have come to a different conclusion?

These are difficult questions to answer. In this chapter, we consider the many strategies that qualitative researchers have developed to incorporate rigor into their work and to establish the trustworthiness, authenticity, and credibility of their findings. They represent the qualitative equivalent of validity and reliability in quantitative research and may fairly be said to have been designed to prevent the type of doubts that Freeman raised about Mead's research.

We consider first the strategies suggested by Lincoln and Guba (1985) to establish trustworthiness, then we cover some additional strategies suggested by others, and, lastly we discuss some of the issues and points of disagreement regarding quality in qualitative research. Not every strategy will be appropriate for every qualitative study. As with reliability and validity in quantitative research, the informed judgment of the researcher is needed to select the appropriate strategies and build them into the research plan.

CREDIBILITY

Equivalent to internal validity, credibility may be established through prolonged engagement and persistent observation, member checking, peer debriefing, negative case analysis, and triangulation.

Prolonged Engagement and Persistent Observation

Thick, rich description is the goal of most qualitative data collection, not thin, limited information that lacks depth or detail, which limits understanding and may lead to premature closure or superficial conclusions on the subject matter of interest (Creswell & Miller, 2000; Schensul, Schensul & LeCompte, 1999). Prolonged engagement and persistent observation allow the time and opportunity to test possible explanations and develop emerging explanations (Long & Johnson, 2000).

There are no standards for the amount of time that should be spent with an individual participant or how long a researcher should be engaged in a setting or society. However, the amount is expected to be extensive. Derek Freeman thought Margaret Mead had not spent enough time in Samoa, nor did he believe she had been as fully engaged in their society as was desirable, although she was there 9 months. It is safe to say that a 2-week stay in the Brazilian rain forest or on a remote island would not qualify you as an expert on the health behaviors of the indigenous people there. Perhaps several months or a year would if you'd studied the existing literature on them and learned their language ahead of time (not small tasks). You would likely need to return to further clarify and recheck preliminary conclusions as well as to ensure that some of what you observed was not a temporary state of affairs.

To bring this closer to home, how long would you need to be engaged with an emergency department staff before you could describe this subculture within health care? Six or eight weeks coupled with in-depth interviewing and perhaps some document review might be sufficient in some cases because you already know the language and the culture of health care, but this depends on what you are studying.

Achieving what seems to be saturation may not be a sufficient criterion for judging prolonged engagement: Simple repetition of previously heard stories or themes or the lack of new coding categories may only mean that the interviews have remained at a superficial level and need to go beyond it. Some qualitative researchers substitute larger numbers of people for increased depth of interviewing with the typically smaller number of participants in a qualitative study. This may be acceptable in some types of surveys, such as a public opinion survey on a health-related behavior such as smoking, but not in a more in-depth study of a topic such as the long-term effects of a child with Down syndrome on the parents and unimpaired siblings. In most instances, when conducting a qualitative study, "'being there' matters" (Freeman, deMarrais, Preissle, Roulston, & St. Pierre, 2007, p. 28).

Conrad, Garrett, Cooksley, Dunne and MacDonald (2006) from Australia used a semi-structured guide to interview 70 adults with hepatitis C in 12 group meetings and 20 individual interviews that were 49 to 80 minutes in length. Data from early interviews were used to inform later interviews. Transcriptions were checked for accuracy. Although the researchers indicated that they were using the grounded theory approach, they noted that their use of matrices as described by Miles and Huberman (1994) was a departure from grounded theory. It also appears that the results were not raised to the theoretical level of abstraction that is the goal of grounded theory. There was little discussion of new or refined theory emerging from the study. They did find that previous undocumented "attacks" were reported and that interviewees feared the stigma attached to their diagnosis and described how some of them dealt with it. The researchers noted several ways in which they addressed rigor and trustworthiness:

- The individual interviews were more in-depth than the group discussion, providing rich description.
- The larger than usual sample made up for the briefer group interviews.
- An audit trail was maintained.
- Verification of findings with participants and a community advisory group was done.

Although it is arguable that the interviews did not constitute persistent observation or produce thick, rich description, the other strategies seemed to be appropriately applied.

Member Checking

Member checking is an interesting approach to establishing the credibility of the results of a qualitative study. The "members" are the participants in the study as well as members of the culture or subculture under study or representatives of the community in which you have been working. There are several ways in which member checking can be done. You can share raw field notes or transcriptions of interviews with members of the community, but reviewing them is an onerous task and may not reveal much for the effort. The coding scheme, if one has been devised, is more limited in volume and might be shared with participants or their representatives. Most common is to share preliminary findings with participants, asking them for feedback and incorporating their feedback into the conclusions drawn. Asking a third party (someone otherwise not involved in the study) to conduct the member checking may be appropriate in some cases, but it prevents the give and take between researcher and participants that is part of the strength of qualitative approaches (Long & Johnson, 2000).

There is some controversy about the value of member checking. Of necessity, reports of findings are summarized, and individual participants may not recognize their contributions to the study (Cohen & Crabtree, 2008; Morse et al., 2002). Further, a goal of much qualitative work is to identify themes and to raise them to higher levels of abstraction. In some cases, the goal will be to develop theoretical propositions and statements. For some participants, information at the higher levels of abstraction is difficult to appreciate or to relate to their own everyday life experience (Morse et al., 2002). However, a researcher who has completed a prolonged engagement with the participants and engaged in persistent observation of them should be able to phrase his or her findings in such a way that the participants may understand it and comment on whether or not these findings resonate with them. It is important to avoid a condescending "they'd never understand," attitude. If you cannot put your conclusions into terms that the participants would understand, perhaps you also do not yet understand them well enough to write about them.

Peer Debriefing

Peer debriefing is a second strategy for seeking evaluative feedback on the preliminary conclusions of your study. In the first instance, member checking, the feedback was sought from the participants in the study who would contribute feedback based upon their personal experience. In peer debriefing, you are seeking feedback from individuals with expertise on (1) the subject of the study and (2) the methodology of the study. It is important to find someone who has some expertise as well as time and motivation to provide a thoughtful critique. While an enthusiastic but uncritical "Atta boy!" or "Atta girl!" is heartening, it really is not helpful.

Seale (2004) relates an example of a published study that might have benefited from this kind of thoughtful critique prior to publication. The study by Lupton (2004) concerns the treatment of the subject of breast cancer in the Australian press. Seale comments that, while it is a highly relevant topic, the report is lacking in credibility. In particular, there are obvious contradictions in Lupton's arguments. For example, women suffering from breast cancer are said by Lupton to be rendered invisible, yet women's magazines frequently publish personal stories. An alliance between organized medicine and the media is suggested by Lupton, but Seale notes there is considerable distrust between them and that a history of the BBC (British Broadcasting Corporation) and health professionals demonstrates frequent clashes between them. Also noted is the failure to report the coding scheme used in the analysis or to report negative cases and that saturation was not adequate. Seale concludes that Lupton's preexisting political values led to a biased presentation of the research.

We can surmise that if Lupton had addressed the issues of trustworthiness of qualitative research during the conduct of the study and in the reporting of the findings, such a critical evaluation would not have been received. In particular, a thoughtful, analytical peer debriefing and clearer statement of Lupton's use of feminist theory might have helped Lupton prepare a more credible research report on an interesting topic.

In contrast Richter, Parker, and Chaw-Kent (2001) addressed several aspects of trustworthiness when they conducted a qualitative study of the needs of 13 high-risk pregnancy patients in Edmonton, Alberta, who had been hospitalized for at least 1 week. They defined high risk as a pregnancy in which the life or health of the mother or infant is jeopardized by a disorder that is coincidental with or unique to the pregnancy (p. 314). Ten of the women were interviewed individually, three in a focus group. Interviews lasted up to 90 minutes.

After the interviews were transcribed, two of the investigators independently conducted thematic analyses. Emerging themes were shared with subsequent participants. A detailed description of how the themes were checked and rechecked is provided. Considerable detail is provided about the women and the reasons for their hospitalization. The researchers addressed Lincoln and Guba's (1985) criteria for credibility, dependability, confirmability, and transferability mentioning prolonged engagement, description of the context of the study, independent coding, and comparison of the results. Among the concerns that emerged were boredom due to the long hospitalization, desire for more privacy, and more flexibility regarding visiting hours, especially for those from rural areas whose families had to travel a long way.

Negative Case Analysis

Part of the richness of qualitative research lies in the complexity of the data gathered. It would be highly unusual for every participant to express the same viewpoint on the subject under study. In fact, if that does happen, it would be important to find out if you are only hearing what they think you want to hear or if they are holding back because the level of trust is still low.

The reporting of negative cases does not weaken your findings. Patton (2002) notes that including them changes the tone of the report, making it more credible because you, the researcher, have made it clear that alternative explanations were considered. In fact, lack of disagreement, data that fit the explanation perfectly and explanations with few or no exceptions are more likely to be received with some skepticism because they are too perfect (Patton, 2002).

Negative cases are those that are counter to what seems to be the prevailing themes or relationships. They need to be reported and carefully analyzed. Several scholars have emphasized that the goal is not to refute these negative cases but to consider their meaning and incorporate them within your conclusions. Here is a simplified example:

> Knowledge of the seriousness of a disease and perceived personal vulnerability are generally thought to motivate people to be screened for such problems as glaucoma, colorectal disease, or Alzheimer's disease. Yet caregivers of individuals with Alzheimer's disease who evidence serious behavioral problems often decline to be

screened for Alzheimer's disease. Is this a contradiction to the proposition that perceived seriousness of the disease and personal vulnerability motivate people to be screened? It might suggest that these caregivers are too frightened by the prospect of developing Alzheimer's disease and, therefore, do not want to know if they are likely to do so. Or, perhaps, it suggests that they are experiencing problems related to Alzheimer's disease for which there are few easy solutions and that this element of hopelessness counters the other potential motivators. You can see that an in-depth analysis of these negative cases could lead to a further refinement of theories regarding health-related behavior.

Triangulation

Triangulation is the use of two or more points of reference to determine the location of a third, as yet unknown, point. A GPS uses a type of triangulation to analyze information from satellites to tell someone his or her location.

In research, triangulation allows cross-checking of both data (including testing for consistencies and inconsistencies) and preliminary conclusions. It also provides for multiple perspectives, which are particularly valuable when addressing a complex subject that no one method or source can provide enough explanation for (Patton, 1999). There are several different ways to triangulate (Patton, 2002):

- Methodological triangulation uses of multiple methods to collect data, such as observation and interviews.

- Source triangulation involves obtaining different viewpoints, such as interviewing patients, families, and caregiving staff.

- Analyst (investigator) triangulation is an independent analysis by more than one investigator, such as having two researchers develop coding schemes independently and then compare the codes produced. Use of multiple investigators as part of a team collecting data is another type of investigator triangulation.

- In theory triangulation, results can be related to multiple theories, but Lincoln and Guba (1985) object to this, calling it "epistemologically unsound and empirically empty" (p. 307), saying a fact is no more sound or believable just because it agrees with more than one theory.

Morse, Bottorff, and Hutchinson (1995) conducted a phenomenological study of patients' experience of illness and injury, focusing on their expressions of discomfort. Although they do not use the term, they triangulated the methods and sources of information used. They obtained data from both interviews and biographical accounts of illness experiences found in the literature. The interviews were conducted with 36 patients and 12 relatives of patients. Experiences drawn from the literature are woven into the narrative on patients' experiences as are the experiences and feelings of the family members interviewed. The experiences of the families and experiences drawn from the literature enrich the patient narrative in an almost seamless fashion that is evidence of the skill of the investigators in presenting their findings.

TRANSFERABILITY

Equivalent to external validity or generalizability in quantitative research, transferability refers to the applicability of the findings to other situations and other people. In quantitative research, samples are often randomly selected and statistics are applied to estimate the extent to which findings can be generalized. This is not done in qualitative research. Instead, the qualitative researcher uses purposeful sampling. A detailed description of the sample and the context in which the study was conducted enables others to decide the extent the findings may be transferred to other individuals and other situations.

Qualitative research is not designed for the purpose of making generalizations as quantitative research aims to do. Instead qualitative research is meant to describe a phenomenon within a certain context. However, qualitative researchers may make connections between their findings and those from other studies, making careful comparisons across settings and people (Freeman et al., 2007).

DEPENDABILITY

Dependability is equivalent to reliability in quantitative research. Here Lincoln and Guba (1985) propose the use of an inquiry audit, drawing upon the work of Halpern (1983). To do this, an *audit trail* must be created while the research study is being done. This is a carefully compiled record of the conduct of the study itself, the investigator's thoughts and the decisions that were made along the way. Halpern proposed six types of materials to be compiled:

- Raw data: All field notes, video or tape recordings, any documents or other items collected

- Data analysis products: Any summaries or ideas that occur to the researcher during the study

- Data synthesis products: Coding schemes created, coded data, themes found, and interpretations made

- Process notes: Descriptions of how data were obtained and how analyses were done

- Reflections of the investigator: The personal notes and reflexive journal kept by the researcher or researchers

- Surveys or questionnaire guides: Any forms used to collect information on participants' ages, gender, occupation, and so forth; semistructured interview guides; and similar materials

There is also a formal process by which a knowledgeable outside individual is brought in to review all of these materials and attest to them. Even if this is not done, creation of the audit trail is an excellent idea and probably should be done for every qualitative study. It helps the researcher provide the *transparency* sometimes missing in reports of qualitative studies, and it allows the reader to judge the rigor of the study and trustworthiness of the findings. Further, it imposes a discipline on the researcher that is very valuable at the end of the study: "helping to systematize, relate, cross-reference, and attach priorities to data that might otherwise have remained undifferentiated until the writing task was undertaken" (Lincoln & Guba, 1985, p. 319). Reporting a summary of the activities in which the researcher participated during a study makes this process more visible or *transparent* and lays it open for examination by one's peers and potential consumers of the research (Davies & Dodd, 2002).

CONFIRMABILITY

Confirmability is equivalent to the effort to maintain objectivity in quantitative research. As with the other criteria, objectivity is never fully achieved even in quantitative research, and qualitative research is sometimes directed toward including the researcher's perspective and reactions rather than neutralizing them. In fact, confirmability is not considered relevant to studies within the phenomenological, feminist, and some other qualitative paradigms (Morse et al., 2002). Instead, the qualitative researchers report the work done, the analyses undertaken, and the conclusions that are reached.

The *reflexive journal,* mentioned in relation to the audit trail, is the final strategy in the Lincoln and Guba work on establishing trustworthiness. The journal should include:

- Schedules, daily activities
- Log of data collections done and methods used
- Personal reflections

While part of the audit trail, the reflexive journal is quite different from the other strategies and quite unlike anything reported in a quantitative study. Before beginning a qualitative study, the investigator records his or her expectations and preliminary ideas about what is going to be studied and what he or she expects to find. This is extremely important as the investigator will want to refer back to these preconceived ideas during and after the study has been completed, asking several questions:

- To what extent have I changed my conceptualization on the basis of the research done?
- What ideas have been modified, revised, recast, or refined based on the new findings?
- Have any of my ideas remained unchanged? If so, is this because they have been confirmed or because I have not yet been able to let go of them despite disconfirming evidence?

As the study begins and progresses through its various stages, the investigator continues to record personal experiences (intimidated by the gang leaders?), feelings (felt sadness seeing the aftermath of a disaster?), and preliminary hypotheses about the subject of interest. Flashes of insight are recorded so they are not lost and so their origins are remembered (for example, a mother comments that friends treat her differently since they learned that her child has an HIV infection, leading to ideas about the extension of stigma to other family members). The journal also helps the investigator keep biases and prejudgments at bay, opening the possibility of seeing things a different way.

In some ways, the audit trail and reflexive journal of the qualitative study are similar to the laboratory notebook kept by bench scientists. In their notebooks, they record experiments and findings as they are done. This is often used to track progress as well as occasionally to document who discovered something new and when it was first noted.

Although the reflexive journal is not a formal part of most quantitative research designs, quantitative researchers could also benefit from recording ideas, preliminary hypotheses, and especially meaningful observations during the study. It is often the flash of insight or a particularly meaningful observation that leads to new avenues of research and exciting discoveries.

ADDITIONAL CRITERIA FOR TRUSTWORTHINESS

A number of refinements to the original Lincoln and Guba framework for trustworthiness have been developed. You'll notice that many are criteria for *judging* trustworthiness rather than strategies for *establishing* trustworthiness. While they need to be considered during the design and conduct of the study, many are meant to be applied when the study is done. Some are comprehensive frameworks and detailed checklists for evaluating qualitative studies. The latter go beyond the purpose of establishing the rigor of a study but can be valuable guides for the qualitative researcher if not applied too rigidly (Borreani, Miccinesi, Bunelli, & Lina, 2004). We will consider just a few that enhance the Lincoln and Guba framework already presented.

A Broader Perspective

Patton (1999) expanded upon the original criteria by adding two additional aspects for consideration in evaluating a qualitative study. His criteria are:

- Use of rigorous methods for collecting high-quality data that is then carefully analyzed
- The credibility of the researcher (Morse et al. [2002] have also said that the research is only as good as the researcher is.)
- Philosophical belief in the value of qualitative inquiry

The first criterion is most like the ones already discussed. The second, credibility of the researcher may include some or all of the following:

- The training received by the researcher
- Extent of the experience of the researcher

- Track record (prior publications and studies conducted)
- Creativity, flexibility, sensitivity, and skill (Morse et al., 2002)
- Presentation of self: The manner in which the researcher makes clear his or her relationship to the topic under investigation (for example, if the researcher also has asthma or has been the victim of a natural disaster) and the researcher's philosophical and/or political position (for example, a feminist perspective or religious conservatism).

Davies and Dodd (2002) provide an example of the flexibility required of a qualitative researcher. While conducting a qualitative study, they initially tried to limit their respondents' stories to their present pregnancy. They found, however, that that is not the way most women talk about their experience and that the women did not see their present pregnancy as an isolated event. So the researchers had to let the women tell their story in relation to other pregnancies and to the birthing process. The result, not too surprisingly, was more interesting than it would have been otherwise.

These criteria also emphasize the importance of learning how to focus, how to observe, and how to interview effectively. Preparation for field work may include learning a new language, preparing for the physical requirements of the setting, and articulating one's initial expectations. The reflexive journal should address the researcher's reaction to the setting and participants. It may be mild (patients who do not adhere to their prescribed medication regimen) to deep and disturbing (women who have killed their children). Patton (1999) offers a few additional points:

- Being value free is actually impossible.
- Excessive closeness to the subject leads others to suspect subjectivity.
- Being absorbed into the group ("going native") endangers the research.
- The researcher strives for a caring, responsive approach to participants, remaining neutral and impartial to the extent possible but recognizing again that being value free is not possible.

Finally, belief in the value of qualitative research (the third criterion) seems to be obvious. However, adaption of a qualitative approach without understanding of all it encompasses is likely to lead to superficial or even misleading results.

Transactional vs. Transformational Framework

The debate on what constitutes quality in qualitative research is not limited to nursing or even to health care. Neither is it limited to the United States, although it is especially lively here. From education, Cho and Trent (2006) suggest a different framework, that of transactional versus transformational validity:

- Transactional validity employs interaction between researcher and participants through such techniques as member checking and triangulation of services.

- Transformational validity focuses upon the research process as a means to effect social change. One way to do this is through collaborative action by the researcher and participants. The researcher would be expected to communicate how he or she has been challenged and transformed through the collaborative interaction with participants (Cho & Trent, 2006).

Transformational validity is a much more radical notion of what constitutes quality in qualitative research. It is, however, particularly relevant to action research and to qualitative research emerging from a political agenda.

Evaluating Credibility

Although focused on grounded theory, the criteria suggested by Charmaz (2005) also offer an expanded view of what constitutes trustworthiness. These criteria are divided into the categories of credibility, originality, resonance, and usefulness. The credibility criteria are of most interest to us in this chapter:

- Are the data sufficient in terms of the range, number, and depth of the observations or interviews?
- Were systematic comparisons made between the observations and categories created?
- Are the links between the data and the conclusions strong or logical?
- Is there enough evidence for the reader to form an independent conclusion? (p. 528)

These criteria, although phrased differently, echo the earlier ones in many ways.

Additional Criteria

The following are a few more selected criteria that build upon what has already been said (Morse et al., 2002; Patton, 2002).

- Methodological coherence: Do the data collection techniques and sampling match the question to be addressed?
- Checking and rechecking: Is there evidence that the researcher has questioned and compared the data and the developing conclusions multiple times and in multiple ways?
- Design checks: Does the researcher specify the time the data were collected? Does the researcher specify the place, people, and setting(s) the data were collected from?
- Researcher's stance: Has the investigator reported his or her own personal beliefs, professional values, and other information that might affect the conduct and analysis of the study?

Issues Related to Evaluating Trustworthiness

A number of the issues and controversies surrounding the evaluation of rigor and trustworthiness in qualitative research have already been mentioned. These and other issues that are frequently raised include the following:

- Use of quantitative research terminology versus a separate language for qualitative criteria—some prefer the terms *validity*, *reliability*, or *rigor*. Others reject these terms and believe that such terms as those proposed by Lincoln and Guba (1985) are more appropriate.
- Should judgment of the quality (authenticity, credibility, and so forth) be the responsibility of the researcher and peer reviewers or the readers of the study report? In other words, who is responsible for evaluating rigor?
- Is qualitative research just a different set of methods, or is it an entirely different paradigm? Is it a craft rather than a philosophy (Seale, 2004)?
- Can a uniform set of criteria be applied to the incredible variety of qualitative approaches?

Not all qualitative researchers are convinced that attention should be paid to establishing the rigor or trustworthiness of study results. Qualitative researchers' opinions on this question can be classified into one of three positions (Cohen & Crabtree, 2008; Rolfe, 2006).

1. Qualitative studies should be judged by the same or similar criteria as quantitative research. This is the drive for rigor in the research and places responsibility for this with the researcher, not the reader.
2. A different set of criteria are needed for qualitative research. Because qualitative research is based upon a different philosophy it should not be judged in the same criteria.
3. There is some question whether or not any predetermined set of criteria are appropriate. Let the reader decide.

Sandelowski and Barroso (2002) have argued that more attention needs to be paid to aesthetic and rhetorical (style of writing) concerns. They urge readers to appreciate variability in reports of qualitative studies and to distinguish between errors of fact that do not undermine the value of the findings such as a study that is incorrectly labeled a phenomenological study when it is really a content analysis and one that has fatal flaws. A reporting error is not fatal if the findings themselves are credible and useful (p. 15). The *meaningfulness* of the work and its artful presentation are essential to the quality of qualitative research (Sandelowski, 1986). Sandelowski links these issues to the tension between the empirical and aesthetic ways of knowing in nursing:

> Valuing this tension and attempting to understand it may serve to create even more relevant and distinctive modes of inquiry in nursing. It may also serve to unify rather than divide nursing scholars. (1986, p. 36)

It is at this juncture that nursing scholars may be able to agree. A comparable state-ment from Morse and colleagues echoes Sandelowski in different terminology: "Elegant inquiry is stunning; the arguments are sophisticated in that they are complex yet elegant, focused yet profound, surprising yet obvious" (2002, p. 15).

CONCLUSION

It is difficult to imagine a nurse scholar or practitioner who could say that the quality of a nursing-related study is not important. However, the researcher may choose from a number of principles, criteria and strategies, deciding the extent to which scientific adequacy, system-aticity, trustworthiness, transparency, qualities of the researcher, theoretical consistency, aes-thetics, literary qualities, and stimulation of social action are desired. This judgment should be based upon the purpose of the study, its philosophical roots, and the approach used.

REFERENCES

Borreani, C., Miccinesi, G., Bunelli, C., & Lina, M. (2004). An increasing number of qualitative research papers on oncology and palliative care: Does it mean a thorough development of the methodology of research? *Health and Quality of Life Outcomes, 2*(7). doi: 10.1186/1477-7525-2-7.

Charmaz, K. (2005). Grounded theory in the 21st century: Application for advancing social justice studies. In N. K. Denzin & Y. S. Lincoln (Eds.), *The Sage handbook of qualitative research* (pp. 507–535). Thousand Oaks, CA: Sage.

Cho, J., & Trent, A. (2006). Validity in qualitative research revisited. *Qualitative Research, 6*(3), 319–340.

Cohen, D. J., & Crabtree, B. F. (2008). Evaluative criteria for qualitative research in health care: Controversies and recommendations. *Annals of Family Medicine, 6*(4), 331–339.

Conrad, S., Garrett, L. E., Cooksley, W. G. E., Dunne, M. P., & MacDonald, G. A. (2006). Living with chronic hepatitis C means 'you just haven't got a normal life anymore'. *Chronic Illness, 2*, 121–131.

Creswell, J. W., & Miller, D. L. (2000). Determining validity in qualitative inquiry. *Theory Into Practice, 39*(3), 124–130.

Davies, D., & Dodd, J. (2002). Qualitative research and the question of rigor. *Qualitative Health Research, 12*(2), 279–289.

❖ A readable essay by two doctoral students pondering the notion of rigor in qualitative research.

Freeman, D. (1983). *Margaret Mead and Samoa: The making and unmaking of an anthropological myth.* Cambridge, MA: Harvard University Press.

Freeman, M., deMarrais, K., Preissle, J., Roulston, K., & St. Pierre, E. A. (2007). Standards of evidence in qualitative research: An incitement to discourse. *Educational Researcher, 36*(1), 25–32.

Geertz, C. (1973). *The interpretation of cultures.* New York, NY: Basic Books.

Guba, E. G., & Lincoln, Y. S. (1998). Competing paradigms in qualitative research. In N. K. Denzin & Y. S. Lincoln (Eds.), *The landscape of qualitative research: Theories and issues* (pp. 195–220). Thousand Oaks, CA: Sage.

Halpern, E. S. (1983). *Auditing naturalistic inquiries: The development and application of a model.* Unpublished doctoral dissertation, Indiana University, Bloomington.

House, E. R. (2008). Qualitative evaluation and changing social policy. In N. K. Denzin & Y. S. Lincoln (Eds.), *Collecting and interpreting qualitative materials* (pp. 623–640). Los Angeles: Sage.

Jerosch-Herold, C., Mason, R., & Chojnowski, A. J. (2008). A qualitative study of the experiences and expectations of surgery in patients with carpal tunnel syndrome. *Journal of Hand Therapy, 21*, 54–62.
   ✧ A detailed section on quality of the data analyzed drawing upon Lincoln and Guba and Miles and Huberman is included in the data analysis section of this article.

Kirk, J., & Miller, M. L. (1986). *Reliability and validity in qualitative research.* Beverly Hills, CA: Sage.

Lincoln, Y. S., & Guba, E. G. (1985). *Naturalistic inquiry.* Newbury Park, CA: Sage.
   ✧ Chapter 11, "Establishing Trustworthiness," is one of the most widely quoted sources on quality of qualitative data. It is also quite readable. There is also an appendix with details on creating an audit trail.

Long, T., & Johnson, M. (2000). Rigour, reliability and validity in qualitative research. *Clinical Effectiveness in Nursing, 4*, 30–37.

Lupton, D. (2004). Femininity, responsibility and the technological imperative: Discourses in breast cancer in the Australian press. *International Journal of Health Services, 24*(1), 73–89.
   ✧ This is the study that Seale critiqued.

Mead, M. (1949). *Coming of age in Samoa.* New York: New American Library of World Literature.
   ✧ Want to judge for yourself? You can read Mead's original study to see if you agree with Freeman's critique.

Meyrick, J. (2006). What is good qualitative research? *Journal of Health Psychology, 11*(5), 799–808.

Miles, M. B., & Huberman, M. (1994). *Qualitative data analysis: An expanded sourcebook* (2nd ed.). Thousand Oaks, CA: Sage.

Morse, J. M. (2003). A review committee's guide for evaluating qualitative proposals. *Qualitative Health Research, 13*(6), 833–851.

Morse, J. M., Barrett, M., Mayan, M., Olson, K., & Spiers, J. (2002). Verification strategies for establishing reliability and validity in qualitative research. *International Journal of Qualitative Methods, 1*(2), 1–19.
   ✧ Noted nurse scholar and Editor of Qualitative Health Research, Dr. Morse and colleagues explain why they support using the terminology of mainstream science in evaluation of quality in qualitative research.

Morse, J. M., Bottorff, J. L., & Hutchinson, S. (1995). The paradox of comfort. *Nursing Research, 44*, 14–19.

Morse, J. M., Niehaus, L., Wolfe, R. R., & Wilkins, S. (2006). The role of the theoretical drive in maintaining validity in mixed-method research. *Qualitative Research in Psychology, 3*, 279–291.

Patton, M. Q. (1999). Enhancing the quality and credibility of qualitative analysis. *HSR: Health Services Research, Part II, 34*(5), 1189–1208.

Patton, M. Q. (2002). *Qualitative research and evaluation methods.* Thousand Oaks, CA: Sage.

Richter, M. S., Parker, C., & Chaw-Kent, J. (2001). Listening to the voices of hospitalized high-risk antepartum patients. *Journal of Obstetric, Gynecologic, & Neonatal Nursing, 36*, 313–318.

Rolfe, G. (2006). Validity, trustworthiness and rigour: Quality and the idea of qualitative research. *Journal of Advanced Nursing, 53*(3), 304–310.

Ryle, G. (1971). *Doing phenomenology: Essays on and in phenomenology.* New York, NY: Routledge.

Sandelowski, M. (1986). The problem of rigor in qualitative research. *Advances in Nursing Science, 8*(3), 27–37.
   ✧ This author argues against having a standard set of criteria for evaluating qualitative research. Brings in viewpoints of many nursing scholars in qualitative research.

Sandelowski, M., & Barroso, J. (2002). Reading qualitative studies. *International Journal of Qualitative Methods, 1*(1), Article 5. Retrieved July 23, 2008 from http://www.ualberta.ca/~iiqm/backissues/1_1Final/pdf/sandeleng.pdf

 ◇ A detailed guide for reading qualitative studies is described and appended to this article. It is worth reading carefully if you want to either write or evaluate (appraise is the term they prefer) a qualitative research report.

Schensul, S. L., Schensul, J. J., & LeCompte, M. D. (1999). *Essential ethnographic methods: Observations, interviews and questionnaires.* Walnut Creek, CA: Altamira Press.

Seale, C. (2004). Quality in qualitative research. In C. Seale, G. Gobo, J. F. Gubrium, & D. Silverman (Eds.), *Qualitative research practice* (pp. 409–419). Thousand Oaks, CA: Sage.

 ◇ Provides an excellent critique of a study that does not live up to the author's criteria for quality in qualitative research.

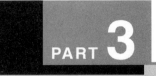

PART 3

Implementation Phase

CHAPTER 12

Research Ethics

The rights of people who participate in research studies and the responsibilities of those who conduct research are the focus of this chapter. The chapter begins with a brief description of some of the troubling events that led to the formal procedures now in place to protect study participants and to guide researchers' behavior. Special procedures for those who are considered vulnerable populations will be discussed as well as the process for obtaining approval for your study, obtaining consent from study participants, and other issues related to the responsible conduct of research.

A TROUBLED PAST

The majority of researchers have always acted in an ethical manner and protected the rights and safety of the participants in their studies. However, there have been some instances where this was not the case. These instances, a few of which will be mentioned here, have made it clear that guidelines for the protection of both human and animal subjects were and are still needed.

Tuskegee Syphilis Study

One of the best known examples of failure to protect the people participating in a research study in the United States is the Tuskegee Syphilis Study. Deception and failure to provide adequate treatment of a serious disease were the primary ethical violations.

This study began in 1932 but continued until the early 1970s. The participants were 399 African-American men, most of whom were very poor and illiterate as well. They probably agreed to participate in order to receive free medical care (some of the advertisements for pharmaceutical studies today still use this as an incentive but provide many more safeguards, including halting the study if a treatment is shown to be harmful, or if a treatment is found that is so effective that it can no longer be withheld from the control group).

The men were recruited because they had syphilis. They were given small doses of the current treatment (bismuth, neoarsphenamine, and mercury), later replaced with aspirin, which is ineffective in the treatment of syphilis. They did not know that the doses were small or ineffective or that participation included agreement to an autopsy. In fact, many of the men entered the military during World War II and were supposed to be treated for their syphilis, but the Public Health Service made them exempt from the treatment. The Public Health Service also kept them from receiving penicillin when it became available in the 1940s.

The study originally brought educational opportunities and prestige to the Tuskegee Institute and its affiliated hospital, generating praise and support from African-American community leaders for this. An African-American nurse was involved in the study as well, but she did not question the ethics of the study, probably trusting in the good will of the researchers and having been taught to do as she was instructed: "we were taught that we never diagnosed, we never prescribed; we followed the doctor's instructions!" (Brunner, 2009, p. 2).

Half the men died of syphilis or related complications despite the availability of an effective treatment for over 20 years before the experiment ended. Brunner (2009) ends this narrative with a strong statement about the violation of trust that occurred. "In light of this and many other shameful episodes in our history, African-Americans' widespread mistrust of the government and white society in general should not be a surprise to anyone" (p. 3). Interestingly, in a study of the effect of the Tuskegee incident, Katz and colleagues (2008) found that far more blacks than whites in four U.S. cities ($N = 1113$) were aware of the Tuskegee study (73% vs. 55%), but the white participants reacted more negatively to it. Katz et al. suggest that this difference may be due to the "daily cultural reality in the black community" (p. 1140).

Although one of the best known, the Tuskegee Syphilis Study was not the only instance of the violation of ethical conduct in research, and African-Americans are not the only group to have experienced this (Epstein, 2008).

A more recent example from Los Angeles:

In 1989 African-American and Hispanic American infants were given an experimental vaccine to prevent measles without full disclosure of the risks involved. The parents had not been told that this vaccine was not licensed in the United States or that it had "potentially lethal" side effects (Moreno-John et al., 2004, p. 1015). Violations of confidentiality have also had adverse effects on Native American groups. One tribe found themselves ostracized after they had been identified as participants in a syphilis study; another tribe's members suffered lower credit ratings after having been identified as participants in a study of alcoholism (Moreno-John et al., 2004).

Another case that drew a lot of media attention was the death of Jesse Gelsinger, a young man who had ornithine transcarbamylase deficiency. Although he knew it probably would not help him, Gelsinger agreed to experimental gene therapy in the hope that what was learned would benefit others. He died within days of receiving the experimental treatments (DeRenzo & Moss, 2006). Investigation following his death raised some serious questions. Apparently Gelsinger did not meet all of the criteria for eligibility for the experimental treatment. It also appeared that he was not told of some of the problems with the treatment that arose in animal studies. DeRenzo and Moss (2006) note that omission of this type of information from the consent is not uncommon, but this case raises questions about what should be done in the future. It was also discovered that some of the investigators had financial interests in the results, suggesting a serious conflict of interest in allowing him to proceed with the treatment. Financial interest and payments from drug and device companies are a concern because they may reduce researcher objectivity (Kaiser, 2009).

Some researchers have also violated the trust of the consumers of research by falsifying data. This has been done in a number of ways. One scientist was found to have painted the skin of the mice used in the study with a felt-tipped pen to make it look as if skin grafts from other mice had been successful (Medicine, 1974). Another was found to have falsely reported what was done with nonhuman primates in seven publications on federally supported research. These animals were supposed to have had their kidneys removed so that the effect of a transplanted kidney could be evaluated, but it had not been done (NIH, DHHS, 2009). In another instance, a team of researchers falsified data in a study on centenarians, creating records for nonexistent participants because they were unable to recruit enough to complete their sample (ORI, 1995).

These violations endanger the health and well-being of the participants and their families, reduce trust in researchers, and raise questions about the reporting of research results. Although relatively infrequent (Resnick, 2007), their impact on the public trust is enormous. They affect all researchers, including those who do not and would not commit such violations of ethical conduct in research.

PRINCIPLES OF ETHICAL CONDUCT IN RESEARCH

Research ethics are the "norms for conduct that distinguish between acceptable and unacceptable behavior" in other words, the standards for conduct when doing research (Resnick, 2007, p. 1). The principles of ethical conduct in research define these standards.

In 1976, the National Commission for the Protection of Human Subjects of Biomedical and Behavioral Research met at the Smithsonian's Belmont Conference Center for 4 days. This conference plus almost 4 years of deliberations resulted in the well-known Belmont Report (1979), which is the primary basis for the principles of ethical conduct in research in the United States. Two other important documents, the Nuremberg Code of 1947 (developed in response to experiments done on concentration camp prisoners during World War II) and the Helsinki Declaration of 1964 (revised in 1975), together with the Belmont Report form the foundation for our discussion of research ethics (all three may be found in the appendix). There are also guidelines that have been issued by the federal government, the American Psychological Association, and many professional organizations that expand upon these fundamental codes.

The three fundamental principles of ethical conduct in human research are (1) respect for person, (2) beneficence, and (3) justice. Beneficence (doing good) is sometimes separated out from nonmaleficence (doing no harm) (as in Johnson, 2004). We will consider each of these three principles separately and then discuss their application to the conduct of a research study.

Respect for Person

There are two parts to this first principle:

1. Individuals should be treated as autonomous agents. The term *autonomous* refers to the ability to make decisions, and the principle refers to honoring those

decisions, unless they are detrimental to others. Lack of respect for persons is shown when a person is denied freedom to act on his or her decisions or when information needed to make a decision is withheld without a compelling reason to do so (NIH, 2009).

2. Individuals with limited ability to make decisions for themselves are entitled to protection. This includes the immature (e.g., young children) and incapacitated (e.g., those with severe dementia) but also those with restricted liberty. Prisoners are an example of this last category. According to the Belmont Report:

> It would seem that the principle of respect for person requires that prisoners not be deprived of the opportunity to volunteer for research . . . [but] under prison conditions they may be subtly coerced or unduly influenced to engage in research activities for which they would not otherwise volunteer. (p. 4)

You can see that achieving the optimum balance between offering prisoners opportunities to participate in research studies without placing any pressure on them (even too generous an incentive can be considered too much pressure) is often difficult to do.

Beneficence and Nonmaleficence

Beneficence, in this case, is not being kind or nice but an obligation to do no harm (nonmaleficence) and to maximize possible benefits. This principle obligates researchers to design their studies to reduce risks and increase any benefit as much as possible. Application of this principle also creates some dilemmas for researchers and members of the institutional review boards (IRBs) who review their research.

Involving children in research studies poses some dilemmas related to this principle. For example, research is needed to test the effect of pharmaceuticals in children: Are they safe? For how long? At what dosage? Yet putting children at risk to test a new drug seems to violate the principle of nonmaleficence. These are difficult choices for researchers and for members of IRBs who review these studies, as they attempt to achieve a balance between protection and participation (Powell & Smith, 2009).

Justice

The Belmont Report (1979) defines *justice* in relation to research as "fairness in distribution" (p. 5). This addresses both the denial of a benefit without a good reason or imposing a burden unequally.

The burden of serving as a participant in research fell primarily on the poor in early research studies (in the 1800s), but the benefit went largely to those who could pay for care. Research on prisoners in Nazi concentration camps in Europe and on minorities such as the African-American men in the Tuskegee Syphilis Study in the United States were examples of flagrant injustice (NIH, 2009; Belmont Report, p. 6). In more recent times, researchers focused largely on white men, leaving women, minorities, and children out of their samples. The injustice in this action was that the results could not be confidently applied to the care of those excluded from the research.

APPLICATION OF THE PRINCIPLES

The application of these principles is a complex matter. A number of formal procedures have been developed to provide guidelines for researchers and to assure their adherence to these guidelines. Many of these guidelines address federal government requirements that must be followed to qualify for federal grants and contracts but are generally applied to all studies done within an institution. Additional guidelines and specific details regarding these guidelines (forms to complete, reporting rules, etc.) are often issued by individual institutions. A separate set of guidelines for approval of pharmaceutical agents and medical devices comes from the Food and Drug Administration (FDA), and an additional set of guidelines for research with animals has been developed that parallels those for the protection of human subjects.

Training

In most cases, there are both local and federal requirements for training in the ethical conduct of research. Usually every member of the research team has to complete the required training. This is in addition to whatever specific training is needed to conduct the study.

The first step in assuring that you abide by the principles of ethical conduct in research is to become acquainted with the federal guidelines and your own institution's rules and guidelines.

Basic Training

The following are topics included in the basic training for researchers:

- *Historical perspectives:* Reasons why current rules and regulations were developed
- *Principles of ethical research conduct:* Based upon the Belmont Report and other codes
- *Compliance procedures:* Application for approval from the IRB
- *Informed consent procedures:* When a written consent is necessary and when it may be waived; content of a consent
- *Risks associated with participation in research:* The types of risks a researcher needs to address in various types of studies
- *Vulnerable populations:* Definition of vulnerable populations and special considerations for their protection
- *Special situations and populations:* These include record review, existing datasets, genetic research, research with pregnant women, employees, and so forth
- *FDA regulations:* FDA rules and regulations, International Conference on Harmonization (ICH) guidelines
- *HIPAA requirements:* Confidentiality of medical records
- *Conflicts of interest:* Sources of potential conflict and what interests and relationships you might need to disclose

- *IRB membership:* Roles and responsibilities of IRB members; composition of an IRB (CITI, 2010)

Courses addressing all of these subjects are available online.

Responsible Conduct of Research

This is an additional level of research ethics content required of those who wish to apply for federal grant support. The following topics are included:

- Research misconduct
- Data management
- Conflict of interest
- Collaborative science
- Responsible authorship
- Mentoring
- Peer review
- Lab animals
- Human subjects (CITI, 2010)

Most IRB coordinators will assist you in accessing the required courses or direct you to the IRB's website for further information. The IRB coordinators are also a good resource for answering questions that may arise as you go through the process of seeking IRB approval for your study. They can also be helpful when questions about consenting procedures or other ethical conduct questions arise during the course of the study.

Application for Approval

This is the next step in the quest to abide by the ethics-related rules and regulations governing research with human subjects.

Institutional Review Boards (IRBs)

Virtually every college, university, research institute, and large healthcare institution has an institutional review board. Smaller facilities may not have their own IRB, but there are alternative means for obtaining a review of your proposed study. The first is to obtain a review from a cooperating academic institution or healthcare facility that has an IRB. The second is to use the ethics committee of your facility as a review committee (this would not meet federal standards in most cases if it were the only review done). The third is to use one of the commercial IRBs that charge a substantial fee to conduct the review. Federal guidelines for membership of IRBs include the following:

- At least five members with varied backgrounds
- Expertise and experience related to the studies reviewed among the members
- At least one scientist member and one nonscientist member

- At least one member who is not affiliated with the parent organization or related to a person who is
- Diverse membership in terms of gender, race, and culture
- Members with sensitivity to community attitudes
- May *not* consist entirely of members of one profession
- Regarding research with vulnerable groups, consider including someone who is knowledgeable about and experienced in working with the group
- When additional expertise is needed, experts may be brought in but do not have a vote (DHHS, 2009; Grace, 2009).

Given the differences in these committees, it is evident that you will need to find out their requirements before preparing your application for approval. Ethics committees are likely to ask you to appear in person. Other IRBs are more likely to base their decision on the written application, submitted in hard copy or online. Be sure to check deadlines for submission and meeting dates to avoid excessive delays. Do consult with the IRB coordinator or committee chair if you are not sure what is expected.

Elements of an Application

Application requirements differ from one IRB to another, but most reflect federal requirements. The following is a list of frequently requested information:

- Title of the proposed study
- Source of funding for the study, if any
- List of investigators and their affiliations. Their specific roles in the study may also need to be described.
- Training for everyone working on the study
- Characteristics of the proposed sample. Reviewers are especially concerned about participation of those who are members of a population that is vulnerable or at heightened risk in some way, such as students, employees (including staff nurses), critically ill, infants, foster children (wards of the state), pregnant women, military personnel, nursing home residents, other institutionalized populations, prisoners, people with moderate to severe dementia, the undocumented (those who are in the country without legal authority), those potentially subject to abuse, and so forth. For some of these groups, the possibility of coercion is a primary concern; for others, it is their welfare and safety; for still others, it is their inability to understand what it is that they are agreeing to do and what the consequences might be.
- Investigator experience, professional licenses, any sanctions or problems related to ethical conduct of research in the past. This is not always asked, but it is particularly important in pharmaceutical studies (WIRB, 2010).
- Conflicts of interest: Any personal or financial interest that any of the investigators might have in the results of the study, such as family member involvement,

stock ownership in a pharmaceutical company or device maker, and so forth. Even the *appearance* of a conflict is of concern and has to be reported. Conflicts are often reported in a separate document.

- Use of investigational drugs, devices, recombinant DNA: These usually require that additional information be supplied.

- Environmental concerns, boating safety, use of radioactive and other hazardous materials: These also usually require additional information.

- Research sites: Places and agencies where participants will be recruited and involved in the study. Most IRBs require letters of agreement from external sites, sometimes even from internal sites.

- Participant safety: The possibility of any type of emergency arising or threats to the participant's health, welfare, or safety needs to be raised and measures to address them need to be specified. This includes adverse reactions to any physical treatment, falls or other injuries, emotional distress, or expression of suicidal intent.

- Data Safety Monitoring Board (DSMB): Described in more detail in Chapter 17, DSMBs are needed for clinical trials and other studies during which adverse events might occur. How complex the monitoring system must be depends upon the type and level of risk of participation in the study. The primary purpose of a DSMB is to safeguard study participants (Ellenberg, Fleming, & DeMets, 2002). Secondary purposes are to track the rate of enrollment, any changes in protocol or in eligibility, or any potentially unfavorable outcomes. In some trials it may become evident that one of the treatments being tested is so much less effective that it is no longer acceptable to keep participants in that treatment group. In others, it may become evident that a treatment has too many adverse outcomes and must be stopped.

- Participant privacy, confidentiality, and anonymity: HIPAA rules are expected to be addressed if access to medical records is involved. Participants can grant permission to the investigators to access their medical record data. Privacy also means conducting interviews on sensitive subjects out of hearing of others, making all the usual provisions for privacy during a physical examination as one would in clinical practice, etc.

    Confidentiality and *anonymity* apply to a wider range of studies. They are not synonymous terms. *Anonymity* means that all identifying information has been removed. Doing this, however, can sometimes pose problems. For example, in longitudinal studies, data are collected at multiple time points but need to be connected to the individual participant. Permanently and irreversibly anonymizing data prevents this (Birmingham & Doyle, 2009). On the other hand, there are times when the data collected is so sensitive or might put the respondent at so much risk that it must be kept anonymous. An example would be the risk of deportation for undocumented aliens. Another would be the responses of employees regarding difficulties with their immediate supervisor.

Confidentiality, on the other hand, is expected and must be maintained to the extent allowed by law. How research data is stored, shared, and published are the main concerns here. There are several ways to maintain confidentiality:

- Electronic data should be password protected. Access to computers on which data are stored can also be restricted.

- Paper records should be kept in locked files. Access to the files should be limited to members of the research team.

- Remove as much identifying material as is reasonable.

- Recordings may be destroyed when the study is completed (WIRB, 2010).

Unless specific permission has been obtained, publication of the results of the study should not contain information that might lead to identification of individual participants. This refers to participating institutions as well unless they request that their contribution to the study be acknowledged.

Identification of individual participants is possible on audio as well as video recording. Permission to make public any recording of this type should be obtained from the participant and specific use (training purposes only, in publications, media releases, and so forth) should be identified.

- Consent procedures: How and where participants will be recruited, screened, consented, and enrolled. HIPAA regulations requiring permission to access medical records need to be considered in planning the selection of possible participants from patient populations. Prescreening in some cases may have to be done by facility staff and permission to be contacted by researchers obtained before anyone on the research team can approach a participant who is a patient. If a guardian, next-of-kin, parent, or other representative of the potential participant will provide consent, this also must be noted. Copies of the consent form are usually submitted with the application for approval. If translated, some IRBs require certification of the accuracy of the translation.

- Recruitment procedures: Recruiting materials, including telephone scripts, brochures, radio, television, and written media announcements are usually reviewed by the IRB for their appropriateness.

- Incentives: A description of any inducement to participants is also needed, including dollar amounts or gift value and when the incentive will be given to the participants (WIRB, 2010).

BASIC ELEMENTS OF INFORMED CONSENT

The section of the Federal Code related to protection of human subjects lists eight basic elements of informed consent:

1. State that the study involves research; explain the purpose of the study, expected duration of participation, and the procedures to be followed. Note if any of the procedures are considered experimental.

2. Describe the foreseeable risks and discomforts a participant could encounter.

3. Describe any benefit to the participant or to others from the research.

4. Note available alternative procedures or treatment.

5. Describe procedures to maintain confidentiality to the extent allowed by law.

6. Note whether or not there is any compensation available should an injury occur and how that may be obtained.

7. Describe to whom and how a participant may direct questions about the study, study participants' rights, and reporting of an injury.

8. A statement (often your IRB will provide a template for this) that participation is voluntary, refusal to participate will not result in any penalty or loss of benefits, and that the participant may withdraw at any time without penalty or loss of benefit. (DHHS, 2009, p. 15)

There are other points that may be included in a consent if applicable to your study:

• Note if there is some risk to the embryo or fetus should the participant become pregnant.

• List circumstances under which the participant's physician or research team may terminate participation (e.g., if the participant is transferred out of the facility, no longer drives, or develops an unrelated illness that precludes participation).

• Alert the participant to any costs that might incur related to being in the study.

• Describe consequences of withdrawal (e.g., access to experimental treatment will end) and procedures for orderly termination of participation.

• Note that investigators will inform participants of any new findings that might affect their willingness to continue in the study.

• Approximate number of participants who will be enrolled.

Written consent forms are usually signed by the participant and the investigator. A witness signature may also be required. In cases where participants are deemed incapable of providing informed consent, the parent, next of kin, or guardian may agree and sign on their behalf. If the consent is longer than a single page, participants may be asked to initial every page to assure that they read all of the pages.

Copies of a set of relatively complex consent forms used in the Framingham Heart studies (Boston University, 2010) covering a physical examination, data extraction from medical records, samples for genetic testing, lung function test, arterial tomography, glucose tolerance test, health history and additional examination of the participant if hospitalized for a stroke are found in the appendix.

A simpler consent form for participation in cognitive screening is seen in Figure 12-1.

There are situations where the requirement for written consent may be waived. The following are some of the circumstances under which the written consent may be waived:

PARTICIPANT CONSENT

1. **Title of research study:** Mild Cognitive Impairment Screening Study

2. **Investigators:** _____

   _____

   _____

3. **Purpose:** The main purpose of this study is to evaluate the ability of a short series of tests and questionnaires to identify mild memory problems in people living in the community. A second purpose is to find out what people think about screening for memory problems.

4a. **Procedures:** If you agree to participate in this study, you will be asked a series of questions about your mood, any problems with memory, usual activities, medical history, medications, healthcare access, background (such as age or education), why you agreed to participate, what your thoughts are about memory problems, and what you would do if the tests indicate you might have a memory problem. You will also be given several tests of memory, attention, calculation, and other mental abilities. All of this should take about 45 minutes. The testing will be done at the Memory and Wellness Center or your church or community center. There is no charge for the testing.

   b. **Alternative procedures:** You do not have to participate in this study or in the screening being offered. Instead, you may go to your own doctor, to a specialist in memory problems or to one of the other memory clinics in your area.

5. **Risks:** Some people who take these tests may develop a concern about their memory. If this occurs, a member of the Memory and Wellness Center staff will be available to talk with you about this concern and provide referrals for further counseling. Otherwise, the risk of participation is no greater than those encountered in daily life or in a routine physical or psychological examination. Neither the state of Florida nor Florida Atlantic University provides insurance coverage in the event of injury.

6. **Benefits:** The benefit to you for participating in this study is in finding out whether the screening tests indicate a need for further diagnostic evaluation. If this occurs,

continues

you will be given information about obtaining further evaluation. You will also receive a small gift (value less than $5.00) for completing the tests. You may refuse to participate in this study without penalty. You may also withdraw from this study at any time without penalty. If you do not complete the tests, however, we will not be able to tell you if the results indicate a possible memory problem or need for further diagnostic evaluation. It is hoped that the results of this study will help us in selecting the best tests for use in screening for memory problems.

7. **Data collection and storage:** The data from this study will be kept confidential. An identification number will be attached to the results from this testing session, and your name will be removed. A separate list of names and identification numbers will also be kept so that we can telephone you for follow-up information and obtain your test results if you decide to go to a Memory Disorder Center for further diagnostic evaluation. All data will be kept in locked files and on password-protected, physically secure computers. Results of this study will not be released in any way that might allow identification of individual participants without your specific agreement unless disclosures are required by law.

8. **Contact information:** For related problems or questions regarding your rights as a subject, the Office of Sponsored Research at Florida Atlantic University can be contacted at (561) 297-0777. For other questions about the study, you should call the investigators, _____ (names) at _____ (phone numbers). You will receive a copy of this consent form for your records.

9. **Consent statement:** I have read or had read to me the preceding information describing this study. All my questions have been answered to my satisfaction. I am 18 years of age or older and freely consent to participate. I understand that I am free to withdraw from the study at any time without penalty. I have received a copy of this consent form.

Signature of Subject: _____   Date: _____

Signature of Investigator: _____   Date: _____

Figure 12-1   Example of participant consent.

- If participation involves only minimal risk (there is always some potential risk, however small, so the term *minimal* should be used, not *no risk*)
- If provision of the waiver will not affect the rights or welfare of participants
- If the research cannot be done without this waiver (DHHS, 2009)

An IRB may provide waivers of consent for certain types of research. Some examples are:

- Existing data, documents, and specimens that can be completely deidentified and/or are publicly available
- Observation of public behavior unless it deals with illegal behavior, sexual behavior, alcohol use, or the person can be identified and/or harmed in some way
- Research on normal educational practices and educational tests unless the participations can be identified
- Quality improvement projects unless individuals can be identified

You can see that minimal risk and protection of individual identity are important factors in deciding whether or not consent can be waived.

Internet research provides an interesting example of alternative consent procedures. The consent form can be e-mailed to potential participants, or it can be posted on the website and participants asked to agree to or to accept the invitation to participate that was approved by the IRB (Whitehead, 2007).

The issue of public versus private communications is an important one in Internet research. People seem to assume that their postings will only be read by members of their "virtual community," yet it is actually possible to electronically trace a communication back to its original source (Whitehead, 2007). Grace (2009) notes that alerting people who post that they are being observed and that their postings are being used in research will probably change the dynamics of the interactions, although this may be necessary to protect their right to be fully informed.

Consenting activities are not completed when a signature on the consent form has been obtained. It is important to make sure all pages are initialed, the signature has been witnessed, and the consent form is placed on file. After that, every time the participant is involved in an activity related to the study, he or she is agreeing to continue in the study. Even in qualitative research, situations arise during the conduct of the study that requires reflection on the principles of ethical conduct in research. For example, when participants begin to reveal very personal information, the researcher may remind the participant of the research context and any limitations on confidentiality that might pertain to the situation (Guillemin & Heggen, 2009; Bhattacharya, 2007). This is called *ongoing consent* (DeRenzo & Moss, 2006). It is considered a continuing process throughout participation in the study because consent may be withdrawn at any time.

Changes in Protocol. Any substantive change in the procedures related to involvement of the participants in the study should be reported to the IRB as an amendment.

ISSUES RELATED TO ETHICAL RESEARCH CONDUCT

Deception

You will recall from the principles of ethical research conduct that the investigators are obligated to be sure each participant is and remains fully informed. Sometimes, however, researchers find that they cannot conduct their study this way. The following is an example:

> A study concerned with whether or not decision making by primary care providers is influenced by the age of the patient was approved despite some deception about its purpose. Participants were told that this was a study of clinical decision making. They were not told that it was a study of age bias in clinical decision making. They were presented with three cases of individuals coming to a primary care clinic. Only the age of the patients was changed for half of the participants. If participants had been told that this was a study about age bias in clinical decision making, this likely would have affected their responses and masked any existing biases.

Breaking Confidentiality

Although it rarely occurs, there are occasions when a legal proceeding makes it necessary to provide data obtained in a research study. There are other instances where it is necessary to take action, such as reporting child abuse, reportable communicable diseases, a suicide threat, or a driver who is found to be unsafe on the road (Btoush & Campbell, 2009; Keogh & Daly, 2009). In some states, reporting such problems is mandatory, in others voluntary. Participants need to be informed if they risk being reported for any reason.

Translations and Literacy

To be fully informed, participants need to have consent information presented in their own language. Translation from English to other languages is not a simple matter because equivalent words are not always present in the language of your participants. At the very least, a translation from English into the second language by one translator, a back translation from the second language back into English by a second translator, and review of the results is needed. Some IRBs also require that the translation be certified.

Literacy is another consideration with some participants. People who cannot read often do not want to reveal this and may pretend to understand the consent or ask to take it home to study it so that a family member can read it for them. It is important to assure that every participant fully understands the information in the consent. The consent may be read to the participant, and the investigator may explain any potentially complex term or ideas in the consent. Use of plain, simple language in the consent is also helpful as is an estimate of the reading level of the language used in the consent form.

Vulnerable Populations

Mentioned several times already in this chapter, vulnerable participants are a special concern to the researcher.

Pregnant Women, Fetuses, and Neonates

Extra protections are required when conducting research involving pregnant women, their fetuses, and neonates. For example, researchers are encouraged to conduct preliminary studies on pregnant animals or nonpregnant women before testing on pregnant women. Risk is to be minimized to the extent possible, and researchers should not have any part in decisions about terminating a pregnancy or judging the viability of a neonate (DHHS, 2009).

Children

Children are persons who have not reached legal age for consent to treatment under the law. Guardians are individuals authorized under state or local law to consent to medical care for the child. Assent is an important consideration in research with children. The federal regulations define assent as affirmative agreement, not just a failure to object (DHHS, 2009, p. 28).

The IRB is expected to take into account the age and psychological state of the children involved in a study. Assent may not be required if participation is considered a direct and important benefit to the child. Parental or guardian permission is required except in special circumstances of neglected or abused children.

Prisoners

An IRB reviewing research involving prisoners should have at least one member who is a prisoner or prisoner representative, and the majority of the board should not have any association with the prison. The risks should not be any greater than would be accepted by nonprisoner volunteers; the benefits or advantages should not be so great that they impair the prisoner's ability to weigh the risks. Selection procedures should be fair and not arbitrarily influenced by prison authorities or other prisoners (DHHS, 2009). Studies done with prisoners should, in general, be on topics of concern in this population.

Illness and Crisis Effects

When potential participants are very ill or in the midst of a major crisis, their ability to concentrate and to comprehend the details of a consent form may be compromised. It is the researcher's responsibility to help them understand the content of the consent and what they are agreeing to (Silva & Sorrell, 1984).

Cognitively Impaired

When planning a study involving participants who are cognitively impaired, investigators need to specify how they will determine the person's capacity to understand the study procedures. If participants do not have the capacity to understand, determination of the legally authorized representative who can provide consent must be specified (WIRB, 2010). Assent of the participant should then be obtained whenever the impaired individual is involved in study activities, an example of *ongoing assent*.

Victims of Intimate Partner Violence

Safety and confidentiality are major concerns when conducting research with individuals who have been the victims of intimate partner violence. In particular, it is essential that the abusive partner be kept unaware of the victim's participation in research because of the danger of exacerbating the violent behavior. Btoush and Campbell (2009) suggest some ways to protect the participants:

- Use a vague title such as "women's health" for the study.
- Arrange a safe way to contact them, and find out if it is safe to leave a message.
- Ask if it is safe for them to be in possession of a copy of the consent that is usually given to participants.
- Keep telephone conversation vague until you are certain no one can overhear it.
- Discuss safety issues during the consenting process.
- Warn the participant that the researcher cannot guarantee confidentiality if the study involves group interviews.
- Provide cash compensation for travel and child care expenses.
- If you are providing information about resources for victims of intimate partner violence, obscure it by making it a part of a long list of other nonspecific resources.

In this and other situations where disclosure of data collected during the study may have adverse consequences for participants or damage their financial standing, employability, insurability, or reputation, a *certificate of confidentiality* may be issued by the National Institutes of Health to protect the data from forced disclosure (NIH, 2010). The certificates protect participants and researchers from forced disclosure such as court orders and subpoenas. Examples of sensitive information that can be protected by these certificates include:

- Data on HIV, AIDS, other STDs
- Information on illegal activities and drug and alcohol use
- Genetic study results
- Information that could lead to social stigmatization or discrimination
- Information on an individual's mental health (DHHS, 2010)

You can apply for a certificate of confidentiality after your study has been approved by the IRB with the application for a certificate specified as a condition of approval.

Information about the certificate, what it protects and what disclosures might be made, should be included in the consent form (DHHS, 2010).

Balancing Protection and Participation

Clearly, it is often difficult to find the optimal balance between protection and participation in research. There are times when researchers feel that IRB decisions limit their ability to conduct research. In fact, there are occasions when members of an IRB are inconsistent or even arbitrary in their decisions. For example, access to potential participants can be so tightly controlled that recruitment becomes very difficult or impossible to achieve (Powell & Smith, 2009). On the whole, however, most IRBs are genuinely concerned about the safety and welfare of participants and at the same time are supportive of researchers' efforts to conduct their studies.

ETHICAL CONDUCT RELATED TO ANIMAL MODEL RESEARCH

Institutional Animal Care and Use Committee (IACUC)

The use of animal models in health-related research is a subject of some controversy. Some groups object vigorously to subjecting animals, especially mammals, to research procedures. Others argue that many lives have been saved because of animal research.

As is the case with human research, there are federal guidelines for animal model research, notably the US Government Principles for the Utilization and Care of Vertebrate Animals Used in Testing, Research, and Training. The Institutional Animal Care and Use Committee (IACUC) parallels the IRB for human subjects as the review committee for animal research (IACUC, 2010). The IACUC also inspects animal facilities at least every 6 months. Membership in the IACUC includes at least one veterinarian, an active researcher, a nonscientific member, and an outside member.

In most cases, the animals are kept in a university or hospital vivarium, and the studies are done in the laboratory (with the exception of studies of wild animals). Veterinary care for the animals is required as is consultation with the veterinarian prior to receiving approval for a study.

Protocol Review

In conducting a review of an application, members of the IACUC focus upon the following:

- Amount of pain and distress and how it is handled. Usually anesthesia, sedation, or analgesia is provided to reduce pain and distress.
- An appropriate numbers of animals used (i.e., no more than necessary)
- The 3 *Rs*: Replacement, reduction, and refinement need to be addressed. *Replacement* refers to using animal tissue instead of live animals, prescreening of

potentially toxic substances before animal testing, or using human volunteers instead. *Reduction* refers to reducing the number of animals used to the least necessary. *Refinement* means decreasing any pain or distress as much as possible (Smith, 2001).

- Description of the study procedures that involve animals
- The investigator's experience and skill related to the proposed study
- Scientific review if peer review by an outside review committee (e.g., an NIH proposal review panel) has not been done.

Application for Approval

Like an application for approval of a study involving human subjects, application for approval of a study using an animal model requires that you address a number of concerns regarding ethical conduct. You can expect to be asked about the following:

- Investigator qualifications: Training and experience with the type of research proposed
- The species and number of animals to be used
- All of the procedures that will involve the animals
- How pain and discomfort will be minimized
- Assurance that the study does not duplicate previous studies unless necessary
- Animal living conditions and veterinary care
- Surgical procedures: Justification if more than one major procedure per animal is proposed. Infection control and pre- and postoperative care must be described.
- Euthanasia: Procedures must follow established guidelines (FAU, 2010; Office of Laboratory Animal Welfare, 2010; Institute of Laboratory Animal Resources, 1996)

You can see that the use of animal models in research is strictly controlled. Researchers are expected to ensure that the research is necessary and that the animals are treated in as humane a manner as possible.

CONCLUSION

The number of rules and regulations concerning ethical conduct of research may seem daunting at first. However, a little patience and careful study of the guidance provided will help you comply with all of these rules and regulations. It will also help to keep in mind that these rules and regulations were developed to define your responsibilities as an investigator and to protect the subjects, human or animal, of your research.

REFERENCES

Basic HHS Policy for Protection of Human Research Subjects. Code of Federal Regulations Title 45, Department of Health and Human Services, Part 46, Protection of Human Subjects, Subpart A. Retrieved April 15, 2010, from http://www.hhs.gov/ohrp/humansubjects/guidance/45cfr46.htm

Bhattacharya, K. (2007). Consenting to the consent form: What are the fixed and fluid understandings between the researcher and the researched? *Qualitative Inquiry, 13*(8), 1095–1115.

Birmingham, K., & Doyle, A. (2009). Ethics and governance of a longitudinal birth cohort. *Paediatric and Perinatal Epidemiology, 23*(S1), 39–50.

Boston University Schools of Medicine, Public Health, Dental, Medicine, and the Boston Medical Center. (2010). *Research Consent Forms. H-22762-The Framingham Heart Study N01-HC-25195 1910G*. Retrieved April 15, 2010, from http://www.framinghamheartstudy.org/research/consentfms.html

Brunner, B. (2009). The Tuskegee Syphilis Experiment. Retrieved April 15, 2010, from http://www.tuskegee.edu/global/story.asp?s=1207586

Btoush, R., & Campbell, J. C. (2009). Ethical conduct in intimate partner violence research: Challenges and strategies. *Nursing Outlook, 57*(4), 210–216.
◇ If intimate partner violence is the subject of your study, you will find this article very helpful.

Collaborative Institutional Training Initiative. (2010). Course in responsible conduct of research retrieved April 15, 2010, from https://www.citiprogram.org/rcrpage.asp?language=english&affiliation=100

Collaborative Institutional Training Initiative. (2010). Frequently asked questions retrieved April 15, 2010, from https://www.citiprogram.org/announcements.asp?language=english

Collaborative Institutional Training Initiative. (2010). Support Center for CITI. Retrieved April 15, 2010, from http://citiprogram.supportcenterpro.com/knowledgebase/

Department of Health and Human Services. (2009). *Findings of scientific misconduct*. Office of Research Integrity. NOT-OD-08-096. Retrieved April 15, 2010, from http://grants.nih.gov/grants/guide/notice-files/NOT-OD-08-096.html

DeRenzo, E. G., & Moss, J. (2006). *Writing clinical research protocols: Ethical considerations*. Amsterdam, The Netherlands: Elsevier.
◇ This is a comprehensive text that addresses many of the ethical issues that arise in conducting research.

DHHS Office of Extramural Research. (2010). *Certificate of confidentiality kiosk*. Retrieved April 15, 2001, from http://grants1.nih.gov/grants/policy/coc

DHHS Office of Research Integrity. (1995). Retrieved April 15, 2010, from http://ori.dhhs.gov

Ellenberg, S. S., Fleming, T. R., & DeMets, D. L. (2002). *Data monitoring committees in clinical trials: A practical perspective*. Chichester, UK: John Wiley & Sons.

Epstein, S. (2008). The 'rise of recruitmentology': Clinical research, racial knowledge, and the politics of inclusion and difference. *Social Studies of Science, 38*(5), 801–832.

Florida Atlantic University Policies and Procedures Manual. (2010). *Institutional animal care and use committee*. Retrieved April 15, 2010, from http://www.fau.edu/research/rcs/files/P1FAUPolicies-Procedure.pdf

Grace, P. J. (2009). *Nursing ethics and professional responsibility in advanced practice*. Sudbury, MA: Jones and Bartlett.

Guillemin, M., & Heggen, K. (2009). Rapport and respect: Negotiating ethical relations between research and participant. *Medical Health Care and Philosophy, 12*(3), 291–297.

Institute of Laboratory Animal Resources. (1996). *Guide for the care and use of laboratory animals* [Institute]. Washington, DC: National Academy Press.

Institutional Animal Care and Use Committee. (2010). *Animal research guidelines and policies, colleges and universities.* Retrieved April 15, 2010, from http://www.iacuc.org/aboutus.htm

Johnson, M. (2004). Real-world ethics and nursing research. *Journal of Nursing Research, 9*(4), 251–261.

Kaiser, J. (2009). Senate probe of research psychiatrists. *Science, 325*(5936), 30.

Katz, R. V., Kegeles, S. S., Kressin, N. R., Green, B. L., James, S. A., Wang, M. Q., et al. (2008). Awareness of the Tuskegee Syphilis Study and the U.S. presidential apology and their influence on minority participation in biomedical research. *American Journal of Public Health, 98*(6), 1137–1142.

Keogh, B., & Daly, L. (2009). The ethics of conducting research with mental health service users. *British Journal of Nursing, 18*(5), 277–281.

Medicine: The S.K.I. Affair (contd.). (1974, June 3). *Time.* Retrieved April 15, 2010, from http://www.time.com/time/printout/0,8816,911353,00.html

Moreno-John, G., Gachie, A., Fleming, C. M., Napoles-Springer, A., Mutran, E., Manson, S. M., et al. (2004). Ethnic minority older adults participating in clinical research: Developing trust. *Journal of Aging and Health, 16*(5), 93S–123S. doi: 10.1177/0898264304268151.

Nagy, T. F. (2005). *Ethics in plain English: An illustrative casebook for psychologists.* Washington, DC: American Psychological Association.

National Institutes of Health. (n.d.). *NIH announces statement on certificates of confidentiality.* Retrieved April 15, 2010, from http://grants1.nih.gov/grants/guide/notice-files/NOT-OD-02-037.html

National Institutes of Health, Office of the Secretary. (2009). *The Belmont report: Ethical principles and guidelines for the protection of human subjects of research (April 18, 1979).* Retrieved April 15, 2010, from http://ohsr.od.nih.gov/guidelines/belmont.html

Office of Laboratory Animal Welfare. (2010). *Public Health Service Policy on Humane Care and Use of Laboratory Animals.* Retrieved April 15, 2010, from http://grants.nih.gov/grants/olaw/references/phspol.htm

Powell, M. A., & Smith, A. B. (2009). Children's participation rights in research. *Childhood, 16*(1), 124–142.

Resnick, D. B. (2007). *What is ethics in research & why is it important?* Retrieved April 13, 2010, from http://www.niehs.nih.gov/research/resources/bioethics/whatis.cfm
   ❖ An interesting discussion of research ethics that includes a few case examples.

Silva, M. C., & Sorrell, J. M. (1984). Factors influencing comprehension of information for informed consent: Ethical implications for nursing research. *International Journal of Nursing Studies, 21*(4), 233–240.

Smith, R. (2001). Animal research: The need for a middle ground. *BMJ, 322*(7281), 248–249.

Western Institutional Review Board. (2010). Content and guide. Retrieved April 15, 2010, from http://www.wirb.com/content/quick_download_forms.aspx

Whitehead, L. C. (2007). Methodological and ethical issues in Internet-mediated research in the field of health: An integrated review of the literature. *Social Science and Medicine, 65*, 782–791.

CHAPTER 13

Participant Recruitment

It is exciting to begin a new research study. With a clearly defined design and institutional review board (IRB) approval in hand, many new researchers think that they have overcome the highest hurdles. In some cases, that may be true, but for many another challenge awaits: recruiting participants to the study.

In this chapter we will consider the process of participant recruitment and enrollment, what motivates people to participate in a research study—the *incentives*, and why they may decline—what *barriers* to participation exist. We will also consider the question of retention, which becomes important if you need to maintain contact and retest or reinterview participants.

RECRUITMENT

Ten Steps to Completing Participant Recruitment and Enrollment

Getting to YES is the title of a popular book on negotiation first published in 1981, now in a second edition and a long running best seller (Fisher & Ury, 1981; Fisher, Ury, & Patton, 1991; Wikipedia, 2009). Our end goal in participant recruitment and study enrollment is also to get to yes. However, participant recruitment involves establishing trust and increasing motivation; it is a process of persuasion rather than negotiation.

Participation in research is *voluntary*. A well-planned, culturally sensitive (stretching the term culture to include people of different ages, genders, health status, and income, as well as race and ethnic group membership) recruitment effort is designed to find and enroll *willing* volunteers. The steps to accomplishing this goal are outlined in Figure 13-1 and described below.

1. *Specify* the people needed for your study. Be as specific as possible about who would be eligible (inclusion criteria) and who would not (exclusion criteria). Figure 13-2 illustrates a simple set of inclusion and exclusion criteria for a cognitive screening study. Every study has its own specific inclusion and exclusion criteria based on the purpose of the study.

2. *Develop* a recruitment plan. Complex studies and studies involving hard-to-reach populations require an especially detailed plan for recruitment. The plan should include the inclusion and exclusion criteria and address the following:

   - The means by which you will access the population
   - Potential barriers (disincentives) to participation

1. **Specify** . . .
The desired sample and the inclusion and exclusion criteria

2. **Develop** . . . .
A recruitment plan focused on potential sources of participants and their characteristics and preferences

3. **Contact** . . .
Potential sources to obtain their support and assistance

4. **Disseminate** . . .
Information about the study to potential participants

5. **Ask** . . .
Potentially eligible people to become participants

6. **Consent** . . .
Explain the study, obtain consent

7. **Screen** . . .
Consented individuals to confirm eligibility using inclusion and exclusion criteria

8. **Enroll** . . .
Involve consented participants in designated role within the study

9. **Retain** . . .
Enrolled participants through incentives, maintaining contact

10. **Report** . . .
The findings of the study to completed participants and those who helped with recruitment

Figure 13-1 Getting to "yes": Steps in participant recruitment, enrollment, and retention.

Source: Inspired by information from Berger, Begun, and Otto-Salaj, 2009; Taylor-Piliae and Froelicher, 2007; Fisher and Ury, 1981.

Inclusion	Exclusion
• Age 50 to 100 • Male or female • Noninstitutionalized (community dwelling) • Able to speak English or Spanish*	• Has been diagnosed as having Alzheimer's disease or a related chronic progressive dementia • Evidence of active psychosis • Current treatment for major depression • Severe hearing or vision loss that would preclude testing

Figure 13-2 Inclusion and exclusion criteria for a cognitive screening study.

Note: *Examiners were bilingual English-Spanish, and the cognitive tests were available in English and Spanish.

- How you will establish trust
- How and what will persuade people to participate

3. *Contact* potential sources of participants. These are the sources that can provide access to possible participants. They often serve as gatekeepers, protecting the privacy of potential participants but also allowing and facilitating access under appropriate circumstances. It is not unusual for the researcher to be asked to provide details about the study and the protection of participants before agreement (sometimes permission) is achieved. For example:

- Access to school-age children and their parents often requires approval of the school system or board of education.
- Primary care practitioners may recommend participation if assured of the safety of their patients.
- Healthcare facility administrators and nurse executives may allow access to patients under their care given assurance of safety for their patients, protection of privacy, and the worthiness of the study.

   In other instances, these initial contacts are community or organizational leaders whose support of the study encourages people to participate. In one example the manager of a public housing unit agreed to become a participant in a study of culture bias in psychological tests. Once she had done this and described her (pleasant) experience to the residents, many of them agreed to participate as well.

There has been research done comparing the productiveness of different sources of participants. For example:

> Carr and colleagues (2009) compared two different strategies for recruiting people into studies of Alzheimer's disease. The first strategy was a 3-hour continuing education course offered to primary care physicians at a conference center. The course was advertised through direct mailing, the Alzheimer's Association, and university outreach. The second strategy was a community health fair advertised through direct mailing, the Alzheimer's Association, and an article in a family magazine. Memory screens and educational sessions were offered. Costs of the two strategies were similar. The first strategy cost $3372; the second cost $3807. Sixty-nine participants were recruited through the community-based strategy; *none* were recruited through the primary care providers who expressed concern about potential risks and fear of losing patients. Direct contact was clearly more effective in this case, but actions could also be taken to allay the physicians' concerns before seeking their assistance in recruiting participants, potentially improving their effectiveness as a source of participants.

4. *Disseminate* information about the study to potential participants. The means through which it is possible to reach people who might be interested in participating range from the highly impersonal but mass appeal of television, radio, newsprint, or the Internet to highly personal one-on-one conversations on street corners for hard-to-reach youth (Auerswald et al., 2004), in clinics for people with a particular health concern, or telephone calls to people identified by a trusted source (a religious leader or agency director, for example) as potential participants.

   Bonk (in press) collected data on the most effective way to disseminate information about a study, asking participants how they heard about the study. The results are graphically shown in Figure 13-3. As you can see, the brochure about the study (Figure 13-4) was most often mentioned by these participants. Use of the Web and health fairs was not as productive in recruiting older adults (Bonk, in press).

   There are some special considerations for recruiting participants via the Internet. Certain groups of people are relatively easy to reach online. This includes college students who have assigned e-mail addresses, members of professional organizations, and members of online support and special interest groups. However, other groups of people are likely to have limited access to the Internet and will be difficult to reach this way. This includes people over age 65, those with lower incomes or levels of education, and some minority groups.

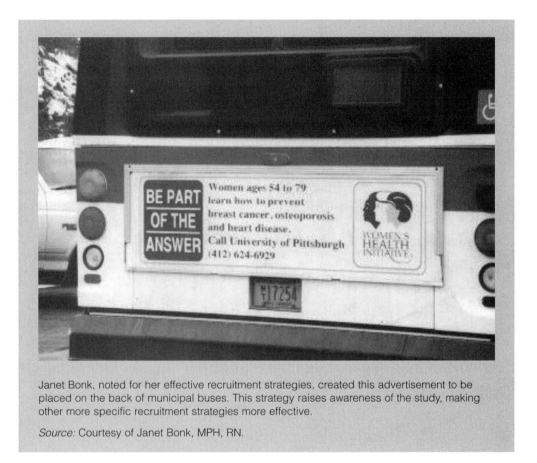

Janet Bonk, noted for her effective recruitment strategies, created this advertisement to be placed on the back of municipal buses. This strategy raises awareness of the study, making other more specific recruitment strategies more effective.

Source: Courtesy of Janet Bonk, MPH, RN.

Others, such as people in rural areas, are more likely to have dial-up service which is slow, making it difficult to respond to a survey. It is also very difficult to obtain a representative sample through Internet-based research (Dillman, Smyth, & Christian, 2009).

5. *Ask* potentially eligible people if they are willing to participate. Again, this may be done through a trusted source such as their primary care provider, social worker, or religious leader in person, by telephone, or via e-mail or regular mail. In general, the more personal and persuasive the approach, the higher the response rate will be. In one example:

> Harris and colleagues (2008) compared four different strategies to recruit older adults for a 1-week physical activity study using accelerometers.

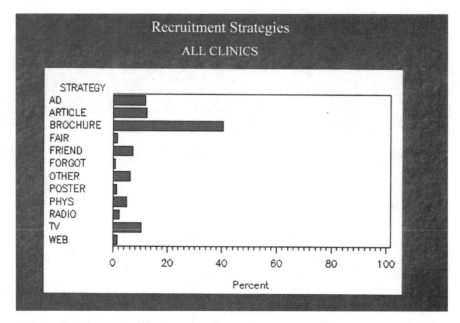

Figure 13-3 Comparative effectiveness of recruitment strategies.

Source: Bonk, J. (2009, January 29). Recruitment and retention of participants for longitudinal studies. Paper presented at the symposium on Longitudinal Studies on Aging, Boca Community Hospital, Boca Raton, FL. Used with permission of J. Bonk.

> Invitations to participate were extended to 560 clients in a U.K. primary care practice (the source of the letter may have been a factor in the relatively good response rate) divided into four groups. All received the letter of invitation. One fourth received nothing more, one fourth received a telephone call from a research nurse, one fourth received a questionnaire along with the letter, and one fourth received both the call and the letter. The response rates were compared. Although 39% in the telephone strategy group either asked not to be telephoned or couldn't be reached, use of the telephone contact increased participation from 38% to 48%. Inclusion of the questionnaire, which had been expected to deter volunteers, did not significantly reduce participation (p. 662).

6. *Consent* is obtained after the study purposes, procedures, risks, and benefits are explained. This procedure and the forms used to obtain consent were described in the Chapter 12 discussion on research ethics.

7. *Screening* to determine an individual's eligibility is done on the basis of the inclusion and exclusion criteria. These criteria can be very simple in which case

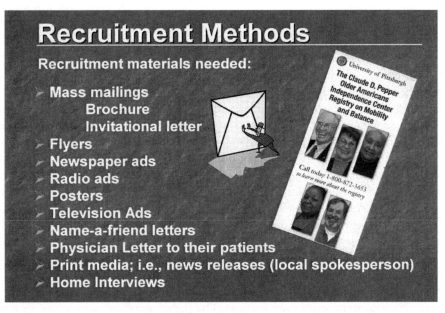

Figure 13-4   A variety of methods may be used for participant recruitment.

Source: Bonk, J. (2009, January 29). *Recruitment and retention of participants for longitudinal studies.* Paper presented at the symposium on Longitudinal Studies on Aging, Boca Community Hospital, Boca Raton, FL. Used with permission of J. Bonk.

this step goes quickly. In other instances such as clinical trials of new drugs, the criteria are complex and quite specific. Often pregnant women cannot participate, for example, or individuals taking other drugs that may interfere with or confound the results are excluded.

8. *Enroll* participants. You have finally gotten to yes and are ready to get the person, now a participant, involved in the study. This may entail random assignment to a treatment group, scheduling of regular treatments, arrangements for blood tests or scans, and so forth. All of these activities should be spelled out in the study protocol.

9. *Retain* participants. Many studies require a series of testing sessions or treatments or both. Longitudinal studies require multiple encounters over years or even decades. Specific strategies to retain participants will be discussed later in this chapter.

10. *Report* the findings of the study to the participants. This last step is often forgotten, leaving participants and your sources feeling unappreciated and unwilling to help you or other researchers again.

Motivators

If there is a "guru" (guide or teacher) of participant recruitment in survey research, that person is D. A. Dillman, who published his first work in the 1970s. Dillman (2000; Dillman, Smyth, & Christian, 2009) adopted a systematic, research-based approach to discovering the strategies that increase response rates to various surveys. His early work concentrated on surveys sent out by mail. Every detail was considered: the importance of personalizing the name and address on the envelope, crafting a cover letter, how to fold the questionnaire, the best order in which to ask the questions, how and when to send reminders, and so forth. Response rates up to 70% could be achieved by meticulously following all of the steps. Today, survey websites, pop-up questionnaires, and automated telephone surveys have transformed survey research although the traditional door-to-door and mailed surveys are still used. The basic challenges of getting a satisfactory response rate and representative sample remain the same.

The reasons people agree to participate in a research study range from a desire to earn some money to doing something that will benefit others. Dillman and colleagues (2009) suggest that social exchange theory is a useful basis for understanding why people do and do not agree to participate in a research study. Based on work by Blau, the theory proposes that "people's voluntary actions are motivated by the return these actions are expected . . . to bring" (p. 22). In other words, they are more likely to agree to participate "when perceived rewards outweigh the costs" (p. 22). Dillman and colleagues point out that they are referring to social rewards, not economic (monetary) rewards. Social rewards may include appreciation, positive regard, feeling important, or feeling that one has done something that will benefit others. The following is a list of major sources of the motivation that underlies agreement to participate in a research study.

Altruism

Even though it may not benefit them personally, many people are willing to participate in a study that they believe will help others. For example, a family caregiver may agree to his very ill wife's participation in a study "so others don't have to go through what she's going through now," or a person who has a chronic illness may agree to participate "to help others." Don't underestimate the power of altruism. For many, it is the main reason they agree to be a part of a research study.

Curiosity

When they learn the subject of a study, some people will agree to participate just to satisfy their curiosity about the questions that may be asked or to find out how well they might do on a test.

Social Reasons

The opportunity to tell one's story or to share a personal experience may be enough to motivate people to participate, particularly if the researcher expresses genuine interest in their experience. Others may agree because their friends have done so.

Information and Diagnosis

Participation in some clinical studies presents an opportunity to obtain results on clinical tests whether a measure of lung capacity, homocysteine levels, or PSA results. Screening studies can provide information about the likelihood of having a specific problem.

Monetary Incentive

A small monetary incentive may be attractive to potential participants, even those who are not low income. Caution must be exercised, however, that the payment is not large enough to be coercive, that is, to entice people to participate for the money even though they would otherwise decline. The money or gift is meant to be a token of appreciation, not payment for work done. It is interesting to note that while providing the incentive beforehand seems to create a desire to reciprocate, giving it to people afterward does not do this (Dillman, Smyth, & Christian, 2009).

Experimental Treatment

Participation in intervention studies often provides an opportunity to access new medications, surgical intervention, or behavioral treatment that is not available otherwise. Usually these are experimental interventions that have not yet been approved or become generally accepted methods of treatment. In these instances, it is especially important that the participant is fully informed about the risks and benefits of the experimental treatment.

It is probably evident by now that a single study cannot offer all of these incentives or appeal to all of the possible sources of motivation listed. Instead, the researcher can review these possibilities for the study under consideration and consider which motivators may be employed to facilitate participant recruitment.

Barriers

"If you build it, they may not come" is the title of an article in which Lee (2009) reports the results of participant recruitment in a 5-year study of an in-home marital enrichment program for couples who adopted special needs children.

> Of the 470 adoptive couples who were eligible for this program, the researchers conservatively expected 90 (about 20%) to participate. They thought that they were offering an attractive opportunity to these couples and quote Stanley (In Lee, 2009, p. 251) as saying that, given the stresses of adopting a special needs child, "If you build it, they will come!" But the couples did not come. Only 27 enrolled; of these 11 dropped out.
>
> An evaluation was conducted to find out why the couples did not come. An ethnographic approach based on observation, documents, interviews, and focus groups was used. Many lessons can be learned from what was discovered. Lee notes, first of all, that the literature did *not* support the idea that adoptive couples wanted this program. In fact, the literature consistently reported adoptive parents' calls for help with

the children, not with their marriage. Many of the parents said the adoption had strengthened their marriage. The couples reiterated this: marital enrichment was not their immediate need. Instead, they needed help with the child (p. 258). Others saw the program's focus on their marriage as threatening. In fact, similar programs adopted nonthreatening titles such as "Healthy Marriages, Loving Children," to emphasize the positive and reduce the fears and anxieties of potential participants (p. 257). A group format with free child care might also have been more successful since the new parents reported feeling isolated and overwhelmed by their new responsibilities.

There are many other factors that may have contributed to the very small number recruited in this study. However, one factor in particular seems to underlie the recruitment problem: failure to do a needs assessment before doing the study (Lee, 2009). The reader may recall that the CBPR (community-based participatory research) design is based upon the principle of involving the population of interest in every step of the research process. Although it is a very time- and energy-consuming process, it does help the researcher to avoid "building" a program that people do not want.

The barriers or disincentives also vary by study and potential participants. The following is a list of common reasons why people decline to participate:

1. *Irrelevance:* If the study seems unimportant, uninteresting, or of no concern to the potential participant, there will be little intrinsic motivation to agree to participate.

2. *Inconvenience:* It is the responsibility of the researcher to facilitate participation in every way possible. Yet some inconvenience is likely to be present in many studies. People who are highly motivated may not be deterred by some inconvenience. A fictionalized example:

> Arthur H. was suddenly quite ill. After a series of diagnostic tests, he was told that he had a rare aggressive form of leukemia for which there currently was no approved treatment. There was, however, an experimental drug being tested at several university health centers around the country. One of the testing sites was about 250 miles from his home. Given the experimental nature of the drug, the mode of administration, and the need to be monitored closely for adverse effects, only individuals who lived within 30 minutes of the medical center were eligible for this clinical trial. He would also need someone with him to monitor his condition and, if necessary, summon help, during the 6-month treatment. After considerable thought, discussion, and budget calculations, Arthur's wife requested a leave of absence from her employer and temporarily relocated with him to an apartment within walking distance of the medical center. For Arthur and his wife, participation in the study meant a chance for life, although at great risk and cost to him and his family.

3. *Cost:* Time, energy, and monetary costs can be powerful deterrents. Reimbursement of monetary costs is reasonable and usually effective. Appreciation of the participant's time investment often is adequate to reduce the deterrence of a substantial time investment. Efforts can also be made to reduce the amount of fatigue resulting from participation. For example, testing may be divided into two or three sessions or a rest period may be provided. This is especially important when participants are ill or frail.

4. *Fear:* There are many different aspects of fear as a disincentive. Undocumented (illegal) immigrants fear being reported to the authorities and facing eventual deportation. Anyone who has used an illegal substance or engaged in other illegal behaviors may also fear that this might be reported to authorities. These fears have a legal basis.

    A different fear is fear of physical harm from taking a relatively untested drug or undergoing a relatively untested treatment. There are also fears with a psychosocial basis. These include fear of looking foolish if one cannot perform a task or offers a poorly considered opinion. More powerful is fear of embarrassment related to revealing very personal information, undergoing physical examination, or fainting when blood is drawn.

While it is possible to gain the potential participants' trust and confidence in the research team through evidencing competence and concern for the individual's safety and well-being, it is also realistic to expect that some people will still decline to participate due to one or more of the reasons listed above.

RETENTION

Enrolled participants are very valuable to the researcher. Often a great deal of time and energy have been invested in recruiting and enrolling them. The participants, too, have already invested their time and energy in your study. Attrition, the loss of subjects, is a loss for everyone involved. It is important to keep track of any participants lost to follow-up so that you can compare their characteristics to those of people retained for differences between the two groups. Attrition may not only affect your sample size but also may leave you with a biased sample that affects analysis of the outcomes (Wilson, Huttly, & Fenn, 2006).

Barriers to Retention

Why do people drop out of a study? Hudson and colleagues (2000) provided a few quotes from older African-Americans commenting on what it was like to be a participant in two of their studies, a community-based study of stress and physical health and a clinic-based study of adherence to hypertension treatment:

- "I began to get tired" (after 30 minutes answering questions)
- "Some of the questions sound like they're repeating in a different way"
- "Some of the scales are kind of confusing" (p. 77).

People can become restless, confused, frustrated, and fatigued by poorly worded, repetitive questions. Some will persist, but others will put the survey down, leave questions unanswered, or click off an Internet survey if the questions asked are not user-friendly.

Physical health problems may be a barrier to retention of participants. Those who are too ill to continue may need to be followed-up in a manner that is respectful of the effects of their illness but that can still capture the most critical information about what has happened to them. Transportation is another problem for older people or those with limited income. Arranging transportation or reimbursing participants (as quickly as possible since some may not be able to afford to wait) may encourage people to return.

Psychosocial stressors may also be barriers. The time needed to complete a follow-up interview may be too demanding for a heavily burdened caregiver or single parent holding two jobs to support the family. Some simply may not be able to continue in the study, but others will continue if the experience is positive and supportive. As mentioned earlier in the case of couples adopting a special needs child, providing child care or a much needed opportunity for an empathetic ear may be the answer.

Painful procedures and embarrassing or offensive questions are formidable barriers to retention. Painful procedures are endured when people hope for a benefit from the experience. Embarrassing questions are tolerated if the interviewer is sensitive and the questions are clearly relevant to the study. Offensive questions, often culturally insensitive questions, are not well tolerated, and the researcher should consider removing them from the study protocol.

Motivators to Increase Retention

Taylor-Piliae and Froelicher (2007) reported an impressive 97% retention rate in their exercise study (Tai Chi) done with older Chinese immigrants. Their list of strategies that were believed to have increased retention is a good place to start in considering motivators. The following are selected from their list and elaborated upon to cover a broader range of situations:

- *A well-designed plan for tracking participants:* Longitudinal study staff often request contact information for one or two people who do not live with the participant but could provide information if the participant moved or were taken ill. Frequent communication through greeting cards, study updates, and newsletters also help to maintain contact. A tracking plan may be quite elaborate in a longitudinal study as much attrition is due to inability to contact participants at a later date.

- *Personalized feedback provided:* This is especially valuable in clinical studies where participants appreciate learning the results of the tests that were done, whether a lumbar puncture, genetic tests, or depression measure, and what the results may mean.

- *Conduct the study in an accessible and comfortable location:* It is helpful to bring the study to the participants, to their homes, schools, places of worship, or community center, if this is easier for them or makes them more comfortable. If this is not possible, provide help with transportation, and make both the waiting area and interview or testing locations as pleasant and comfortable as possible.

- *Personal attention and encouragement:* The extent to which participants feel respected, important, and welcome is very important. This caring, attentive environment can overcome most physical limitations in the study location.

- *Incentives:* Small monetary payments are well-tested motivators although there are some indications that they do not constitute the primary or only reason for remaining in a study (Garner, Passetti, Orndoff & Godley, 2007). Other incentives may be small gifts, t-shirts, certificates of participation, and holiday or birthday greetings (which serve several purposes including maintaining contact).

- *Respect for cultural values, beliefs, and norms:* These will differ with every group and need to be assessed while planning the study. Some examples are:

  ○ Taylor-Piliae and Froelicher (2007) began their program after the Chinese New Year celebration had ended to accommodate their participants.

  ○ Younger, more acculturated members of ethnic minority groups may find questions about traditional beliefs insensitive. For example, African-American college students were critical of being asked if they avoided splitting the pole or if they had seen people "fall out" (from a questionnaire designed by Landrine & Klonoff, 1995) while older African-Americans were not offended by them.

  ○ Recruitment for a study of the effects of a specially designed exercise routine for individuals with advanced Alzheimer's disease had been relatively successful in nursing homes with a primarily European American resident population. However, when the researchers began recruitment in two nursing homes with a primarily Hispanic American resident population, they encountered a noticeable lack of interest on the part of the families who would provide consent. Use of Hispanic American graduate research assistants had not helped, so the researchers called a meeting of the entire research team to discuss the situation. Through observation of the transactions between research staff and families of potential participants, input from key informants who understood the cultural beliefs and norms of these families and search of the literature, several possible explanations were generated and a new, more successful approach to recruitment was implemented (Williams, Tappen, Buscemi, Rivera, & Lezcano, 2001). The families had expressed concern about disturbing their loved one's rest and comfort (*tranquilidad*). Many thought it would be best to leave them in peace and solitude (*soledad*). They also expressed considerable skepticism that anything could be done. There may also have been some feelings of guilt over placing a loved one in a nursing home rather than caring for him or her at home. To allay these concerns and present the proposed intervention in a more culturally congruent framework, the researchers reduced their emphasis on the possible superiority of the proposed intervention. Instead, they assured families that most residents appreciated the contact with research staff. They also met with multiple family members either at home or at the nursing home and offered the option of a Spanish language version of the consent form even if family members were fluent in English. The percent agreement from families that were contacted doubled when these culturally sensitive adaptations were employed.

The experience of these researchers emphasizes not only the importance of cultural *sensitivity* but also more generally of incorporating an understanding of the potential *participants*, their needs and concerns, into the recruitment plan.

- *Maintaining communication:* This motivator overlaps with many of the others. Greeting cards and study newsletters with summaries of study findings are common ways to stay in touch and express appreciation. Participants may also be encouraged to contact members of the study team to discuss concerns (Shatenstein, Kergoat, & Reid, 2008) if appropriate.

Dillman, Smyth, and Christian (2009) warn against using a negative, demanding, or patronizing tone in any communications or instructions to study participants. Reminders to return questionnaires also should be positive and appealing with some variation from one message to the next.

As was true of the barriers and incentives for recruitment, these barriers and motivators to remain in the study are not all appropriate for all studies. Various combinations of them will be appropriate for a specific study. Here is an example:

Garner et al. (2007) surveyed 145 adolescents age 12 to 18 who had completed a study of outpatient treatment for substance use. The monetary incentive ($40 for each interview and an extra $10 for completing it in a timely manner) was rated the top motivator by 77% of those surveyed. A very close second at 75% was the understanding that their participation was important. The next most important factors in the ratings were wanting to finish something they'd started, convenient mode of data collection (it didn't take too much time and could be done by telephone), and they trusted that the information they provided would not be shared with parents, counselors, or others. Ninety-five percent said they were glad they had participated. Most thought the study was worthwhile and believed it would help others.

A positive experience, trusted research staff, relevant and potentially beneficial study purposes, convenience, and modest incentives together can motivate participants to remain in a study.

CONCLUSION

In 1989, Diekmann and Smith commented that few if any research textbooks addressed participant recruitment (Dillman's work was one of the few exceptions). Berger, Begun, and Otto-Salaj remarked on the same situation in 2009. Attention to issues of recruitment, especially recruitment of hard-to-access individuals, is now increasing very rapidly.

Participant recruitment is both an art and a science. In-depth understanding of the potential participant and the context in which the study will be done is essential. What works in one context (e.g., telephone calls) may be considered rude or may be met with frequent hang-ups in another. A number of researchers have now reported their successful and unsuccessful strategies. Some have even set out to compare the effectiveness of different strategies empirically and reported their results. Epstein (2008) calls this emerging area of applied research *recruitmentology*, reminding us that, that while it can be hard work to recruit and retain research subjects, we cannot do our research without them.

We have just begun to systematically draw upon our understanding of trust, persuasion, and motivation from disciplines such as psychology, nursing, sociology, anthropology, marketing, and public relations to improve our ability to reach people and persuade them to participate. Given the importance of participant recruitment and retention, we are likely to do much more of this in the future.

REFERENCES

Auerswald, C. L., Greene, K., Minnis, A., Doherty, I., Ellen, J., & Padian, N. (2004). Qualitative assessment of venues for purposive sampling of hard-to-reach youth: An illustration in a Latino community. *Sexually Transmitted Diseases, 31*(2), 133–138.

Berger, L. K., Begun, A. L., & Otto-Salaj, L. (2009). Participant recruitment in intervention research: Scientific integrity and cost-effective strategies. *International Journal of Social Research Methodology, 12*(1), 79–92.

Bonk, J. (in press). A road map for recruitment and retention of older participants for longitudinal studies. *Journal of the American Geriatrics Society.*

Carr, S. A., Davis, R., Spencer, D., Smart, M., Hudson, J., Freeman, S., et al. (2009). Comparison of recruitment efforts targeted at primary care physicians versus the community at large for participation in Alzheimer disease clinical trials. *Alzheimer Disease and Associated Disorders.* Retrieved from http://www.ncbi.nlm.nih.gov/pubmed/19571728

Diekmann, J. M., & Smith, J. M. (1989). Strategies for assessment and recruitment of subjects for nursing research. *Western Journal of Nursing Research, 11*(4), 418–430.

Dillman, D. A. (2000). *Mail and internet surveys* (2nd ed.). New York: John Wiley & Sons.
   ✧ Just about anything you might want to know about persuading people to participate in a survey can be found in this book.

Dillman, D. A., Smyth, J. D., & Christian, L. M. (2009). *Internet, mail and mixed mode surveys.* New York: John Wiley & Sons.
   ✧ As you can see by the title, this updated edition by Dillman and colleagues has more information on research using the internet and its limitations.

Epstein, S. (2008). The rise of "recruitmentology": Clinical research, racial knowledge and the politics of inclusion and difference. *Social Studies of Science, 38*(5), 801–832.

Fisher, R., & Ury, W. L. (1981). *Getting to YES: Negotiating agreement without giving in.* New York: Penguin.

Fisher, R., Ury, W. L., & Patton, B. (1991). *Getting to YES: Negotiating agreement without giving in.* New York: Penguin.

Garner, B. R., Passetti, L. L., Orndoff, M. G., & Godley, S. H. (2007). Reasons for and attitudes toward follow-up research participation among adolescents enrolled in an outpatient substance abuse treatment program. *Journal of Child and Adolescent Substance Abuse, 16*(4), 45–57.

Harris, T. J., Carey, I. M., Victor, C. R., Adams, R., & Cook, D. G. (2008). Optimising recruitment into a study of physical activity in older people: A randomised controlled trial of different approaches. *Age and Ageing, 37*(6), 659–665.
✦ Readers might find the telephone script from this study to be of interest: it can be found in the supplementary materials at Age and Ageing *online.*

Hudson, S. V., Leventhal, H., Contrada, R., Leventhal, E. A., & Brownlee, S. (2000). Predicting retention for older African Americans in a community study and a clinical study: Does anything work? In S. E. Levkoff, T. R. Prohaska, P. F. Weitzman, & M. G. Ory (Eds.), *Recruitment and retention in minority populations: Lessons learned in conducting research on health promotion and minority aging* (pp. 67–78). New York: Springer.

Landrine, H., & Klonoff, E. A. (1995). The African American Acculturation Scale II: Cross-Validation and Short Form. *Journal of Black Psychology, 21*(2), 124–152.

Lee, R. E. (2009). "If you build it, they may not come": Lessons from a funded project. *Research in Social Work Practice, 19,* 251–260.
✦ This is a very interesting analysis of the factors contributing to an unsuccessful recruitment effort.

Pinn, V. W., Harden, J. T., & Blehar, M. C. (2002). *Outreach notebook for the inclusion, recruitment and retention of women and minority subjects in clinical research* [NIH Publication No. 03-7036]. Washington, DC: DHHS, National Institutes of Health.

Shatenstein, B., Kergoat, M.-J., & Reid, I. (2008). Issues in recruitment, retention, and data collection in a longitudinal nutrition study of community-dwelling older adults with early-stage Alzheimer's dementia. *Journal of Applied Gerontology, 27*(3), 267–285.

Taylor-Piliae, R. E., & Froelicher, E. S. (2007). Methods to optimize recruitment and retention to an exercise study in Chinese immigrants. *Nursing Research, 56*(2), 132–136.
✦ A report of a very successful recruitment and retention effort.

Wikipedia. Getting to Yes. Retrieved October 2, 2009, from http://en.wikipedia.org/wiki/Getting_to_YES

Williams, C. L., Tappen, R., Buscemi, C., Rivera, R., & Lezcano, J. (2001). Obtaining family consent for participation in Alzheimer's research in a Cuban-American population: Strategies to overcome the barriers. *American Journal of Alzheimer's Disease and Other Dementias, 16*(3), 183–187.

Wilson, I., Huttly, S. R. A., & Fenn, B. (2006). A case study of sample design for longitudinal research: Young lives. *International Journal of Social Research Methodology, 9*(5), 351–365.

CHAPTER 14

Data Collection: Testing and Observation

After all the planning is done, approvals have been obtained, and participants are being recruited, it is time to begin collecting data. The type of data you decide to collect and how you go about collecting it will have a great impact on its value in the analysis, reporting, and application phases of your research study.

If you consider the entire spectrum of nursing research, from the highly subjective nature of phenomenology to the highly controlled nature of a clinical trial or animal study, you will begin to appreciate just how many options are available to you in terms of the type of data to collect and how to collect it. The data may be highly structured or free flowing; it may be identical for every participant involved in the study or may be quite variable depending upon the participant's individual experience and situation. You may have a lengthy interaction with each participant or a very brief one. The interaction may be close and personal or entirely impersonal, intrusive or unobtrusive, pleasing or even painful. The participant in fact may no longer be alive as in historical research or a psychological autopsy after suicide, or the individual may be just entering existence as a newborn. You may have only a handful of participants or thousands.

To address this great variation yet remain focused upon the most important principles of data collection, we will begin with general principles related to the testing that is done in some studies and then proceed to observation, interviews, online data collection, and the use of secondary and archival data. Some of these methods, such as testing, generate primarily quantitative data; others, such as interviewing, may generate quantitative data, qualitative data, or both.

We will begin with the initial planning and preparation for data collection, including selection of measures, and then consider procedures for specific data collection modes. Specific approaches to testing and observation will be discussed in this chapter; interviewing in the next chapter; and online, secondary, and archival sources in the following chapter.

INITIAL PREPARATION FOR DATA COLLECTION

A disorganized approach to data collection is likely to lead to wasted time and discarded data. A forgotten question in the sociodemographic section (how could we have forgotten to ask them their age?), inaccurately recorded observations, or mishandled specimens mean you cannot fully describe your sample or completely analyze your results.

IRB Approval

It is assumed that the procedures and measures to be used have already been reviewed and approved by the appropriate IRB or IACUC committee. This means you have already selected measures and outlined your procedures. However, you may at this point realize that your choice of measure was not the very best (recruitment activities may have made you aware of the limited health literacy of your sample or participant reluctance to collect urine for 24 hours, for example) or a new measure better suited to your population may have just been published. Any substantive change must be submitted to the IRB or IACUC for approval. However, these amendments to the original protocol are usually simple to submit and relatively quickly approved unless full board review is required for a vulnerable population or the change raises new questions about your study.

Selection of Measures

We have already considered reliability, validity, and trustworthiness issues in considerable detail. The following is a list of additional considerations to review when selecting the measures for your study.

- *Reliability:* Has reliability been reported? Has it been at acceptable levels? Was it tested with similar populations under similar circumstances? If these are quite different, reliability may need to be thoroughly tested in this new study.

- *Validity:* The questions regarding reliability apply to validity as well. In addition, you must be certain the instrument actually measures what you need to measure. The Health Opinion Survey is an interesting example. If you chose this instrument on the basis of its title, you might expect that it measures people's perception of their health status, but it does not (McDowell & Newell, 1996). This instrument was created as a screening test to distinguish mentally healthy from neurotic individuals in the community. It has no theoretical base but was created empirically from answers provided by ill and well respondents (i.e., neurotic and nonneurotic individuals). The questions are interesting, asking respondents if they smoke, have cold sweats or dizzy spells, tremble, or have trouble sleeping. Physical symptoms and a vague name were deliberately chosen by its originator to disguise the purpose of the scale. Health Opinion Survey (HOS) results do distinguish neurotic and nonneurotic individuals, but it is not clear what an HOS score means. It works, but it is not clear why or how it should be interpreted (McDowell & Newell, 2006, p. 18). It has been suggested that it reflects degrees of stress experienced by the respondents. Its use is not recommended, but it is a good example of the type of measure to avoid using.

- *Trustworthiness:* If the data to be obtained are qualitative, have your data collection procedures been found to have rigor in previous studies? What is your plan to establish trustworthiness in the present study?

- *Sample characteristics:* There are a number of reasons why use of a particular measure may pose problems with your sample. A few possible participant characteristics to consider are:
  - ◦ Limited vision or hearing: Large print may be used on questionnaires that will be completed by individuals with low vision.
  - ◦ Difficulty with balance, strength, or mobility
  - ◦ Difficulty with fine motor movement such as drawing, holding a pencil or pen, or filling in dots on a computer-read test form
  - ◦ Illness and resulting fatigue, pain, distress, or delirium may limit ability to understand and respond.
  - ◦ Participant age, gender, educational level, ethnicity: Questions or tasks may be inappropriate, culturally biased, or be too difficult for some participants.
- *Difficulty level:* A difficult test may generate too much anxiety or frustration in a severely impaired participant.
- *Time and energy requirements:* Time and/or energy demanding tests or tasks may overwhelm ill or frail participants.

Rater Training

Practice using the selected measures is necessary before beginning data collection. Familiarity with the questions or tasks makes the session proceed more smoothly and allows the rater to focus on the participant's response and on entering the results accurately. If you are not collecting your own data, training of raters (data collectors or examiners) should include the following:

- Background information on the measures being used: Why they are important, how results may vary from one person to the next, how the results will contribute to the outcomes of the study
- Assuring consent and rights of participants to decline tests, skip questions, or withdraw altogether
- Confidentiality: Importance of not discussing people or their problems outside the research setting or with those who are not members of the research team as well as protection of written and electronic data
- Safety precautions related to the testing situation, whether preventing falls in mobility testing or infection when employing multiuser equipment such as pulmonary function analyzers
- Approach to participants: Making them comfortable, explaining procedures, monitoring discomfort
- Emergencies: What types of emergency situations might arise and how to handle them

- Adverse events: What constitutes an adverse event and how to handle them, also to whom they are reported, and within what time frame

- Guidelines for test or questionnaire administration

- Practice in administration of the tests

- Importance of accurate, objective scoring, and interrater and intrarater reliability

- Accuracy in recording results

- "Housekeeping" issues such as handling of completed forms, filling in missing items (such as the participant's ID on every page), recording time, date, and other information

Creating and Assembling Forms and Test Packets

Each study requires its own forms: codebooks (explained in the descriptive data analysis chapter), participant tracking forms (ID, consent dates, pretest dates, and so forth), examiner tracking (hours, participant contact), consent form files, reports for funders, adverse event reports, reports to the cooperating facility, and so forth. Names and ID numbers may be kept in separate files to protect confidentiality.

Test packet creation and assembly requires some thought. Sociodemographic information (name, date, identification number, address, occupation, race, language, education, income and so forth) are usually placed first. However, very sensitive information such as income and immigration status may be placed at the end, allowing more time to develop rapport with the participant and a higher comfort level with answering questions of a personal nature. Occasionally, it is necessary to ask for additional screening information to verify eligibility for the study. It may also be necessary to do a brief vision or hearing screen to be certain participants' results are not affected by sensory impairments. These tests need to be done before proceeding with the remainder of the tests and should be placed near the beginning of the test packet. In some instances, different forms of a test will be used for people of different educational levels or different functional levels but they should be used with some caution as this complicates analysis of the results.

Each test or questionnaire used should be formatted for ease of use, readability and ease of scoring. Some copyrighted tests may not be altered without permission—this is usually made clear by the producer of the test. You also want to be sure that all permission and fee requirements have been addressed.

Tests of a similar nature may be grouped together for ease of administration. However, in some cases, there is an *order effect* that needs to be considered in assembling the test packet. For example, reading a passage about heart disease may remind a participant of information that had been forgotten and could affect results on a knowledge test placed later in a test packet. In some cases, tests are assembled within packets in two or three different orders to allow evaluation of an order effect. Performing several similar tasks may also affect scores. For example, individuals may perform better on a second request to interpret a food label than on the first due to a *practice effect*. For this reason, any redundancy in test items also needs to be carefully evaluated.

Test Administration

In some instances, test administration is so complex that special courses are offered to prepare examiners (there is even a "spit camp" to train people to collect salivary cortisol samples correctly). If this is the case with tests that are part of your study test battery, it is certainly worthwhile to complete the course before administering the test.

In most cases, however, understanding the purpose and approach of the test and adequate practice with guidance from an experienced researcher is sufficient.

We will address some general considerations in test administration and then consider the special requirements for three different types of testing: functional tests, physical assessments, and collection of biological specimens.

General Considerations

The following are considerations relevant to most testing situations:

Motivation: Your introduction to the testing session and explanation of the value of the study may encourage the participant to complete the session.

Privacy: People can be very self-conscious about exposing any limitations or physical abnormalities. Affording privacy is not only respectful but puts them at ease.

Comfort: The temperature of the room, comfortable seating, good lighting, and quiet help the person concentrate by reducing distractions.

Physical limitations: In some cases, the testing is designed to identify physical limitations. In other cases it is important to ensure that physical limitations such as poor vision do not artificially lower scores.

Order: Be sure that questions or tasks are presented in the correct order. Do not skip around.

Timing: In some cases, the speed with which a task is completed is of interest. You might need to practice timing to be sure it is recorded accurately.

Fatigue: Adults or children who are sick, disabled, or frail may fatigue easily. It is important to be alert to increasing fatigue; in some instances, it is necessary to break the testing into separate sessions.

Frustration: If the tasks presented are too difficult, participants may want to skip them or withdraw from testing altogether. It is important to be alert to frustration levels and to have a plan for dealing with it.

Depression: Like physical illness, the presence of depression may affect participant response to questions and performance on the tasks presented.

Personal Approach

A warmly supportive approach on the part of the examiner is recommended. It is not necessary to be cold, mechanical, or emotionless to be objective and professional in your role as data collector. It is possible to engage in relaxed conversation during the session without distracting attention from the testing or slowing down the session. You can encourage the person with neutral statements such as "good," "fine," or "you're doing well." In most cases, it is not appropriate to comment on the quality of the performance or the correctness of a response, but you can acknowledge the effort with these neutral phrases. It is also not appropriate to provide hints or prompts unless they have been incorporated into the test. It is important to avoid any demeaning or condescending comments, to use "honey" or "dear" with an older person, or to be artificially sympathetic (Lezak, 1983). A genuine expression of empathy if a task is difficult or a test is painful may be appropriate and appreciated, however.

TESTS OF FUNCTION

The term *function* is used in many different ways: cognitive function, social function, physical function, self-maintenance, even health status and emotional function. Within the conceptual framework known as the disablement process, for example, the term *function* refers to any limitations on performance, while *disability* refers to specific role and task limitations. *Impairment* refers to the physical abnormality that underlies these limitations and is due to some type of disease process (Granger, 1984; Verbrugge, 1991) (see Figure 14-1).

An example where the term *function* is used a little more loosely than is done in the disablement framework, Kleinman and colleagues (2009) describe an interviewer-administered measure of function designed specifically for individuals with schizophrenia, the SOFI (Schizophrenia Outcomes Functioning Interview). The SOFI encompasses four domains of functioning defined as follows by the researchers:

Disease
Active pathology
⇓
Impairment
Physical abnormalities
⇓
Function
Limitations on performance
⇓
Disability
Specific role and task limitations

Figure 14-1   Disablement process.

Source: Granger, 1984; Verbrugge, 1991.

- *Living situation:* Ability to access residence without supervision, autonomy in scheduling

- *Independent activities of daily living:* Money management, travels independently, self-care, treatment adherence

- *Productive activities:* Parenting, working, school attendance

- *Social functioning:* Social network, appropriateness of social interaction (p. 278)

Two versions, patient and informant, were created. Agreement between patient and informant using ICCs (see the reliability chapter for an explanation of ICCs) ranged from .65 for social functioning to .78 for living situation.

Not only are different types of function measurable, there are also different perspectives from which to approach measurement of this important dimension of everyday life and different types of criteria upon which to judge functional versus nonfunctional status:

- *Testing actual performance versus report of performance:* Ratings for a well-known functional measure, the FIM (Functional Independence Measure) (Granger & Hamilton, 1992), are based upon observation, patient interview, and/or health record. It is usually completed by a therapist, physician, or nurse. The individual's degree of disability is conceptualized as an indicator of need for care and assistance (McDowell & Newell, 1996). Although rehabilitation oriented, it includes items related to memory, social interaction, and communication. In contrast, the DAFS (Direct Assessment of Functional Skills) (Loewenstein et al., 1989) tests performance on a range of skills thought to be especially affected by cognitive impairment. It includes tasks such as time and date orientation, using the telephone, making change, writing a check, and interpreting road signs.

- *Capacity versus usual performance:* Depending upon the purpose of the measurement, the participant may be asked if he or she is *able* to perform a function or if he or she *actually* performs the task (Moinpour, McCorkle, & Saunders, 1989). For example, many older married men may be capable of preparing a meal but rarely do so because their wives assume responsibility for meal preparation. In the case of individuals with emotional problems, whether or not they actually perform the task or activity may be of more interest than their physical capacity to do so.

- *Self-report versus informant report:* When the individual of interest has limited capacity to respond accurately to questions of function (due to young age, illness, or communication or cognitive limitations) an informant is often used. Considerable research has been done on self- versus informant-report suggesting that they are similar but not equivalent. For example, Sheffler and colleagues (2009) compared child and parent reports of upper extremity function, pain/comfort, and social functioning. Four hundred eighty-nine children (< 12 years of age) and adolescents (≥ 12 years of age) who had a unilateral congenital below-the-elbow deficiency and their parents were interviewed. About two thirds of the children used prostheses. The parents underestimated the children's reports of upper extremity function and reports of social functioning (particularly the adolescents). They overestimated their children's scores for comfort. The researchers concluded that parent-report cannot be considered a true proxy for self-report by their children.

- *Appropriate to the group being evaluated:* The very basic ADLs (activities of daily living), which include bathing, dressing and grooming, are too simple for most physically and cognitively intact populations. The IADLs (independent activities of daily living) are much more appropriate for adults with a temporary or mild impairment. Physical function measures may address the very basic skills such as transfers in bed and bed to chair; somewhat more difficult tasks such as sit to stand, balance, and 6-minute walks; or challenging tasks such as multiple sit to stand, balancing with eyes closed, and walking longer distances. It is important to select the appropriate level or you will encounter *floor* effects (too hard for too many participants so you have many zero scores) or *ceiling* effects (too easy so too many get perfect scores) that limit variance and your ability to detect change.

PHYSICAL ASSESSMENT MEASURES

There are a variety of physical assessment measures designed to be used in research. Many studies combine the results of testing and observation of the individual subject. Clinical expertise is necessary to administer most of these measures. Assuring participant comfort and safety, accurate timing, and accurate recording of results are important considerations in administration of these measures.

The following are some examples of studies employing physical assessment measures:

McFetridge-Durdle and colleagues (2009) measured the hemodynamic response to standing from a seated position in 17 women age 18 or older with chemical sensitivity (five also had chronic fatigue syndrome and three also had fibromyalgia). Activity levels of the women were measured using a pedometer from waking to bed time for 14 consecutive days and reported as average steps per day. American Heart Association guidelines were used for blood pressure measurement, one sitting and one standing. Impedance cardiography measures were obtained using a monitor that produces three signals including an electrocardiogram and analyzes them to produce the following:

- Thoracic fluid status
- Left ventricular function
- Blood ejected with each beat
- Vascular resistance
- Force of ventricular contraction

- Preejection period
- Left ventricular ejection time (p. 269).

Obtaining these signals requires placement of two bands around the neck and chest and placement of three electrodes, two on the chest and one behind the right ear. Participants were asked not to eat for 2 hours before the tests and not to drink fluids that contained caffeine for 4 hours before the test. The hemodynamic responses evidenced a normal pattern, but the responses were observed to be muted in comparison with results on a healthy sample.

D'Alonzo and colleagues (2009) compared two practical procedures for assessing fat mass in large numbers of participants, skin fold thickness (SKF) and bioelectrical impedance in Black, White, and Hispanic [sic] sedentary women age 17 to 44. They point out that excess total body fat is a better operational definition of obesity than BMI because an increase in muscle mass increases BMI and may incorrectly be interpreted as overweight or obesity while others may be over fat (obese) at "normal" BMI levels (p. 274). Handheld BIA (bioelectrical impedance) analyzers are commercially available. BIA may be affected by exercise, menstrual cycle, and fluid intake. It is less uncomfortable for obese participants because it uses arm electrodes and accurate measurement of skin folds requires some technical expertise with the calipers. BIA is done at two to seven body sites and the results are entered into population-specific formulas. The researchers found a high correlation ($r = .98$, $p < .001$) between the two measurements. They note, however, that formulas to calculate SKF in Asians are not yet well developed.

The APACHE II (a revised version of the Acute Physiological and Chronic Health Evaluation) was designed to measure severity of illness in intensive care unit patients and has been found to be a strong predictor of patient survival (Wagner, Knaus, & Draper, 1983; Knaus et al., 1985). The score is calculated from such patient information as age, hematocrit, serum creatinine, Glasgow coma scores, arterial pH, temperature, respirations, and heart rate. One of its uses is to compare patient outcomes across intensive care units. However, the type of patient found in different units (case mix) and differences in transfer and discharge practices can affect mortality rates and weaken the validity of the comparison (Trujiliano, 2009; Rowan et al., 1993).

BIOLOGICAL TESTS

Increasing emphasis on the use of physiological measures or biomarkers of health makes it important to consider which ones may be appropriate in your research. Most commonly collected specimens are blood, urine, saliva, sputum, and stool, but many other body fluids and tissues are potential sources of valuable data. These may include vomit, body cavity fluids (e.g., from ascites), hair and nail clippings, spinal fluid, and biopsied tissues.

Collecting Specimens

The following are general considerations in collecting specimens for laboratory analysis:

- Follow directions for collection, preservation, and transport of specimens precisely. Failure to do this will likely lead to distorted results or no data at all, both of which are very costly.

- Avoid contamination of the specimen. Improper cleaning of the site or handling of the specimen may produce false results. Blood may be contaminated by intravenous fluids, urine by vaginal secretions. If tubes for collecting blood are filled in the wrong order, the needle that enters the tube may pick up some of the powder or liquid within and transfer it to the next tube.

- Maintain specimens at the correct temperature. Most need to be refrigerated or frozen promptly, but there are some exceptions. Cryoglobulins must be kept at body temperature. You may have seen a technician tuck a collection tube of warm blood in his or her armpit and hurry to the lab with it—this is done to keep it at body temperature (L. Marchand, personal communication, April 19, 2010).

- Use the correct collection container. Laboratories usually supply the collection containers—don't make substitutions without checking with them.

- Process collected specimens according to directions. For example, blood often needs to be centrifuged before sending to the lab.

- Collect the correct amount. Do not skimp. Data collection for research purposes needs to be done at the correct time; going back to collect a specimen a second time disrupts the study flow as well as distresses the participant.

- Check the appropriate timing of the collection of specimens. Some results, such as HbA1C and CBC, do not vary appreciably over the day. Others, such as cortisol and other hormone levels vary considerably over the day, so the timing of data collection for them is critical.

Provide clear instructions to the participant. Participants need to know if they should refrain from eating, smoking, brushing their teeth, douching, and so on before the test is done. A heavy meal eaten shortly before blood is drawn may also affect the results. Fat globules displace other blood components in the serum and may distort the results.

Storage and Transport Before a Test Is Done

As indicated above, it is important to store and transport specimens in the correct containers and at the correct temperature.

Any delay in preserving the sample is a potential cause for concern. For example, the glucose level in a blood sample declines rapidly, approximately 15–25 mg an hour, because the red blood cells continue to consume the glucose. Once the specimen is spun down, this no longer occurs. Unless preserved correctly, the red blood cells will begin to break up and may release substances such as potassium into the serum, distorting the results of the analyses.

Specimens being sent to reference labs in other parts of the country are often packed in dry ice, but it is important that the specimen itself not come in contact with the dry ice. Absorbent material should be packed around the specimens in case of a leak that could present a hazard to the people handling the package.

A few examples of nursing research studies using biological data:

Fukuda and colleagues (2008) collected 10 ml of urine from 118 healthy female day shift nurse volunteers in 15 ml sterile collection tubes between 6 a.m. and 8 a.m. Samples were stored at 4°C until centrifuged and frozen at 80°C. Assays for urinary cytokines such as angiogenin (ANG), cortisol, and creatinine were done. The results were compared with scores on the Nursing Stress Scale (NSS) and well known Profile of Mood States (POMS) administered at the end of the shift, between 5 p.m. and 7 p.m. Participants were divided into high- and low-stress groups based on these scores. They found urinary ANG and cortisol levels significantly higher in the high-stress group. The researchers suggest that measurement of urinary ANG could be used to distinguish high and low levels of stress noting also that an increase in ANG production increases risk of cardiovascular disease (p. 189).

Kawano and colleagues (2009) collected saliva and breast milk samples from 22 new mothers during a home visit 2 weeks after a normal delivery. Participants were asked not to eat, drink, or brush their teeth for 30 minutes before saliva was collected. They rinsed their mouths with distilled water and rested 5 minutes before the saliva was collected on the cotton swabs. Samples were collected between 10 a.m. and 4 p.m. to avoid extremes in diurnal variations. Breast milk was collected manually by the investigator in sterile test tubes. Samples were stored at 4°C for transport to the lab, then centrifuged and frozen for most of the analyses. A portion of breast milk was drawn off for leukocyte count before freezing. A relationship between levels of secretory immune globulin or leukocyte count in breast milk and salivary cortisol was not found. The researchers suggest that diurnal variations and the interval between stress and biomarker response may have affected the results.

Newlin and colleagues (2008) conducted a secondary analysis of pretest (baseline) data from a clinical trial involving 109 black women age 21 to 74. BMI (body mass index) was calculated from their height in meters and weight in kilograms using the formula weight ÷ height^2. Overweight was defined as a BMI equal to or greater than 25; obesity as a BMI greater than 30, and extreme obesity equal to a BMI greater than 40. Glycemic control over the previous 12-week period was operationally defined as uncontrolled if the HbA1c was equal to or greater than 7.0 based upon standard laboratory analysis of venous blood samples. Religious well-being and spiritual well-being were measured with the two subscales of the Spiritual Well-Being Scale completed by participants. Holding demographic and physical characteristics constant, religion and spirituality were found to be significantly related to glycemic control using hierarchical linear regression analysis.

Analysis of biological specimens is often combined with other types of data in health related research. An example:

> Warren and colleagues (2008) followed 212 young (6 to 24 months) children recruited from a WIC clinic for 18 months. They collected information on the types of fluids consumed (sweetened or not), use of fluoride toothpaste, nighttime bottle feeding, and presence of *Mutans streptococci* in cultures of saliva. At the end of the study, they found 39% of those who had been 18–24 months at the beginning of the study had caries on poststudy examination. The presence of *Mutans streptococci* at baseline and consumption of sweetened drinks were risk factors for development of caries. This study used three data collection methods: physical examination, questionnaires, and laboratory cultures.

Statistical Analysis

Analysis of biological data may be simple when the result is dichotomous, such as malignant vs. normal tissue or positive culture vs. negative culture for *C. difficile*. Some results, such as glycosolated hemoglobin values, may be handled as a continuous variable. Other results, however, such as diurnal variations in cortisol levels, may need to be handled as a time series (Zbilut, 2009) or with other, more complex, strategies. For these, you may want to consult with a biostatistician.

OBSERVATION

Observation is often the first data collection method used when exploring a new research topic. Naturalistic or unstructured observation is probably one of the most common paths to the development of new ideas in research, leading to moments of insight that are further developed and eventually tested.

Observation may be highly structured or unstructured, but it should always be systematic and purposeful. The observer may be a participant in whatever activity is under observation or entirely outside the activity, even obscured behind one-way glass or entirely separated from the participants as the viewer of videotaped interactions.

The more structured types of observations typically generate quantitative data while unstructured or naturalistic observation typically generates qualitative data. The qualitative data are usually reported in narrative form, but they can also be organized by subject matter and can be coded and quantified in some but not all instances. Coding and quantifying would be inappropriate in a phenomenological study, for example.

Structured and Semistructured Observation

Structured observation is usually done with a set of codes, checklists, or guides that specify what is to be observed and recorded. Recording may be done either by hand or electronically but should be done immediately. Observations are usually done at regular intervals such as every 10 seconds, every quarter hour, and so forth. The observer/data collector is not likely to be an active participant in whatever activity is being observed, partially by necessity since recording may require all of the observer's time and attention but also to avoid "disturbing" the activity by changing it in any way.

Coding Forms

Many times, an existing observational code may be used or adapted for the specific setting and activity. If an appropriate existing one can be found, this is the preferred strategy because creation of a new coding scheme is time consuming and requires additional attention to the validity and reliability of the data generated. At the very least, the new form should be reviewed by experts and pilot tested before use.

> Cardona and colleagues (1997) were concerned about the amount of time nursing staff of a locked dementia unit spent responding to resident outbursts, particularly physically aggressive behaviors. To study this problem, they adapted a data collection instrument previously used by Hendrickson and colleagues (1990) in an acute care setting. Tasks unique to this unit such as traffic flow through the locked doors and behavior management were added. The modified instrument (see Figure 14-2) was piloted by the researchers on 13 8-hour shifts. Additional modifications were made to facilitate recording and to combine some of the categories, particularly those related to paperwork, and the instrument was piloted a second time. Direct patient care (e.g., bathing), indirect patient care (e.g., documentation) and nonpatient activities (e.g., breaks, meals) were the three major categories of staff activity. Staff were observed for a full 8½-hour shift. Their activities were recorded every 15 minutes. One data collector observed three staff members per shift (one recording was made every 5 minutes). Only day and evening shift staff activities were observed, but both weekday and weekend activities were observed. Random selection without replacement was used to select the days for observation. The five investigators did all of the data collection. The data obtained were analyzed quantitatively.
>
> This is an example of a highly structured observational study. Given the use of five data collectors, it was also important to test and report interrater reliability. To do this, two observers collected data on the same shift on the same three staff members but did not discuss either their observations or the data recorded on several days.

This particular type of observational data collection may be classified as work sampling, but it can be used to record activities of long-term care residents, children at play, and others of interest to the researcher. The same type of recording form was created for the purpose of determining the various functional areas of a new day center building that had the most use (lobby area, conference room, outdoor areas, art room, and so forth) and the character of the activity occurring (fully engaged, partially engaged, unengaged; sitting, standing, walking, or sleeping; solitary or group activity) by staff, participants, and visitors (see Figure 14-3). It was adapted, modified, and piloted in the same manner as the work sampling form in Figure 14-2, but in this case day care participants, staff, and visitors' use of the various areas is recorded.

DATA COLLECTOR'S NAME ________ STAFF (pls circle one) NA LPN RN DATE ________

	03:30	03:45	04:00	04:15	04:30	04:45	05:00	05:15	05:30	05:45	06:00	06:15	06:30	06:45	07:00	07:15	07:30	07:45	08:00	08:15	08:30	08:45	09:00	09:15	09:30	09:45	10:00	10:15	10:30	10:45	11:00	11:15	11:30	11:45
I. BEDSIDE PATIENT ACTIVITIES																																		
1a. Feeding																																		
2b. Bathing/Cleaning/Dressing																																		
3c. Procedures/Therapies																																		
4d. Medications																																		
5e. Education/Support—Patient																																		
6f. Education/Support—Family																																		
7g. Assessment/Rounds (nonpatient)																																		
8h. Mobility/Transfers																																		
9i. Behavior Management																																		
10j. Agitation, breaking up fights																																		
11k. Leave unit with patient(s)																																		
II. OTHER PATIENT CARE																																		
12l. Charting																																		
13m. Orders																																		
14n. Other Documentation																																		
15o. Nonreport interaction telephone																																		
16p. Nonreport interaction in person																																		
17q. Shift Change Report (rounds or tape)																																		
18r. Prepare Therapies																																		
19s. Other (e.g., making beds)																																		
III. NONPATIENT																																		
20t. Locked Door Management																																		
21u. Leave Unit																																		
22v. Personal Time																																		
23w. Breaks, Meals																																		
24x. Other																																		
	1	2	3	4	5	6	7	8	9	10	11	12	13	14	15	16	17	18	19	20	21	22	23	24	25	26	27	28	29	30	31	32	33	34

COMMENTS:

Figure 14-2 Observation coding form: Work sampling study.

Source: Cardona, 1997, with permission.

Data Collector | Date:

Side: North (L) | South (R) | Comments:

	8:00			8:15			8:30			8:45			9:00			9:15			9:30			9:45			10:00			10:15			10:30		
	St	Part	Vis	St	Part	Vis	St	Part	Vis	St	Part	Vis	St	Part	Vis	St	Part	Vis	St	Part	Vis	St	Part	Vis	St	Part	Vis	St	Part	Vis	St	Part	Vis
Sidewalk																																	
ACTION																																	
SIT																																	
STD																																	
WLK																																	
ASLP																																	
INTERACT																																	
SOL																																	
GRP																																	
ENGAGED																																	
FULLY																																	
PARTLY																																	
UNENGAGED																																	
Bench																																	
ACTION																																	
SIT																																	
STD																																	
WLK																																	
ASLP																																	
INTERACT																																	
SOL																																	
GRP																																	
ENGAGED																																	
FULLY																																	
PARTLY																																	
UNENGAGED																																	
Lobby/Hall/Total																																	
ACTION																																	
SIT																																	
STD																																	
WLK																																	
ASLP																																	
INTERACT																																	
SOL																																	
GRP																																	
ENGAGED																																	
FULLY																																	
PARTLY																																	
UNENGAGED																																	

Notes: st = staff; part = participant; vis = visitor; std = stand; wlk = walk; aslp = asleep.

Figure 14-3 Observation recording form: Day center study.

Source: Courtesy of Ruth Tappen.

Although they called it naturalistic observation, Holditch-Davis and colleagues (2001) used structured observation to collect data on mother–infant interactions during home visits when the infants were 12, 18, and 24 months old. They recorded the type of mother interaction every 20 seconds as the following:

- Directing negative affect toward child
- Directing positive affect toward child
- Playing with child
- Talking with child
- Interaction (touch, talk, play) (p. 7).

In this case, there is some overlap between the categories. The researchers noted that it took 3 to 6 months of practice before acceptable interrater reliability was achieved.

To compare various nursing homes' proportions of bedfast residents, Bates-Jensen and colleagues (2004) used hourly direct observation of residents during the daytime hours, recording whether they were in or out of bed and what they were doing. They defined bedfast operationally as having been observed to be in bed during 80% or more of the hourly observations (p. 267). They found that all the homes had underestimated the number of bedfast residents they had: those who had reported 0% to 4% bedfast residents actually had an average 8% bedfast residents based on the direct observation data.

This study demonstrates the value of direct observation when compared to self-report, which is often based upon an estimate (sometimes just an "educated guess") that can be highly subjective and inaccurate. The disadvantage, of course, is that direct observation is labor intensive, particularly in comparison with self-report.

The *degree of interpretation* required in some observational data collection is a reason to look very closely at the validity of the results and their meaning. An example is staff interpretation of behaviors thought to evidence pain in individuals with advanced dementia. Chen, Lin, and Watson (2010) found fair to moderate agreement among RNs in their assessments of pain but poor agreement among nurse aides (NA). Further, there were differences between reports of pain by the individuals themselves compared with RN and NA assessment:

- Individual self-report: 30% reported pain
- Registered nurse assessment: 18% thought to have pain
- Nurse aide assessment: 20% thought to have pain (p. 46)

The researchers suggested RNs and that NAs may not recognize some of the pain cues and may not trust the report of people with dementia. They also noted greater agreement when the individual's impairment was not as severe, suggesting a greater ability to communicate pain to staff. Training of the staff raters improved agreement.

An extreme example of how much caution may be needed when interpreting observed behaviors is the effect of masked facial expression in individuals with Parkinson disease. Mikos and colleagues (2009) warn that their diminished expressivity should not be interpreted as decreased emotional experience, yet it is easy to see how this could happen with untrained observers.

Naturalistic Observation

The work of Piaget (1969) is a classic example of systematic, purposeful observation that led to new insights regarding infant and child intellectual development. Piaget used naturalistic observation and some informal experiments to understand intellectual development in infancy by studying his own three children:

> He would sit by the crib and make careful notes of the child's play; or he would direct his attention to the child's eye movements and try to determine the direction of the child's gaze. (Ginsberg & Opper, 1969, p. 27)

These patient, detailed observations over long periods of time led him to discover phenomena such as the different types of reasoning done at different stages of a child's development. Imposing too much structure on these observations could have limited, even made it impossible, to notice and record the behaviors that led to his insights.

The informal experiments that followed the observation were designed to test some of Piaget's ideas. For example, Piaget held son Laurent age 3½ months and noted that Laurent looked at him and searched but did not attempt to nurse. When placed in his mother's arms but not touching her breast, he immediately opened his mouth wide, evidence of anticipation of feeding (Ginsberg & Opper, 1969).

Observation is also used in conjunction with other methods, especially interviews. Ethnography is a good example of research that often employs a combination of interview and naturalistic observation. Body language, gestures, and the settings within which activities occur often provide additional valuable information (Angrosino, 2005).

Some issues related to use of naturalistic observation as a research method follow.

Active vs. Nonparticipation

There is a continuum in the degree to which the investigator or data collector participates in the activities under observation. Each has pros and cons to consider in making your choice but the ultimate decision is primarily influenced by the specific situation and purpose of the study.

Active participation. This is frequently the choice of investigators who are conducting a study within their own environment, often a work setting but also as part of a support group, a day center, a community group or similar settings. The advantage of full participation is acceptance by the group (those being observed), fostering a high-comfort level and low self-consciousness. The disadvantage is, unfortunately, equally powerful. Being a part of the group means identifying with them, even eventually beginning to think like them. It is very difficult to mentally step back and observe at the same time. Spradley (1980) cautions that "the more you [already] know about a situation as an ordinary participant, the more difficult it is to study it" (p. 61). In fact the less you already know, the more of the unspoken norms, rules, beliefs, and values you will see when engaging in naturalistic observation.

Moderate participation. This is the middle ground between full, active participation and remaining on the sidelines. It strikes a balance between being an insider or an outsider. It allows the investigator time to record observations but reduces the sense of "being watched" on the part of the participants.

Nonparticipation. At this level, the investigator or data collector is an observer. This doesn't mean absolute silence or refusal to make eye contact, but it does mean being a quiet, unobtrusive presence. The advantage is that you can focus your attention on the observations being made, thinking about what is happening, what it may mean, and recording both your observations and your thoughts. At first, participants may react to being observed and try to be on their best behavior, but in most instances they revert to their usual behavior after they become accustomed to your presence.

Entering the Field

Permission to observe people is not always easy to obtain. In comparison with a clinical trial, questionnaire, or even an interview, potential participants cannot be certain exactly what you will see or how you will interpret it. This means that they will need to have a high level of *trust* in you and other members of your team. It may take considerable time and negotiating skill to gain entry, particularly if members of the group or community have reason to distrust outsiders. The extent to which the investigator differs from potential participants may also influence the decision to allow entry, whether it is a matter of age, gender, race, sexual preference, or other characteristic (Gray, 2009). Introduction by a member of the group you wish to study is often very helpful (Fetterman, 1998).

Documenting the effort to gain entry, the response of the potential participants, and your own reactions is recommended because this negotiation marks the beginning of your observation of the group of interest.

Creating a Framework for Your Observations

Observation done for research purposes is both systematic and purposeful. You cannot observe everything that is happening in most situations. Your purpose in conducting the study provides the general framework or guide to what you want to observe. More detailed direction will be developed as the study progresses.

> For example, upon entering a dementia-specific day center, the researcher observed the general environment and routines to provide background (context) before focusing on the types of communication that occurred between clients and staff and client to client, which was the purpose of the study. This research was conducted at two day centers. A sample from the contextual descriptions:

OBSERVATIONAL NOTES: CONTEXT[1]

Center I   February 23   Entered at 9:15 a.m.

Obs: It's warm in here. I can smell coffee, toasting bagels, hear scraping of knives—staff buttering bagels; sometimes they add jelly. Most clients have arrived, are sitting and watching food being prepared. Low buzz of conversation, mostly staff asking clients what they'd like to have, handing it to them, and calling them by name; little client to client conversation. Clients sipping OJ or coffee, picking up bagel and nibbling. Center manager's desk sits against the far wall. It's crowded. Old tables, folding metal chairs. Hard for clients to move around. Staff are continually rearranging tables and chairs as activities change.

Imp: Feels cozy, comfortable, quietly congenial. This atmosphere may not last the day, but this is how the day begins.

Center II   March 3   Entered 10:00 a.m.

Obs: It's quiet as I walk in. Lots of open space. New, contemporary décor in peach and blue (though seats are covered in plastic). Four to a table, big chairs. People playing with dominoes, cards—all solitary pursuits. A staff member moves quietly among the tables, calls people by name, brings them magazines, other games. There is a separate rectangular room with recliners lined up against the two long walls, big flat screen TV at far end. Clients come in to "watch the news" at noontime. Glassed in office has one person at computer, her back is to the main room.

Imp: No warmth, not just physical temperature but in staff voices, feel of room (formal), response (lack of) of clients. Not sure why yet, but does not feel as comfortable as Center I despite much nicer furniture, more space to move around. Feels empty.

Although only a sample, the difference in the two centers begins to emerge from these descriptions. These samples do not present the whole picture: more detail would be needed to enable the reader to understand each center. Note separation between observations (obs) and subjective impressions (imp), which is important. Also the abbreviated comments; short forms of words can be used to facilitate recording impressions and observations.

The following is a general list of physical environment and participant characteristics that provide context and contribute to the "thick description" that is the goal of much qualitative research:

---

[1]Obs = observation; Imp = impression.

Time and date: Record time entered and left the field, also the date to preserve sequence of observations.

Physical space description: Layout, traffic flow, furnishings, other objects, color, temperature, sounds, odors

People: Characteristics of people observed, age, gender, race, ethnic group, commonalities, dress, and so forth

Actions and interactions: Activities observed; how people, objects, and environment interact or do not interact

Emotional climate: Any evidence of the feeling states of the people observed

Implicit understandings, norms, expectations: Interpretation of actions, interactions, apparent goals, purpose

Sequencing: Patterns to actions, interactions

Timing: Tempo, rhythms, energy levels

Events: Larger-scale interactions that occur (Gray, 2009; Spradley, 1980)

This list just provides a starting point. The purpose of your study and unique features of your setting and characteristics of the people observed will direct the specifics of your naturalistic observations.

Recording Observations and Field Notes

You cannot record everything you observe, even if you adopt a nonparticipant role. Keep the purpose of your study in mind as you record what you see. You may use video or audio recordings, with permission, but will still have to develop either a coding form or observation framework for analyzing the data. The effect of video recording also needs to be considered before using it.

Notes taken on site are usually brief and abbreviated, whether handwritten or typed into a word-processing program. To the extent possible try to record important comments verbatim rather than paraphrasing. Rich detail (thick description) is the goal, not generalizations or summaries. Table 14-1 shows an example of the difference between summarized generalities and rich detail from the study of staff–client and client–client communication in an adult day center.

It is evident that there is little data to analyze in the summarized observation, but there is rich detail to be analyzed in the expanded observation, which is a typed version of notes taken at the center while the interchange was occurring. Note the difference between recording what was observed and recording impressions. These need to be clearly separated in your documentation. It is essential that you distinguish statements made by participants (paraphrased or verbatim quotes), objective observations (description of what you see *without interpretation*), your interpretation of the observed situation, and your subjective response to what is observed. Furthermore, separate notations of insights, theoretical explanations, and possible hypotheses should be recorded. Be sure to date each entry.

TABLE 14-1   Summarized vs. Detailed Observational Notes

Date April 14	Summarized Observation	Detailed Observation
Time: 10:45 a.m.	New client attended today	Newcomer (her first day at the center)
Site: Center I	She was very quiet but may have been a little overwhelmed by the new surroundings. A full-time attendee approached her and questioned her about arrangements to be picked up at the end of the day.	First saw her speaking with social worker in a corner of the main room. Heard social worker ask, "Tell me what kinds of problems you are having with your memory?" Did not hear her answer or remainder of their conversation but saw that newcomer was answering quietly, social worker nodding. At end of conversation, social worker brought her to a table and pulled out a chair for her to sit with others at the table. Did not introduce her [perhaps because the group was singing at the moment?]
		Old timer: a full-time attendee, RL arrives early, brought by daughter who works full-time, picks her up at closing time. She is an energetic lady, a "handful" for staff sometimes though not aggressive verbally or physically. As soon as social worker left the main room, RL got up from her chair and walked over, took empty seat next to the newcomer, asked her how she got there. "My son brought me." "Is he going to pick you up?" "I don't know. I guess . . ." "Does he know when to pick you up?" Newcomer took a deep breath, seemed to be getting ready to answer "If he doesn't get here in time, they'll lock the doors and you'll be here all night." Newcomer sits there, blinking rapidly, hands clasped tightly in lap, says nothing [It appears that no staff heard this conversation. No one turned toward them, no one corrects RL.]
		Imp: Wonder if RL scared the newcomer.
		Evidence of concerns of adult day center attendees. Evidence of attendees' awareness of their limitations and dependence on others?

Spradley (1980) offers a helpful list of the types of data that should be recorded:

1. *Condensed notes:* These are your on the spot notes, abbreviated to save time and to record as much as possible.

2. *Expanded account:* As soon as possible (preferably immediately) after leaving the field, fill in as many details as you can to expand upon the original condensed notes.

3. *Personal journal:* Here you record your "experiences, ideas, fears, mistakes, confusion, breakthroughs, and problems," related to your observational data collection (Spradley, 1980, p. 71). These are your reactions and feelings.

4. *Analysis and interpretations:* Here is where you note patterns that emerge from the data, your own insights and theorizing, analysis of the meaning of what you have observed, the implications for the people involved, connections to what you have read, and so forth.

Using Video Recordings

An advantage of video recordings is that they are a permanent record of your observations. They may be reviewed as many times as you want, paused, reversed to recheck what you thought you saw, and so forth. They can also be used for more than one analysis:

> Solberg and Morse (1991) analyzed 40 hours of video recordings made of four male infants who had had chest surgery. The recordings were begun 12 hours postoperatively and continued for 4 hours. The infants had been intubated so were unable to cry aloud. This was a secondary analysis of the recordings that had originally been done to study infants' pain response. The purpose of the secondary analysis was to examine comforting strategies used by their caregivers during periods of distress. Distress was operationally defined as evidenced by such behaviors as frowning, movement of legs, and crying-related movements. The end of a period of distress was operationally defined as being marked by "a quiet state, a drowsy state, or by falling asleep" (p. 80).

Duration of periods of distress was measured in seconds. Both the infants' and caregivers' behaviors were noted as were patterns of interaction between them. Thirty periods of distress and 98 episodes of comforting were noted. The comforting strategies included patting, kissing, rocking, squeezing, and vocalizations. The researchers noted that the comforting strategies were not always effective and that the infants were often handled without regard to the location of their incisions.

There are disadvantages to using video recordings as well. It is difficult to follow people who are moving around, as in the day center example. The recordings may not pick up subtle facial expressions or quiet vocalizations unless volume and distance from the individual are carefully set to do this. They also do not pick up room temperature or odors. But most important is the effect of recording on both the observer and the observed. The more naturalistic observations are difficult to obtain with video until participants become accustomed to the recording equipment and go back to their usual behavior, while the task of recording may distract the observer from the main goal—observation.

CONCLUSION

Whether you are collecting blood samples, completing an observational code sheet, or doing field work with a group entirely new to your experience, be sure to keep your mind engaged and open to new connections between what you already know and what you are observing and/or hearing. Discovery can go hand in hand with even the most structured research protocol for data collection if you remain open to this possibility.

This chapter addressed testing and observational methods of data collection. The next chapter will address the use of interviews to collect data.

REFERENCES

Angrosino, M. V. (2005). Recontextualizing observation: Ethnography, pedagogy and the prospects for a progressive political agenda. In N. K. Denzin, & Y. S. Lincoln, *The Sage handbook of qualitative research* (pp. 729–745). Thousand Oaks, CA: Sage.

Bates-Jensen, B. M., Alessi, C. A., Cadogan, M., Levy-Storms, L., Jorge, J., Yushii, J., Al-Sumarcai, N. R., & Schnelle, J. F. (2004). The minimum data set bedfast quality indicator. *Nursing Research, 53*(4), 260–272.

Cardona, P., Tappen, R. M., Terrill, M., Acosta, M., & Eusebe, M. I. (1997). Nursing staff time allocation in long-term care: A work sampling study. *Journal of Nursing Administration, 27*(2), 28–36.

Chen, Y-H., Lin, L-C., & Watson, R. (2010). Validating nurses' and nursing assistants' report of assessing pain in older people with dementia. *Journal of Clinical Nursing, 19*, 42–52.

D'Alonzo, K. T., Aluf, A., Vincent, L., & Cooper, K. (2009). A comparison of field methods to assess body composition in a diverse group of sedentary women. *Biological Research for Nursing, 10*, 274. doi: 10.1177/1099800408326583.

Denzin, N. K., & Lincoln, Y. S. (2005). *The Sage handbook of qualitative research*. Thousand Oaks, CA: Sage.

Denzin, N. K., & Lincoln, Y. S. (2003). *Collecting and interpreting qualitative materials*. Thousand Oaks, CA: Sage.

Fetterman, D. M. (1998). *Ethnography: Step by step*. Thousand Oaks, CA: Sage.

Fukuda, H., Ichinose, T., Kusama, T., Yoshidome, A., Anndow, K., Akiyoshi, N., et al. (2008). The relationship between job stress and urinary cytokines in healthy nurses: A cross-sectional study. *Biological Research for Nursing, 10*, 183. doi: 10.117/1099800408326583.

Ginsberg, H., & Opper, S. (1969). *Piaget's theory of intellectual development: An introduction*. Englewood Cliffs, NJ: Prentice-Hall.

Granger, C. V., & Hamilton, B. B. (1992). UDS Report: The uniform data system for medical rehabilitation report of first admissions for 1990. *American Journal of Physical Medicine and Rehabilitation, 71*(2), 108–113.

Granger, C. V. (1984). A conceptual model for functional assessment. In C. V. Granger & G. E. Gresham (Eds.), *Functional assessment in rehabilitation medicine* (pp. 14–26). Baltimore: Williams & Wilkins.

Gray, D. E. (2009). *Doing research in the real world*. Los Angeles: Sage.

Hendrickson, G., Doddato, T. M., & Kovner, C. T. (1990). How do nurses use their time? *Journal of Nursing Administration, 20*(3), 23–28.

Holditch-Davis, D., Miles, M. S., Burchinal, M., O'Donnell, K., McKinney, R., & Lim, W. (2001). Parental caregiving and developmental outcomes of infants of mothers with HIV. *Nursing Research, 50*(1), 5–14.

Kawano, A., Emore, Y., & Miyagawa, S. (2009). Association between stress-related substances in saliva and immune substances in breast milk in puerperal. *Biological Research for Nursing, 10*, 350. doi: 10.1177/1099800409331892.

Kleinman, L., Lieberman, J., Duke, S., Mohs, R., Zhao, Y., Kinon, B., et al. (2009). Development and psychometric performance of the schizophrenia objective functioning instrument: An interviewer administered measure of function. *Schizophrenia Research, 107*, 275–285.

Knaus, W. A., Draper, E. A., Wagner, D. P., & Zimmerman, J. E. (1985). APACHE II: A severity of disease classification system. *Critical Care Medicine, 13*(10), 818–829.

Lezak, M. D. (1983). *Neuropsychological assessment.* New York: Oxford University Press.

Loewenstein, D. A., Amigo, E., Duara, R., Guterman, A., Hurwitz, D., Berkowitz, N., et al. (1989). A new scale for the assessment of functional status in Alzheimer's disease and related disorders. *Journal of Gerontology, 44*, 114–121.

McDowell, I., & Newell, C. (2006). *Measuring health: A guide to rating scales and questionnaires.* New York: Oxford University Press.

McDowell, I., & Newell, C. (1996). *Measuring health: A guide to rating scales and questionnaires.* New York: Oxford University Press.

McFetridge-Durdle, J. A., Routledge, F. S., Sampalli, T., Fox, R., Livingstron, H., & Adams, B. (2009). Hemodynamic response to postural shift in women with multiple chemical sensitivities. *Biological Research for Nursing, 10*, 267. doi: 10.1177/1099800408324251.

Mikos, A. E., Springer, U. S., Nisenzon, A. N., Kellison, I. L., Fernandez, H. H., Okun, M. S., et al. (2009). Awareness of expressivity deficits in non-demented Parkinson disease. *Clinical Neuropsychologist, 23*, 805–817.

Moinpour, C. M., McCorkle, R., & Saunders, J. (1989). Measuring functional status. In M. Frank-Stromberg (Ed.), *Instrument for clinical nursing research* (pp. 23–45). Norwalk, CT: Appleton & Lange.

Newlin, K., Malkins, G. D., Tappen, R., Chyun, D., & Koenig, H. G. (2008). Relationship of religion and spirituality to glycemic control in black women with type 2 diabetes. *Nursing Research 57*(5), 331–339.

Piaget, J. (1969). *The child's conception of the world* (J. Tomlinson & A. Tomlinson, Trans.). Totowa, NJ: Littlefield, Adams & Company.

Rowan, K. M., Kerr, J. H., Major, E., McPherson, K., Short, A., & Vessey, M. P. (1993) Intensive care society's APACHE II study in Britain and Ireland-II: Outcome comparisons of intensive care units after adjustment for case mix by the American APACHE II method. *BMJ, 307*, 977–981.

Sheffler, L. C., Hanley, C., Bagley, A., Moliter, F., & James, M. A. (2009). Comparison of self-reports and parent proxy-reports of function and quality of life of children with below-the elbow deficiency. *Journal of Bone and Joint Surgery, 91*, 2852–2859.

Solberg, S., & Morse, J. M. (1991). The comforting behaviors of caregivers toward distressed postoperative neonates. *Issues in Comprehensive Pediatric Nursing, 14*, 77–92.

Spradley, J. P. (1980). *Participant observation.* Ft. Worth, TX: Holt, Rinehart & Winston.

Trujiliano, J. (2009). Stratification of the severity of critically ill with classification trees. BMC *Medical Research Methodology, 9*, 83.

Verbrugge, L. M. (1991). Physical and social disability in adults. In H. Hibbard, P. A. Nutting, & M. L. Grady (Eds.), *Primary care research: Theory and methods.* Rockwell, MD: DHHS, PHS, Agency for Health Care Policy and Research.

Wagner, D. P., Knaus, W. A., & Draper, E. (1983). Statistical validation of a severity of illness measure. *American Journal of Public Health, 73*(8), 878–884.

Warren, J. J., Weber-Gasparoni, K., Marshall, T. A., Drake, D. R., Dehkordi-Vakil, F., Dawson, D. V., et al. (2008). A longitudinal study of dental caries among very young low SES children. *Community Dentistry and Oral Epidemiology, 37*, 116–122.

Zbilut, J. P. (2009). Biosignatures of health. *Biological Research for Nursing, 11*, 208. doi: 10.1177/1099800409341176.

CHAPTER 15

Data Collection: Interviewing

In this second of three chapters on data collection, we examine the use of interviews to collect data. As with observation, the interview may be highly structured following a predetermined sequence using predetermined questions, or it may be unstructured, guided by the responses of the participant as the interviewer follows the conversational threads and potential themes of the interview. In either case, interviewing done for the purpose of research must be systematic and purposeful; that is, it should be well planned with a clear goal or objective in mind. Interviews are usually conducted with an individual participant, but you may also have occasion to interview a family, community group, or members of a focus group together.

The power of the interview lies in the opportunity for the participant to contribute to the direction that the study will take. Often the researcher does not know beforehand all of the important issues or responses that will arise. Open-ended interviews allow these new ideas to emerge, while closed-ended questions do not allow any opportunity for them to emerge, especially if presented as a paper and pencil or online questionnaire.

Another strength of the interview is the ability to capture the individual's experience in his or her own words. This makes it possible to convey the results to one's readers in the voices of the participants. An example:

Following hurricane Andrew, which leveled parts of Miami-Dade County, Florida, many people suffered post-traumatic stress disorder. Hearing how they experienced the hurricane and its aftermath in their own words helps an outsider understand what the experience was like:

"The whole house shook. We hid in the closet in the bathroom because it was the only room that didn't have windows."

"We left the house at the last minute and went to a shelter. But they didn't allow pets so we left our dog in the house. We never found her."

"BN [newscaster] got us through the hurricane. I couldn't go through another one without his voice on the radio."

"I can't stand wind anymore. Whenever I hear the wind, it reminds me of going through Andrew."

"It's raining in my kitchen. We can't find a tarp to cover the missing part of our roof."

"We lost all our photos, pictures of the kids as babies. Everything else can be replaced but not the photos."

"We are living in a trailer parked where our house was. We will rebuild."

"I can't live here anymore."

Notice that, while the responses are different, there is an underlying congruency in the tone of these statements. The purpose of unstructured interviewing is to collect this type of information and then analyze it either descriptively, interpretively, or both. The focus of this chapter is on the data collection; analysis will be discussed in Chapter 21. We begin with structured and semistructured interviews, and then consider unstructured interviews and the conduct of focus groups.

STRUCTURED AND SEMISTRUCTURED INTERVIEWS

Unlike structured observation, which often employs a well-developed coding format, structured and semistructured interviews are often based upon investigator-created interview guides. The most structured interview closely resembles an examiner-administered questionnaire, clearly defining the topic of interest and sometimes even putting boundaries on the responses from the participant. Semistructured interview guides, on the other hand, employ specific but open-ended questions and allow freer responses from the participant (see Figure 15-1).

Structured	Semistructured	Unstructured
Closed-ended questions	Open-ended questions	Broader, open-ended questions
Limited participant responses	Responses are usually brief, a sentence or two	Guided participant responses
Short responses, may even be "yes" or "no"	Moderately flexible, responses to different questions may overlap	Rich, in-depth descriptions obtained
Predetermined questions and forced choice response categories	Interview guide	Free-flowing dialogue, reflexive stance of interviewer
Interviewer takes neutral stance, often uses script	Interviewer has some discretion to prompt or reword question	Highly flexible interview session, follows thread of interviewee responses
Analysis done upon completion	Interviewer often takes notes about the context and interaction for later analysis	Data collection and analysis occur simultaneously

Figure 15-1   Continuum of interview approaches.

Source: Based on Fontana and Frey, 2005; Morse, 2001.

Constructing the Questions

In *structured interviewing*, a set of specific questions is used. In the most structured interview, a set of possible responses is also created (resembling a multiple choice question). This should only be done if you are certain of the range of responses that will be elicited and if you plan to analyze the results quantitatively. Along with the questions and response choices, a script for introducing the study and for prompting the participant may also be written. The idea behind preparing the questions and writing a script is to leave nothing to chance (Fontana & Frey, 2005). The downside of this most structured approach is that discovery of new perspectives, ideas, and insights is unlikely to occur. Simply allowing additional comments and encouraging the interviewer to make notes on participant reactions, comments, and observations allows for some discovery but also for greater understanding of the responses to the closed-ended questions.

Semistructured interviews employ open-ended questions that a person can answer in a few phrases or sentences. This kind of interview is used when the researcher cannot predict all the possible responses but wants to keep responses focused upon a specific topic. Consider a few examples:

Kearney (2010) used the Reaction to Diagnosis Interview (RDI), which was designed to elicit mothers' resolution of their child's psychiatric diagnosis. The RDI consists of five questions derived from the Adult Attachment Interview. The interview is conducted by trained interviewers and videotaped for later transcription. Interview duration was several minutes to a half hour.

Duxbury and colleagues (2010) used what they called pragmatic questions to interview nurses and patients after medication rounds. Examples of questions:

- For nurses: How do you feel about the medication round you have just completed? Were there any issues that needed to be dealt with after the round?

- For patients: What did you find useful or helpful about the way you have just received your medication? Are there any ways that the medication round could be improved upon? (p. 55)

Clearly, these are open-ended, semistructured questions because they are very specific and focused but do not anticipate what the responses might be as is done with structured interviews.

On a similar topic, Bolster and Manias (2009) observed and then interviewed nurses and patients concerning person-centered care. The specificity of their focus is evident in examples of the questions used:

- For nurses: How would you define person-centered care in relation to medication activities?

- For patients: How do you feel about the type and amount of information you have been given about your medications while you have been in the hospital (p. 5)?

Stevens (2010) interviewed children age 7 to 11 years old at school using a topic guide. Before beginning the interview, a leaflet explaining the study was read with the child and the child's assent was obtained. The researcher began by asking the child about both acute and chronic health problems and then how they affected the child's life. Prompts such as: "How does this affect you at school?" and "Why did it make you feel like that?" (p. 4) were used to elicit more information. The purpose of these interviews was to inform the development of a preference-based measure of health-related quality of life.

Piloting the Interview Guide

It is essential to pilot test the investigator-created questions before use in a research study. A question that is clearly understood by a researcher immersed in the topic of interest may not be clear at all to a participant. Additionally, the question may not be worded well or it may not elicit the desired response. An example:

A novice researcher interested in how acute care nursing staff respond to families of dying patients created a semistructured interview guide for staff nurses. At a research seminar, he presented the opening question to his classmates: Please describe how you respond to family expressions of concern about a dying patient.

The class was quiet for a moment, thinking about how they would answer this question. Then one classmate spoke, "How many hours do you have to listen to my answer? Do you know how many dying patients I've cared for?" Classmates agreed: this question was too broad and needed to be modified. The novice researcher presented a new question at the next seminar: Think about the last dying patient you cared for. How did you respond to the family's expressions of concern about the patient?

Classmates approved the new question. "This would take me just a few minutes to answer," said one. "Consider preceding this with a question about the context in which the nurse was caring for a dying patient. You might also want to add a question about what family members were present and how they felt about the situation." The novice researcher thanked his classmates for their suggestions. "Asking you to comment on my interview guide was really a good idea. It was like prepiloting my interview guide. I'm going to revise it as you suggested and pilot it before beginning my study."

The example illustrated the use of peer review. There are several other ways to pretest a structured or semistructured interview guide. For example you can convene a *panel of expert researchers* to review and critique the questions. If you do this, be sure to ask them to suggest alternative wording. *Behavior coding* analyzes problematic responses, such as answers that do not respond to the question, skipped questions, and incomplete answers, in order to revise them. Another helpful strategy is called the *think-aloud* technique. This is done with a few participants who are asked to think out loud instead of silently as they compose answers to your questions, sharing their thought processes with you. You can also ask them to paraphrase each question in their own words (Singleton & Straits, 2001). You could be surprised how participants interpret your question and how they decide upon an answer. This is not a matter of honesty versus dishonesty but of the clarity of the question, their comprehension of your question and differences in perspective.

Conducting the Structured or Semistructured Interview

Deviation from the script and the prepared questions is discouraged when using a structured interview. Interviewers are expected to ask the questions in the order presented and to use the prompts and probes supplied in the script. During a semistructured interview, the interviewer is expected to:

- Read the question.
- Use prompts such as "Tell me more" if needed.
- Refrain from expressing an opinion or sharing a personal experience (Singleton & Straits, 2001, p. 70).

Semistructured interviewing allows the interviewer more opportunity to explore answers for clarification or ask for a more in-depth response. The order of the questions is not considered critical, but all of them should be asked and responses recorded unless the participant is unable or unwilling to answer. The interviewer may also share a brief story or interject an encouraging or empathetic comment but should not share personal opinions. Interpretive comments may be added to the written record but should be clearly noted as such. Less structured interview guides usually end by asking the participant if he or she has any additional comments to make. Responses may be written and/or recorded and transcribed later.

UNSTRUCTURED INTERVIEWS

The open, free-flowing, relatively unstructured interview lies at the heart of qualitative data collection. Technically even the most open-ended interview for research purposes has some structure. It has, for example, a beginning, end, and a purpose, however broadly stated. The interviews are usually a dialogue, not a monologue, although a good interviewer may only have to ask a few open-ended questions to launch the interview and then add expressions of interest and understanding to keep the dialogue moving. The good qualitative interviewer will be an expert listener and keen observer.

The purpose of qualitative, unstructured interviews is to collect data that enables the researcher to "understand the experience and interpret the everyday world of the respondent and to communicate the respondent's experience, in all its rich detail, to others" (Morse, 2001, p. 318). To do this, you need respondents who have the experience sought and can reflect on it and articulate it to the interviewer (Morse, 2001).

We will consider general guidelines for conducting an unstructured interview in this chapter. More specifics related to ethnographic, grounded theory, and phenomenological interviewing and analysis, which are inextricably intertwined, will be discussed in Chapter 21.

It is especially difficult to describe qualitative data collection without reference to data analysis because they are done in tandem, if not simultaneously, in much of qualitative research. In fact, it is difficult to imagine collecting this type of data without beginning to think about the themes that are emerging, the concepts that could be constructed, or the descriptions of others' experiences that could be written.

Conducting an Unstructured Interview

These interviews are unstructured only in comparison with the structured and semistructured interview. They are not formless or chaotic as the term *unstructured* might suggest to the new researcher. Instead they are shaped by the interaction between interviewer and interviewee, evolving as the relationship and the substance of the dialogue progress.

Although these interviews do have some of the characteristics of a social conversation, there are several important ways in which they differ:

- Interviewing has a specific purpose. The interviewer is seeking information from the interviewee on a defined subject, however broadly defined it may be.

- Information flow is primarily, although not solely, from the interviewee to the interviewer (Gubrium & Holstein, 2005).

- Most of the talking is done by the interviewee, and most of the listening is done by the interviewer.

- The session is often recorded. Notes are usually made by the interviewer.

- There is a formal agreement between interviewer and interviewee that is made before the interview begins.

- Analysis, interpretation, and written reports reflecting the results of this and other interviews will be done.

Thought of in this way, you can see that you will be learning a great deal from the interviewee. This does not mean that the participant has nothing to gain from the interview. Many interviews end with the interviewee thanking the interviewer (as well as the other way round) for being a good listener, for providing an opportunity to share an experience, for helping him or her to think about the meaning of the experience, and for an opportunity to achieve closure (Spradley, 1979).

Even so, Fetterman (1989) reminds us that each participant is doing us a favor by answering our questions. In turn, it is especially important to demonstrate your respect for each participant, no matter who or what he or she may have done. It is also important to watch for any signs of boredom, fatigue, or feelings of having been insulted and to respond to these quickly.

Opening the Interview

Most interviews begin with an introduction to the study and some warm-up time with a little social conversation (Schensul, Schensul, & LeCompte, 1999). Kvale (2007) points out that these first few minutes are decisive (p. 55). This is done to provide orientation (purpose of the study, subject of the interview, recording the interview, right to decline answering a question, and so forth) and establish rapport with the interviewee, but it should not take too much time.

The interview may be organized in several different ways. Spradley (1979) suggests beginning with a *grand tour* question, one that is very general but directs attention to the subject of the interview. Here are a few examples drawn from Spradley (p. 87):

- Could you describe a typical day in . . . ?
- Tell me what you did yesterday from the time you woke up.
- Tell me how you . . .
- Could you draw a map of . . . ?

Mini-tour opening questions are similar but focus on a smaller unit of experience. For example, you could ask nurses to describe medication distribution or admission procedures instead of an entire shift. Or you can ask people with diabetes how they monitor their blood glucose levels or balance diet and exercise with work, home, or school responsibilities.

These broad questions are followed with more specific ones that ask the interviewee to elaborate, explain, compare and contrast, provide examples, and so forth.

There are several other ways to sequence your questions. You can use time, starting with the beginning of an experience ("Tell me how you first discovered you might have diabetes.") and moving forward in time. Or you can begin with a simple question and progress to more complex ones or with more concrete questions ("What symptoms do you have when an asthma attack occurs?") to the more abstract ("What do you think triggers your asthma attacks?"). With topics that are especially sensitive, it is usually best to begin with the least threatening or embarrassing aspects and proceed to the more personal, intimate details later in the interview.

Continuing the Interview

Kvale (2007) recommends keeping your questions as brief and simple as possible. There are a number of different types of follow-up questions appropriate to continuing the interview. The information sought and the purpose of the interview will guide your selection from this list:

- Prompts and probes: Could you tell me more about that? Do you have another example?
- Asking for specifics: Is there a time of day the attacks are most likely to occur? Does it happen more often in one place than another?

- Guiding the interview (changing direction or topic): Let's talk now about how you feel when an attack occurs.

- Ask for clarification: In what sense is this difficult?

- Checking your interpretations: Did you mean that . . . ? So you feel really frightened when you can't "catch your breath"?

- Pauses: These allow time for reflection, so do not rush to fill silence (Gobo, 2008, pp. 196–197; Kvale, 2007, pp. 60–61).

Completing the Interview

This is the debriefing phase. There are a few additional points to remember about ending the interview effectively:

- Review important points, and allow time for the interviewee to clarify if necessary.

- Ask the interviewee if he or she has anything else to add or additional comments.

- Be sure to express your appreciation for the interviewee's participation.

Some interviewees will share some of the most interesting information after recording has stopped so take your time ending the interview. Once the interview has ended, write down your thoughts and impressions as soon afterward as possible (Kvale, 2007).

FOCUS GROUPS

Originally a market research strategy used to evaluate such things as a new beverage or the positions of a political candidate, focus groups have become very popular in behavioral research (Morgan, 2001). There are a number of variations in the way they are conducted and some subtle differences arise out of the research purpose and the population of interest, but the basic focus group strategy has clearly been built upon the original market research approach.

Focus groups employ group discussion to explore a specific topic (Kitzinger & Barbour, 1999, p. 4). The emphasis is on *encouraging interaction* between group members while a more structured "generic" group interview would employ specific questions asked of each group member in turn—a semistructured interview done in group format.

Purpose of a Focus Group

Focus groups are designed to elicit members' experiences, perspectives, wishes, and concerns. Additionally, the researcher can learn how these perspectives are constructed and expressed through the group process (Kitzinger & Barbour, 1999). Differences in perspective among participants can be discussed and interpreted by the group, an advantage over trying to interpret differences found across individual interviews after they have been completed. Also, members of the group can influence the direction of the session, making this approach responsive to interests and concerns of the group (Soklaridis, 2009, p. 722). The following is an example of very straightforward use of focus groups that used a semistructured approach:

Plummer and colleagues (2006) used both focus group and individual interviews to explore physical therapist assessment strategies and clinical decision making related to poststroke unilateral neglect. Five focus groups were conducted, one of which was composed of new, relatively inexperienced therapists and four with experienced therapists. They used a structured interview guide composed of opening questions about their experience with stroke patients' unilateral neglect, transition questions ("Are there different types of unilateral neglect?"), key questions ("How do you assess unilateral neglect in a patient you suspect has this condition?"), questions about their training, and a closing question (p. 105). The researchers noted that the inexperienced therapists could not distinguish between diagnosing neglect and determining the type of neglect (sensory, motor, spatial, and so forth). Each group session lasted 90 minutes. Participants provided informed consent and were asked to keep the discussion confidential although the researcher is unable to assure this once people leave the group. In their analysis, the researchers noted that the functional implications of unilateral neglect for the patient were not usually assessed and that both hypothesis testing (often begun when reading the medical record before seeing the patient) and pattern recognition (looking for cues such as the patient's arm hanging over the side of the chair) were employed in making their decision.

The next example illustrates the use of focus groups with more emphasis on the interaction between group members:

Mkandawire-Valhmu and Stevens (2009) recruited 72 women attending one of four HIV clinics in Malawi to join focus group discussions of living with HIV. The average age of these women was 33. The women had from 4 to 7 years of education on average although 7 had never gone to school. Forty were married at the time of the study. Two were newly diagnosed with HIV. As the discussions proceeded, the women talked about many issues related to HIV: stigma, abandonment, assault, trying to avoid reinfection, and encouraging others to be tested (including their husbands). They also discussed difficult decisions such as the choice between avoiding exchanging sex for money or having money to feed their children and how to convince their husbands to use condoms. The researchers comment that the conversations "seemed to help women transfer the blame from themselves to broader, structurally imposed circumstances in their lives that were often out of their control, such as economic dependence on their husbands and the ubiquity of oppressive gender roles" (p. 7). The researchers make it clear that they maintained a postcolonial feminist perspective. In the focus groups, the women shared ideas for handling these issues and provided strong support to each other. The researchers note that both the research team and the participants benefitted from the focus group experience.

There is a stark contrast between the type of focus group, the topic under discussion, and the characteristics of the participants in these two examples. In the Malawi example, the focus groups were held on the days the women attended the clinic, using the long waiting times to advantage. They also tried to finish early enough so that the participants, many of whom walked to the clinic, could reach home before dark. The subject matter was literally of life and death importance to these participants. In the physical therapy example, the participants may have felt somewhat threatened or embarrassed that they did not know how to distinguish the different types of unilateral neglect, but this certainly did not have the personal importance that avoiding HIV reinfection or feeding one's children would have.

Combining Focus Groups and Individual Interviews

You may have noticed that a combination of focus groups and individual interviews were used to collect data in the unilateral neglect study (Plummer et al., 2006). This is a useful combination for a number of reasons. The primary one is that people divulge different types of information under different circumstances. Being part of a focus group populated by people with a mutual, difficult-to-discuss problem (breast cancer, HIV, sexual dysfunction, drug misuse) may give reticent individuals the support and encouragement needed to describe their experiences and express their concerns. This may have occurred in the Malawi groups.

Focus groups also provide data on the interaction between people and how status, gender, education, and other characteristics may affect a person's role in the group and how the interaction proceeds. Michell (1999) provides a good example of the different information that came out of focus groups and out of individual interviews and the value of taking note of the patterns of interaction as well as the content of the discussions. Combined, they paint a more complete picture:

> In a study of adolescent lifestyles, Michell and colleagues interviewed thirty-six 11-year-old and thirty-nine 12-year-old students. Seventy-six individual interviews were done, and 21 focus groups were held at baseline. Ten months later, 23 more interviews and 17 more focus groups were conducted. In the focus groups, the researchers noticed that the lowest status girls were withdrawn, even mute. When interviewed individually, however, they disclosed experiences of bullying and victimization that they were understandably reluctant to bring out in the group. While the 11-year-olds talked about all being friends with each other, there was evidence that they were beginning to divide into groups and could identify other students as being in the top, middle, or lower status group. The lower group girls acknowledged their status and how it felt to be lower status only during the interviews, not during the focus groups.

Conducting Focus Groups

Selecting a Meeting Place

There are some good reasons to remove people from their regular environment when conducting focus groups, particularly to reduce distractions and work demands and to attempt to reduce the hierarchical distance between managers and staff, practitioners and patients, and teachers and students. However, the considerations for holding the group sessions in the field—where the participants live and work—also have some merit (Madriz, 2003). Advantages of going to the field include the following:

- Convenience for the participants
- Higher comfort level in familiar surroundings
- Opportunity to observe the social environment

Selecting Participants

Like many other choices in design and implementation of research, selection of participants should reflect the purpose of the study. In general, it is best to restrict participation to those who have had the experience of interest to the study. Including others who have not shared this experience not only dilutes the richness of the data obtained but may also dampen willingness to divulge sensitive information. On the other hand, people new to the experience (newly diagnosed, for example) bring a different perspective from those who have a longer term involvement, and their interaction together is likely to bring out both perspectives. A group of participants who are too alike or who know each other too well may not generate the type of interaction desired.

Opening the Session

This is the critical point in the life of a focus group. The following are some points to remember:

- Tell the group the discussion is being recorded or notes are being taken if that is the case.
- Remind the group of the purpose of the session and of the research study being conducted.
- Remind the group that they should keep any information shared within the group confidential but that you cannot guarantee this.
- Encourage active participation (Edmunds, 1999).
- Begin with an open-ended but focused question, what Spradley (1979) might call a "mini-tour" question.

Maintaining Interaction

This is equally as important as an effective opening but usually easier to do if the topic is of importance to the participants.

- Help the group stay on topic, but allow, even encourage, them to bring up additional issues related to the topic. If side conversations occur, ask participants to "hold their thought for a moment," or remind them that people can only pay attention to one speaker at a time and you can only record one speaker at a time (Edmunds, 1999).

- Use encouraging nonverbal expressions of interest to keep the conversation moving along.

- Follow up on initial descriptions of participants' experiences with prompts to elaborate on important points, compare points of difference and agreement, and so forth.

Transcribing Notes and Recordings

Be sure to make notes on both the content and the group interaction. Verbatim (word-for-word) transcription is usually needed for analysis, but your notes on observed nonverbal responses and group climate will also be valuable in completing the analysis.

Analyzing the Results

Again, both group processes and content should be analyzed. Vicsek (2010) lists some issues that often arise in analysis of focus group results:

- *Format to use in quoting participants:* Frequently, verbatim samples of a piece of an interaction are included in reports and published articles to illustrate and support the thematic discussion. A little smoothing—adding commas, omitting the hesitations—can be done if it does not change the meaning, but it is important to preserve as much of the language of the participants as possible without completely losing or confusing the reader.

- *Quantification:* Information about the number of participants involved, size of the groups, average age, and other pertinent characteristics such as gender distribution, income, and education can be reported quantitatively. An entirely numerical analysis, however, is usually not appropriate. As Vicsek (2010) says, what can we conclude if the word *crime* comes up 30 times in one group and not at all in another? Very little unless we understand the context in which the discussion occurred (perhaps someone's wallet was stolen while attending the last group meeting) and whether or not the subject was discussed without using the word *crime*. Vicsek is referring to the use of content analysis, which is further discussed in Chapter 21. Quantitative data of this type can be useful in some instances, however. For example, the monopolizing of the discussion of one or two individuals can be illustrated through word counts for each participant.

- *Including the group context and interaction:* As we have seen in the examples, the group process can be affected by what is said by the participants. This should be included in the analysis and reporting of results. Lehoux and colleagues (2006) have suggested some aspects to report:

  1. Compare the researcher's purpose with the apparent goals of the participants (this requires some interpretation of participants' comments and behavior).

  2. Frequency of different types of interaction: Changing their minds, deferring to others, ignoring comments made by certain group members, questioning, supporting, and so forth

3. The apparent effect of these interactions on the content of the discussion (this also requires some interpretation)

4. The effect of the moderator, for example, the differences and similarities between the moderator and group members and the way in which the moderator led the discussion (p. 2102)

- *Generalizing to larger populations:* This is a difficult question in qualitative analysis. Vicsek (2010) suggests considering *existence generalization,* which is generalizing "the existence of a certain response, but not its distribution," meaning without any "claim that this is the whole range of responses" (p. 126). In many cases, this may prove to be a comfortable middle ground between generalizing to the larger population as a whole and not generalizing at all.

CONCLUSION

From highly structured, scripted question-and-answer sessions with forced choice responses to free-flowing dialogue, interviews are a valuable approach to data collection. Although it is true of other approaches as well, it is here that it is most apparent how much researchers *learn* from the participants. Interestingly, it is also following an interview, particularly the unstructured interview, that participants are most likely to say they enjoyed the experience and gained a great deal from it. The skill of the interviewer is an important factor here. It may take some practice to become a skillful interviewer, but it is certainly worth the effort.

REFERENCES

Bolster, D., & Manias, E. (2009). Person-centred interactions between nurses and patients during medication activities in an acute hospital setting: Qualitative observation and interview study. *International Journal of Nursing Studies.* doi: 10.106/j.ijnursta.2009.05.021.

Duxbury, J. A., Wright, K., Bradley, D., & Barnes, P. (2010). Administration of medication in the acute mental health word: Perspective of nurses and patients. *International Journal of Mental Health Nursing, 19,* 53–61.

Edmunds, H. (1999). *The focus group research handbook.* Chicago, IL: NTC Business Books.

Fetterman, D. M. (1989). *Ethnography: Step by step.* Thousand Oaks, CA: Sage.

Fontana, A., & Frey, J. H. (2005). The interview: From neutral stance to political involvement. In N. K. Denzin & Y. S. Lincoln (Eds.), *Collecting and interpreting qualitative materials* (pp. 695–728). Thousand Oaks, CA: Sage.

Gobo, G. (2008). *Doing ethnography.* Los Angeles: Sage.

Gubrium, J. F., & Holstein, J. A. (2005). From the individual interview to the interview society. In J. F. Gubrium & J. A. Holstein (Eds.), *Handbook of interview research* (pp. 3–32). Thousand Oaks, CA: Sage.

Kearney, J. A. (2010). Women and children exposed to domestic violence: Themes in maternal interviews about their children's psychiatric diagnoses. *Issues in Mental Health Nursing, 31,* 74–81.

Kitzinger, J., & Barbour, R. S. (1999). Introduction: The challenge and promise of focus groups. In R. S. Barbour & J. Kitzinger (Eds.), *Developing focus group research: Politics, theory and practice* (pp. 1–20). London: Sage.

Kvale, S. (2007). *Doing interviews*. Los Angeles: Sage.
    ✧ A readable, helpful guide to conducting research interviews.
Lehoux, P., Poland, B., & Daudelin, G. (2006). Focus group research and "the patient's view." *Social Science & Medicine, 63,* 2091–2104.
Madriz, E. (2003). Focus groups in feminist research. In N. K. Denzin & Y. S. Lincoln (Eds.), *Collecting and interpreting qualitative materials* (pp. 363–388). Thousand Oaks, CA: Sage.
Michell, L. (1999). Combining focus groups and interviews: Telling how it is; telling how it feels. In R. S. Barbour & J. Kitzinger (Eds.), *Developing focus group research: Politics, theory and practice* (pp. 36–46). London: Sage.
Mkandawire-Valhmu, L., & Stevens, P. E. (2009). The critical value of focus group discussions in research with women living with HIV in Malawi. *Qualitative Health Research.* doi: 10.1177/1049732309354283.
Morgan, D. L. (2001). Focus group interviewing. In J. F. Gubrium & J. A. Holstein (Eds.), *The Sage handbook of interview research* (pp. 141–159). Thousand Oaks, CA: Sage.
Morse, J. M. (2001). Interviewing the ill. In J. F. Gubrium & J. A. Holstein (Eds.). *Handbook of interview research* (pp. 317–330). Thousand Oaks, CA: Sage.
Plummer, P., Morris, M. E., Hurworth, R. E., & Dunai, J. (2006). Physiotherapy assessment of unilateral neglect: Insight into procedures and clinical reasoning. *Physiotherapy, 92,* 103–110.
Schensul, S. L., Schensul, J. J., & LeCompte, M. D. (1999). *Essential ethnographic methods*. Walnut Creek, CA: Altamira Press.
Singleton, R. A., & Straits, B. C. (2001). Survey interviewing. In J. F. Gubrium & J. A. Holstein (Eds.), *Handbook of interview research* (pp. 59–82). Thousand Oaks, CA: Sage.
Soklaridis, S. (2009). The process of conducting qualitative grounded theory research for a doctoral thesis: Experiences and reflections. *Qualitative Report, 14*(4), 719–734.
Spradley, J. P. (1979). *The ethnographic interview*. New York: Holt, Rinehart and Winston.
    ✧ If you can get past a few dated examples, Spradley's work is one of the most readable, helpful guides for conducting an ethnographic interview.
Stevens, K. J. (2010). Working with children to develop dimensions for a preference-based, generic, pediatric, health-related quality-of-life measure. *Qualitative Health Research.* doi: 10.1177/1049732309358328.
Vicsek, L. (2010). Issues in the analysis of focus groups: Generalisability, quantifiability, treatment of context and quotations. *Qualitative Report, 15*(1), 122–141.

CHAPTER 16

Internet, Secondary Analysis, and Historical Research

It is not always necessary to enter a new setting, recruit participants, and collect new data. In some cases, participants can be approached, surveyed, and even given help online. There are also rich reservoirs of existing data available to the researcher who knows how to find them. In this chapter we will discuss online research, secondary analysis of existing databases, and historical research. Each of these methods of data collection has its advantages but also poses some challenges for the researcher.

INTERNET-BASED RESEARCH

As increasing numbers of people gain access to the Internet through work, school, or at home, Internet-based research will probably grow exponentially. While there are many types of research that cannot be done via the Internet and some populations are unlikely to be accessible electronically (such as infants or the critically ill, although even these can be monitored remotely) in coming years, it is likely that more and more research will be done online.

Uses of the Internet

There are several ways in which the Internet may be used to support and/or conduct research. These are:

- *Access to resources:* Search capabilities on the Internet provide access to published work, information about other data sources such as historical archives, research-related services, and communication with other researchers.

- *Participant recruitment:* Online support groups, professional organizations, or special interest group websites and blogs are just a few of the ways that participants can be recruited over the Web.

There are also Internet-based panels that have been created to provide access to potential participants for research. The advantage of these panels is that members have already supplied basic sociodemographic information about themselves so that an appropriate, if not exactly representative, sample may be obtained by sorting through the membership rolls and contacting those who meet eligibility criteria. An example:

West and colleagues (2006) recruited participants from existing Internet panels of adults in the United States, Canada, Britain, and France for a study of smoking cessation. This was done through Harris Interactive, which has created panels in 125 countries. Members of these panels receive incentive points for participation that can be accumulated and redeemed for gifts. Information on smoking was available for the U.S. panel. For Canadian, French, and British recruitment, an online screening questionnaire was sent to potentially eligible participants. Those who were eligible and agreed to participate had to acknowledge consent online (p. 1353).

This is an example of an opt-in volunteer panel that is maintained over time whose members are periodically invited to participate in a study (Fricker, 2008).

Another example is Knowledge Networks (www.knowledgenetworks.com), which is a Web-enabled service providing access to a probability sample of 50,000 Americans including about 3000 adolescents age 13–17. Those who were randomly selected but did not have computer capability were given a laptop and free Internet service. A Latino panel has also been developed. If you think that a sample like this or a portion of this type of sample is what you need, be sure to inquire about the costs.

There are several other ways to recruit participants via the Internet.

Pre-Recruited Panels

Prerecruited panels are actually not recruited via the Internet but through the mail, telephone, in person, through organizations, at work, at school, and so forth. It is possible to develop a probability sample this way. Once recruited, panel members are directed to an Internet site to participate in the study. These sites may be internally created in large organizations with information support services, or the sites may be created by an outside source such as Survey Monkey (www.surveymonkey.com).

List-Based Sampling

Members of an automated electronic mailing list (LISTSERV, for example), a professional organization, or an online support group may be contacted through an e-mail message sent to all members or a selected number of the members. Large employers, universities, and other large organizations may also use their own e-mail lists to recruit participants assuming appropriate IRB approval.

Harvested E-Mail Addresses

E-mail brokers sell lists of e-mail addresses that have been "harvested" from postings or visitors to selected websites. Response rates are low for these lists, and characteristics of those solicited are virtually unknown. Some review boards may consider this an unethical way to recruit research subjects (Fricker, 2008).

Self-Selected Surveying

A banner or link placed on a website visited by people known to have the characteristics sought for your sample may reach a substantial number of potential participants. To participate, those who are interested just click on the link to your study.

Intercept Surveys

These are the pop-up surveys that appear when you enter or leave a website. Because pop-ups can be blocked and there is no information on who responds and who does not, this approach has serious limitations (Fricker, 2008).

Participant Testing and Interviewing

Computer-assisted testing (CAT) has a long and generally successful track record and some attractive features. Questionnaires may be designed to allow participants to skip questions if they are not applicable. For example, if you do not smoke, then questions about number of packs a day or type of tobacco used (cigar, cigarette, filtered, and so forth) are not applicable and will not come up on the screen. Even more helpful is the ability to accurately time participant responses, providing data on response time including any hesitations that may occur. Attention tests are also amenable to electronic presentation. Another example is the useful field of vision tests that are especially important for drivers who may be visually or cognitively impaired. Finally, complex scoring of results can be done automatically, and data (the results) can be generated in analyzable form. None of these electronic capabilities require Internet access, but they can all be made available via the Internet. An example of an ongoing research study that has capitalized on Internet capabilities:

> Project Implicit (2010) is an ongoing Internet-based research study. Participants are presented with a series of paired words such as *young* and *good* or *old* and *good* and asked to respond to them in various ways such as agree-disagree, right-wrong, and so forth. The time it takes to respond to each pair is measured. The underlying assumption of the Implicit Awareness Test is that it takes longer to respond when you are uncertain about the association than it does when the two words in the pair are closely associated in your mind. The researchers explain that there is information we are unwilling (perhaps embarrassed) to share, such as how much you eat or how much you drink or an opinion that is counter to popular belief. There are also things we are even afraid to tell ourselves. "It is well known," the researchers say on their website, "that people don't always 'speak their minds,' and it is suspected that people don't always 'know their minds.'"

For further information about the details of constructing surveys on the web, see Best and Krueger (2004), and Dillman (2000) in the reference list.

Intervention on the Web

Certain forms of intervention that you might want to evaluate can be provided via the Internet. Online counseling and support are an example of commonly used Internet-based interventions.

Although not found to significantly reduce substance use, the approach used by Alemi and colleagues (2010) is interesting. These researchers provided computers and 1 year of

Internet service to both the experimental and control group participants in the study. Members of the experimental group also were given access to online counseling. Participants were recruited from four underserved populations: a South Dakota Indian Reservation, family court in New Jersey, a probation office in Virginia, and clinic in Washington, D.C.

Educational intervention may also be provided via the Internet.

For example, Kingston and colleagues (2009) describe the creation of mental health "first aid" (MHFA) guidelines for lay people who are trying to help someone with a drinking problem. They first used a Delphi technique to obtain input from clinicians, caregivers, and consumers (people with a past history of problem drinking) on what should be in the guidelines. In a Delphi study, each member of the expert panel provides commentary and/or ratings that are then collated and reported to the entire panel. Members of the panel are then asked to provide a new round of comments and ratings. The researchers used an online evaluation survey to evaluate the usefulness of the guidelines. An e-learning version of the MHFA course on a CD is available for those who cannot attend a live course (www.mhfa.com.au).

There are a number of other ways in which people can be helped via the Internet. This includes a wide variety of psychoeducational interventions, peer support, and counseling. It also includes electronic monitoring of various physiological parameters and provision of individualized help and treatment recommendations from doctor to patient or nurse to patient via electronic communication.

Quality Considerations

Many of the concerns regarding the quality of data obtained from Internet-based research revolve around questions of sampling and participant responses. As indicated earlier, most of the recruitment strategies that are suitable for Internet-based research do not produce the probability samples that are desirable for most quantitative studies. They do, however, make it possible to reach some otherwise hard-to-reach groups such as gay groups and homebound patients and their caregivers. Other than the large probability samples that have been developed by commercial entities, Best and Krueger (2004) suggest two other ways in which a probability sample can be developed for Internet-based research: (1) if you have a complete listing of the people who constitute your population, such as students in one university or staff of one or several hospitals or home health services; or (2) if you define the population of interest as those who visit a particular website. Either of these approaches seriously limit your ability to generalize your findings.

There are certain segments of the population that are particularly difficult to access via the Internet. People with limited incomes often cannot afford either the equipment or the Internet service needed. The oldest-old often have little experience with Internet-based activities and require considerable preparation to participate. Also, those who live in rural areas where dial-up service is still the norm may be quite restricted in terms of what they can do online. Large files, such as those with multiple photographs or elaborate graphics, require inordinate amounts of time to download using dial-up service.

A second important question about the quality of data collected via the Internet concerns validity. This question was addressed in a study conducted by Seale and colleagues (2009) who compared online posting and responses to in-person interviews (both yielding qualitative data) from people with breast or prostate cancer and visitors to an online sexual health advice site. The interview transcriptions were obtained from DIPex (www.healthtalkonline), an organization of qualitative social researchers. The Internet postings came from two popular UK breast and prostate cancer websites and to Dr. Ann's Virtual Surgery (www.doctorann.org) focused on adolescent sexual health. Analysis was done using Wordsmith Tools software, creating a list of all the words used and comparing the online responses with the interview responses for frequency of keyword use. Significant differences were found. An example is the word *penis*, used 4048 times online but only 7 times in the interviews. They also noted that most of the interview responses used past tense while online the immediate future was a predominant focus. Intimate or embarrassing information was revealed more often on the Web, suggesting a "subjectively experienced" private environment on the Web (p. 7). The researchers suggest that people being interviewed are less likely to reveal intimate details, but that interviewers have an opportunity to probe for additional details. They also noted the opportunities to give and receive information and emotional support via the Internet. They suggest that Web forums may be a valuable source of data on sensitive topics.

Acceptability

Are people willing to participate in online research? This is a question addressed in a study done by Vereecken and colleagues (2009). They recruited 862 parents of children in 56 nursery schools for a nutrition study. A paper and pencil questionnaire was used for initial data collection. A subsample of 88 was asked to complete a paper and pencil food diary as well, yielding 39 completed responses (44%). The remainder were asked to do this on the Web (N = 467) yielding 217 completed (46%) ones. But of those given a choice between paper response and online response, only 5 out of 58 parents chose online over paper. The researchers speculate this was because of the time required to start up the computer, learn new software, and the assumption that it would be easier to complete the paper version. Those who did use the online forms found them user-friendly, however. Addressing concerns about sampling biases in online research, they reported that those dropping out of online participation were more likely to be fathers, smokers, of lower social status, and having lower levels of nutritional knowledge.

Using flyers, e-mails, and announcements, Bracken and colleagues (2010) recruited nursing staff for an online survey of intimate partner violence and abuse. They achieved a 52% response rate, higher than most mailed surveys. A $10 cafeteria voucher was provided as an incentive.

Ethical Concerns

Questions of privacy and what constitutes public information are complicated in Internet-based research. For example, Eynon and colleagues (2008) note that although a chat room is open to the public, participants "may feel they are part of a trusted community" (p. 26) and willingly reveal intimate details. Is it ethical to use this "public" information for research? Surveys and studies such as Project Implicit provide information about the nature of the study, and usually request electronic consent to participation.

The use of existing communications shared with other visitors to a website poses considerable challenge to protection of human subjects. If researchers inform visitors to the website that the exchanges are being observed and recorded, this may suffice in some instances. However, it remains difficult to assure that every visitor to the site is fully informed. Consultation with your IRB coordinator and reference to the latest published standards are recommended during the planning phase to be sure you are following ethical guidelines and that you will not encounter a denial of approval from your IRB.

SECONDARY DATA ANALYSIS

There is a wealth of already collected data available to interested researchers. Secondary data analysis is a reanalysis of existing datasets asking a different question or taking a different focus. The data may be quantitative or qualitative, although secondary analyses are more common in quantitative work (Gray, 2009).

Data collection is expensive in terms of both time and money. The primary analysis of a dataset often does not exhaust the information or insights that may be extracted from it. In recognition of the remaining (residual) value of existing datasets, the National Institutes of Health (2010) now requires a statement regarding plans for data sharing for any proposal requesting $500,000 or more per year. Reanalysis of existing datasets is one way to increase the return on investment of scarce research dollars.

Sources of Datasets

There are a number of official government-sponsored or government-created datasets available at local, state, and national levels. The US Census is one of the best known, but there are many others such as NHANES (National Health and Nutrition Examination Surveys), a national database that has produced a rich variety of reports. Examples of secondary analyses using existing large databases include the following:

> Belay and colleagues (1999) used national surveillance data from the CDC's (Centers for Disease Control and Prevention) national voluntary reporting system to evaluate the change in incidence of Reye's syndrome in children under 18. Under this reporting system, physicians provide information on cases to their local (often county) or state health department or directly to the CDC for the NRSSS (National Reye's Syndrome Surveillance System) database. The researchers from the CDC found a peak of 555 cases of Reye's syndrome in 1980, the year that the association between aspirin and Reye's syndrome was first reported. Since then, there has been a steady decline down to 2 cases annually in 1994 to 1992. These data suggest that the publicity about the aspirin-Reye's syndrome link was successful in changing the practice of recommending aspirin to treat fevers in children under 18.

Snapp and Donaldson (2008) conducted a post hoc (secondary) analysis of data from the 1988 National Maternal Infant Health Survey (NMIHS) on the effects of exercise in women with gestational diabetes mellitus (GDM). Older age of the mother and higher BMI were associated with GDM. Those with GDM who engaged in moderate exercise (such as walking 30 minutes three times a week) were less likely to have a large-for-gestational-age newborn. The researchers note that insulin and related drugs were not yet used to treat GDM in 1988, effectively eliminating a potentially confounding variable in the analysis.

Taira and colleagues (2009) conducted a secondary analysis of data from the National Trauma Data Bank (NTDB). This is a dataset of hospital admissions for traumatic injury from 700 trauma centers. "Off-hours" admission was defined as having occurred between 6 p.m. and 6 a.m. or on the weekend. Mortality, length of stay in the ICU, and hospital length of stay were the outcomes. An off-hours admission for burns was not found to predict mortality, contrary to findings from other ICU patient populations.

Large clinical trials may also produce rich datasets that can be reanalyzed to answer new questions. For example:

Albertson and colleagues (2009) conducted a secondary analysis of data from the Dietary Intervention Study in Children. The 660 children were age 8 to 10 when enrolled in the study and were followed for about 7 years. The researchers compared the relationship of eating ready-to-eat cereal with the children's blood lipid levels, BMI, and daily nutrient intake. They found that eating cereal was positively associated with nutrient intake in both girls and boys, and with lower blood lipids and lower BMI in the boys, concluding that there are several benefits to eating cereal. For the original study the children selected had serum LDL cholesterol levels between the 80th and 98th percentile for their sex and age and were encouraged to eat cereal as well as fruits and vegetables. In this secondary analysis, results on children in the treatment and comparison groups were combined.

You can see that this secondary analysis was quite different from the primary analysis of the effect of the intervention. It was so different, in fact, that the treatment and comparison groups were combined in the secondary analysis.

Databases from smaller studies can also yield data for secondary analysis. For example:

Mulder and colleagues (2010) enrolled 62 women who were breastfeeding their infants in a psychometric study of the Mother Infant Breast Feeding Progress Tool. Of these 62 mother and infant dyads, there was sufficient information to analyze data on 53 dyads. They reanalyzed the data obtained to examine differences between those infants who lost greater than 7% of their birth weight during their first 2 days of life and those who did not. They found the higher weight loss group (11 infants) had more feedings and significantly more voids than did the other infants, suggesting that the weight loss is primarily due to loss of fluid, perhaps due to diuresis, rather than inadequate breastmilk. They also note that, since this was a secondary analysis, the data relevant to this research question were somewhat limited.

As indicated earlier, qualitative databases may also lend themselves to secondary analysis. An example is the Solberg and Morse (1991) study described in Chapter 14 on testing and observational methods of data collections.

Advantages and Disadvantages to Secondary Analysis

It may seem that undertaking a secondary analysis is relatively easy to do. After all, it is a shortcut to obtaining a completed database, isn't it? Both the recruitment and the testing of participants are done already, and the data has been cleaned and entered into a database so many steps have already been completed.

Actually, while there are some very good reasons to do a secondary analysis, there are also a number of potential pitfalls you should be aware of before using this method of data collection. A list of both the advantages and disadvantages can be found in Table 16-1.

TABLE 16-1	Advantages and Disadvantages to Secondary Analysis
Advantages:	• Eliminates several steps in the research process, saving time and money
	• Additional use of existing databases
	• Often provides larger databases than you would otherwise have the resources to accumulate
	• Databases have been cleaned.
	• Quality of the data is often high, reflecting the expertise of those who directed the work
	• Usually there is some evidence for acceptable reliability and validity of the data.
Disadvantages:	• It is often difficult to find a database containing the desired information.
	• The sample may not be exactly what is most desirable for the new research question. For example, the sample may not be ethnically diverse or the diagnoses may be mixed.
	• Much of the information in large databases is based upon a single question rather than on in-depth questions or testing.
	• Data often are not in the ideal form for the planned analysis. Variables also may not be in desired form. For example, age may have been treated as a categorical variable instead of a continuous (interval level) variable, which limits analysis.
	• Data may not be set up in the manner needed to conduct analysis. Complex transformations may be needed
	• The software used to create the database may not be entirely compatible with your statistical analysis software.

Not one of these disadvantages is enough to cause you to abandon the idea of conducting a secondary analysis. However, if too many of them pertain, it may take weeks or even months to complete the transformation and the subsequent analysis.

Accessing Existing Databases

Understandably, there are often restrictions on the use of existing databases, including protection of participant identities and safely discarding (erasing) the data when the analysis is done. Some databases, such as Medicare information, may be costly to obtain, but the majority are available at low or no cost to qualified researchers.

You may need to learn how to use a new software package or at least spend some time understanding the set up and variables contained in an acquired database. However, if the database contains valuable information that you can extract and analyze to address your research question, then it is certainly worth the effort involved.

HISTORICAL RESEARCH

There seems to be a little bit of that famous fictional detective Sherlock Holmes in historical researchers as they search existing archives, unearthing forgotten documents, interviewing people who were on the scene of an important event, or browsing the Internet for clues to the history of nurses and the nursing profession. Some of what they uncover can make us proud of our professional heritage: the nursing leaders who rallied and protested on behalf of women's rights or on behalf of their half-starved, poorly educated clients and were independent practitioners before we used the term *nurse practitioner*. Other historical records can shock and appall us as we read of systematic discrimination against nurses of color or downright silly nursing practices such as moving flowers outside patient rooms at night.

Historical researchers work primarily with mute evidence (Hodder, 2003, p. 155). Their role is to give voice to this evidence and the people it represents through their review, analysis, and interpretation of these materials.

There are three major phases to historical research: discovery, appraisal, and synthesis (Cramer, 1992). But first, as with all research, a topic must be selected and a title created.

Selecting a Topic

There are a few things to consider when selecting a topic for a historical study:

- How much preparation you have to conduct a historical study
- Familiarity with the historical era being considered
- Potential contribution this study could make
- What is already known or not known about this topic (Fitzpatrick, 2007)

You may want to do some literature searches and read and talk with other researchers before you decide upon a topic, especially if you are new to historic research.

Compose a Title

Although every research report and article has a title, titles are especially important in historical research. The following are some of the reasons why:

- The title informs the reader of the subject of the report.
- Creative titles can also entice the potential reader to read further (Lewenson, 2008, p. 31).
- Titles help the researcher stay focused. It is so easy to go astray when doing historical research—there are so many interesting stories in the documents you read that it is hard to stay on topic. Reminding yourself of the title can help. Lewenson (2008) adds a caveat, however: if the title is too creative, it may make it difficult for interested researchers to find your study. So do not go overboard with your title but do make it interesting.

Your first attempt to compose a title is unlikely to be your last. As the study evolves and you begin the interpretive phase, you may want to shift the focus of the title as well.

Discovery

This is the search phase. Once a general topic has been identified and preliminary title composed, the next step is to find the needed information. The emphasis should be on primary sources, such as original documents, records, or interviews about the event or person under study, rather than secondary sources.

Sources

Historical researchers have a variety of possible sources that may provide the information needed.

Interviews.　If the individuals who were involved in the event of interest are still alive, they may be willing to be interviewed. This is called oral testimony or oral history. The interview is often recorded so that it may be preserved. Personal diaries and written testimony may also be used. The information obtained is often compelling. It is also a means for letting the voices of the ordinary person be heard. For example, much of what nurses do occurs in people's homes or behind closed curtains in a patient room (Miller-Rosser, Robinson-Malt, Chapman, & Francis, 2009, p. 477). Oral testimony reveals these experiences.

Archives.　Archives are repositories of original, unpublished records and documents. Records include materials produced by official (government) entities, businesses, or other organizations. Documents may be personal papers, letters, diaries, photographs, recordings, and other materials. These materials are organized by source or provenance rather than alphabetically or by subject matter and in original (chronological or in the order found) order where possible (Library and Archives Canada, 2010). For example, the early records of two hospitals would not be combined but kept separately and in order of their creation, not alphabetical order.

Archives differ from libraries in several important ways. Libraries hold published materials, which are primarily secondary sources. Archives hold original materials; many are fragile and easily damaged. For this reason, archives may require the researcher to bring only pencil and paper into their reading rooms. Materials are listed in guides to their holdings (finder's guides), but they are not always cross-indexed as is done in libraries. Materials may be accessed by mail, telephone, or in person by appointment. However, many archives are minimally staffed and unable to provide much assistance by mail or over the telephone. Copies of some materials may be available for loan but not originals (Library and Archives Canada, 2010). It is best to have become thoroughly acquainted with the information available from secondary sources (including the background or context related to your topic) before reviewing primary sources. The following is an example:

> The movement for licensure of nurses occurred at a time when women were also lobbying to gain the right to vote, own property in their own name, and keep the wages they earned. Birnbach (2010) investigated the origins of nurse licensure laws in the United States. North Carolina, New York, New Jersey, and Virginia were the first four states to create the registered nurse (RN) designation. She visited the state nurses' association offices of these four states. Many of the documents, such as minutes of meetings and letters written by leaders of the movement related to their efforts to have these laws enacted were handwritten, rather than typed. Then she traveled to state archives in each of the four states to review the related legal records. To do this, it is usually necessary to make an appointment ahead of time and to show your credentials upon arrival. Birnbach also retrieved news articles and professional journal articles on the subject (secondary sources). Secondary source information helped put these efforts in perspective: US history, law, women's rights, education of nurses, and so forth.

The website maintained by the American Association for the History of Nursing (2010) has a list of many of the archives of nursing and health care-related materials in the United States. A few examples:

- Museum of Nursing History, Philadelphia: Books, letters, documents, photographs, pre-1920 caps and uniforms
- History of Nursing Archives, Boston University: Personal and professional papers of nursing leaders, early text books
- National Library of Medicare, Bethesda, Maryland: Pictorial documentation of nursing and nursing association material
- Crile Hospital Archives, Parma, Ohio: Documents related to the history of African-American nurses located in a former US Army hospital

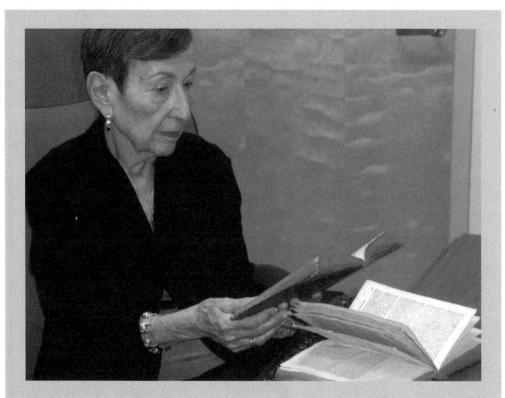

Nurse historian Dr. Nettie Birnbach is shown here examining history books from the early 1800s.

Source: Courtesy of Ruth M. Tappen, EdD, RN, FAAN.

- Alan Mason Chesney Medical Archive at Johns Hopkins, Baltimore, Maryland: Papers of almost 200 individual nurses including Isabel Hampton Robb, Adelaide Nutting, and Dorothea Orem.

There are some ethical considerations in use of documents related to personal health information that may be found in records and documents. The Health Insurance Portability and Accountability Act (HIPAA) rules prohibit release of this information without the person's permission, which is often difficult to obtain. In some cases, waivers may be obtained from the overseeing IRB or data may be deidentified (Lusk & Sacharski, 2005). Deidentification can be a labor intensive task with nonelectronic data. In some cases, the identification of the individual is critical to historical research. In this instance, a request for a waiver is preferable.

1. *Photographs:* There are several different ways to use visual materials (Harper, 2003), such as photographs in qualitative research. Photographs may be used to tell a story, as in a narrative. They can be used to document events, behavior, or settings. They also may be used to interpret events, behavior, and settings. An example of the use of photographs to supplement other historical information.

> Dowdall and Golden (2007) conducted a broad sociohistorical study of Buffalo State Hospital. Opened in 1880, it was first named Buffalo State Asylum; in 1974 it was renamed the Buffalo Psychiatric Center. Annual reports, data on over 4000 patients, meeting proceedings, and articles were reviewed, but the researchers noted that "the sense of everyday life in a complex organization" (p. 346) was missing from all of this data. In their search, they found 800 photographs that they sorted and then analyzed in what they called a "layered analysis," to describe their "ever deeper probing into the images themselves" (pp. 348–349). First, they eliminated duplicates, then long-distance exterior shots of the buildings. They noted that there were more photographs of male patients than females, many showing them at work on various tasks, yet there were actually more women than men in the institution. A stark contrast between an early photo of clean, quiet hallways and a later one of crowded hallways full of patients illustrates the crowding that occurred later. Crowding, illness, and glum expressions in the photographs suggest an environment that was more custodial than therapeutic.

2. *Statistics:* Although historical research is primarily qualitative, statistics are often included. For example, in the Buffalo State Hospital study, the researchers noted that more men appeared in the photographs, but hospital records indicated that there were more female patients than male patients. In honor of the Greek muse of history, Clio, this inclusion of statistical data is sometimes called "cliometrics" (Tuchman, 1998, p. 233).

Some of the ethical considerations in using images of individuals who are still alive are quite complex. Harper (2005) suggests that when taking a photograph would be distressing, rather than pleasing, to the subject(s) or violate their norms, it should not be done.

Appraisal

This is the analysis phase of the study, sometimes called historical criticism or literary analysis. All of the data that has been accumulated is now evaluated for its quality and then for the information that has been obtained.

Quality of the Data Obtained

Efforts need to be made to authenticate primary source material and accuracy of the interpretation. Handwriting, common expressions of the time and corroborating evidence provide some authentication. Rules for estimating the quality (trustworthiness) of the data include the following:

- Two independent primary sources that corroborate establish a *fact*.

- One primary source corroborated by a secondary source with no contrary evidence also *establishes fact*.

- Data from one primary source with no substantial contradictory evidence or from two primary sources with only minor disagreement establishes *probability*.

- If the data are only from secondary sources but provide corroboration and/or neither fact nor probability can be established, then we only have a *possible connection* (Fitzpatrick, 2007, pp. 383–384).

Secondary sources also need to be evaluated, which may be even more difficult. General acceptance of the author's work, agreement with other secondary sources, and credibility of the work are partial evidence of credibility.

Organizing the Information

There are several different ways to organize the information obtained into what will become the historical narrative. Time sequence, from the earliest events to the latest ones or to a culmination of the activities described, is a common one. An alternative is to organize the information geographically (what occurred in the United States compared to Great Britain, for example) by topic or categories such as patient-staff-administration experiences or by the activities of the primary actors (nursing leaders, for example). Two examples:

> Boschma and colleagues (2009) analyzed the central ideas of the six editions of an early, influential fundamentals of nursing textbook, *Harmer and Henderson's Principles and Practice of Nursing*. The narrative was organized sequentially, from the first to the sixth edition.
>
> Winship and colleagues (2009) analyzed oral history and archival materials from three pioneers in psychiatric nursing, Hildegard Peplau, Annie Altschul, and Eileen Skellern. Their report is organized as a description of the ideas of each scholar individually followed by a discussion in which they "triangulated" what they found to form what they called a "collective biography" (p. 505).

Fitzpatrick (2007) lists several frequently used frameworks for analysis and interpretation of historical materials:

- *Great person:* This approach focuses on influential people. An example would be a biography of one or more nursing leaders.

- *Political or economic forces:* The focus here is on the social forces and their effects on historical events. An example would be the passage of the Medicare and Medicaid legislation or the effects of the Great Depression.

- *Social forces:* The influence of social forces on historical events. For example, the women's rights movement has had many effects on the nursing profession.
- *Psychological framework:* A more controversial approach that tries to explain the thinking of the people involved. An example would be an analysis of the reasons why Florence Nightingale opposed licensure for nurses (Birnbach, 2010).

Synthesis

This is the stage during which the organized information is synthesized and interpreted by the researcher. This is the work that gives meaning to the information collected. No longer is the work simply a collection of facts or anecdotes or a recitation of a sequence of events. Instead, it now becomes a commentary on a historical event or leader, what it meant at the time, and what it tells us about the present time and future. Returning to the Buffalo State Hospital example, the researchers began with a recitation of plain facts: 800 photographs, more men than women pictured, and so forth. They proceeded to interpretation, noting the crowding, idleness, and glum expressions of the patients pictured. Finally, they synthesized their observations and interpretations, concluding that the photographs depicted a custodial environment, not a therapeutic environment.

CONCLUSION

The data collection strategies discussed in this chapter are a departure from the more common testing, observation, and interviewing strategies. Each one raises different questions about the quality of the data obtained, access to participants, and the protection of human subjects.

There is still a lot to be learned about the strengths and weaknesses of Internet-based research and questions to be answered about the ethics of using existing data that are felt to be private yet are publicly available. Secondary data analysis probably should be done more often than is currently the case. Although there are challenges to using data collected for another purpose, secondary data analyses often generate a rich yield for the effort expended. Historical research addresses entirely different questions and uses different data collection methods. It requires a sense of context and continuity unlike that of the other data collection strategies. As different as they are, each contributes to our understanding of the patients, clients, their families, and the environment in which nurses provide care.

REFERENCES

Albertson, A. M., Affenito, S. G., Bauserman, R., Holschuk, N. M., Eldridge, A. L., & Barton, B. A. (2009). The relationship of ready-to-eat cereal consumption to nutrient intake, blood lipids, and body mass index of children as they age through adolescence. *Journal of the American Diabetic Association, 190*(9), 1557–1565.

Alemi, F., Haack, M., Nemes, S., Harge, A., & Baghi, H. (2010). Impact of online counseling on drug use: A pilot study. *Quality Management Health Care, 19*(1), 62–69.

American Association for the History of Nursing. (2010). Historical methodology. Retrieved April 13, 2010, from http://www.aahn.org/methodology.html
◇ A helpful website that will direct you to a number of valuable sources for historical research.

Belay, E. D., Bresee, J. S., Holman, R. C., Kahn, A. S., Shariari, A., & Schonberger, L. B. (1999). Reye's syndrome in the United States from 1981 through 1997. *New England Journal of Medicine, 340*(18), 1377–1382.

Best, S. J., & Krueger, B. S. (2004). *Internet data collection.* Los Angeles, CA: Sage.
◇ Helpful detail on the conduct of internet-based research.

Boschma, G., Davidson, L., & Bonifaces, N. (2009). Bertha Harmer's 1922 textbook—The principles and practice of nursing: Clinical nursing from an historical perspective. *Journal of Clinical Nursing, 18*, 2684–2691.

Bracken, M. I., Messing, J. T., Campbell, J. C., LaFlair, L. N., & Kub, J. (2010). Intimate partner violence and abuse among female nurses and nursing personnel: Prevalence and risk factors. *Issues in Mental Health Nursing, 31*, 137–148.

Cramer, S. (1992). The nature of history: Meditations on Clio's craft. *Nursing Research, 41*(1), 4–7.

Dillman, D. A. (2000). *Mail and Internet surveys: The tailored design method.* New York: Wiley.

Dowdall, G. W., & Golden, J. (2007). Photographs as data: An analysis of images from a mental hospital. In S. Sarantakos (Ed.), *Data Analysis* (Vol. 4, pp. 345–372). Los Angeles: Sage.

Eynon, R., Fry, J., & Schroeder, R. (2008). The ethics of Internet research. In N. Fielding, R. M. Lee, & G. Blank, *The Sage handbook of online research methods* (pp. 23–41). Los Angeles: Sage.
◇ This handbook has a number of informative chapters on internet-based research.

Fitzpatrick, M. L. (2007). Historical research: The method. In P. L. Munhall (Ed.), *Nursing research: A qualitative perspective* (pp. 375–386). Sudbury, MA: Jones and Bartlett.
◇ A helpful introduction to the study of nursing history.

Fricker, R. D. (2008). Sampling methods for web and e-mail surveys. In N. Fielding, R. M. Lee, & G. Blank (Eds.), *The Sage handbook of online research methods* (pp. 195–210). Los Angeles: Sage.

Gray, D. W. (2009). *Doing research in the real world.* Los Angeles: Sage.

Harper, D. (2005). What's new visually? In N. K. Denzin and Y. S. Lincoln (Eds.), *The Sage handbook of qualitative research* (pp. 747–762). Thousand Oaks: CA: Sage.

Harper, D. (2003). Re-imagining visual methods: Galileo to neuromancer. In N. K. Denzin & Y. S. Lincoln (Eds.), *Collecting and interpreting qualitative materials* (pp. 176–198). Thousand Oaks: CA: Sage.

Hodder, I. (2003). The interpretation of documents and material culture. In N. K. Denzin & Y. S. Lincoln (Eds.), *Collecting and interpreting qualitative materials* (pp. 155–175). Thousand Oaks, CA: Sage.
◇ Thoughtful essay in interpretation of "mute evidence."

Kingston, A. H., Jorm, A. F., Kitchener, B. A., Hides, L., Kelly, C. M., Margan, A. J., et al. (2009). Helping someone with problem drinking: Mental health first aid guidelines—A Delphi expert consensus study. *BMC Psychiatry, 9*(79). doi: 10.1186/1471#244x-9-7.

Lewenson, S. B. (2008). Doing historical research. In S. B. Lewenson & E. K. Herrmann (Eds.), *Capturing nursing history* (pp. 25–43). New York: Springer.

Library and Archives Canada. (2010). *Using archives: A practical guide for researchers.* Retrieved January 14, 2010, from www.collectionscanada..ca/04/0416_e.html
◇ What to look for, where to look for it, how to access archival material. This is a very practical guide for the beginning historical researcher. Provides suggestions on how to obtain information by mail, telephone, or in person.

Lusk, B., & Sacharski, S. (2005). Dead or alive: HIPAA's impact on nursing historical research. *Nursing History Review, 13*, 189–197.
◇ HIPAA regulations pose some difficulties for historical researchers.

Miller-Rosser, K., Robinson-Malt, S., Chapman, Y., & Francis, K. (2009). Analyzing oral history: A new approach when linking method to methodology. *International Journal of Nursing Practice, 15,* 475–480.

Mulder, P. J., Johnson, T. S., & Baker, L. C. (2010). Excessive weight loss in breastfed infants during the post partum hospitalization. *Journal of Obstetric, Gynecological & Neonatal Nursing, 39*(1), 15–26. doi: 10.111/j.1552-6909.2009.01085.x.

National Institutes of Health. (2010). *NIH data sharing policy and implementation guidance.* Retrieved April 20, 2010, from http://grants.nih.gov/grants/policy/data_sharing/data_sharing_guidance.htm

Project Implicit. (2010). Retrieved April 20, 2010, from https://implicit.harvard.edu/implicit

Seale, C., Charteris-Black, J., MacFarlane, A., & McPherson, A. (2009). Interviews and Internet forums: A comparison of two sources of qualitative data. *Qualitative Health Research,* 1–12. doi: 10.1177/104973209354094.
  ✧ Interesting study but also an informative introduction that reviews issues related to Internet research.

Snapp, S. A., & Donaldson, S. K. (2008). Gestational diabetes mellitus: Physical exercise and health outcomes. *Biological Research for Nursing, 10,* 145. doi: 10.1177/1099800408323728.

Solberg, S., & Morse, J. M. (1991). The comforting behaviors of caregivers toward distressed postoperative neonates. *Issues in Comprehensive Pediatric Nursing, 14,* 77–92.

Taira, B. R., Meng, H., Goodman, M. S., & Singer, A. J. (2009). Does "off-hours" admission affect burn patient outcome? *Burns, 35,* 1092–1096.

Tuchman, G. (1998). Historical social science: Methodologies, methods and meanings. In N. K. Denzin & Y. S. Lincoln (Eds.), *Strategies of qualitative inquiry* (pp. 225–260). Thousand Oaks: CA: Sage.

Vereecken, C. A., Covents, M., Haynie, D., & Maes, L. (2009). Feasibility of the young children's nutrition assessment on the web. *Journal of the American Diabetic Association, 109,* 1896–1902.

West, R., Gilsenan, A., Costs, F., Zhou, W., Brouard, R., Nonnemakec, J., et al. (2006). The ATTEMPT cohort: A multi-national longitudinal study of predictors, patterns and consequences of making cessation; introduction an evolution of internal recruitment and data collection methods. *Addiction, 101*(9), 1352–1361.

Winship, G., Bray, J., Repper, J., & Hinshelwood, R. D. (2009). Collective biography and the legacy of Hildegard Peplau, Annie Altschal and Eileen Skellern; the origins of mental health nursing and its relevance to the current crisis in psychiatry. *Journal of Research in Nursing, 14*(6), 505–517.

CHAPTER 17

Intervention

Not every research study has an intervention, but if your study does, it will feel as if you have finally come to the very heart of your research study when you begin the intervention phase. Here is where you actually do what you have been thinking and talking about for what may have seemed like quite a long time.

Whenever you change, add to, or take away something from the care that is being given or from the environment of the subjects or participants, you are providing an *intervention*. Another term for intervention is *treatment*. The possibilities for intervention in health-related research are mind-boggling in their range and variety. For example, you might repaint prison walls pink to see if the change in color reduces the incidence of physical violence among inmates. You could wrap newborns snugly or let them wave their arms and kick their feet freely to see which approach reduces crying more effectively. You might try music specifically composed to have a calming effect to see if it reduces preoperative anxiety. Or you could become involved in the comparison of invasive and noninvasive devices to measure blood glucose, a test of a new herbal formulation, or in pharmaceutical research. The interventions evaluated in some research studies have been remarkably creative. A few examples of this creativity include the following:

- Painting the stairways next to the escalator in a Swedish airport to look like piano keys increased the number of people who walked instead of riding the escalator (Moore, 2009).

- Feeding junk food to rats resulted in a response similar to that of addiction: after 40 days the rats would not eat more nutritious food, even though they were starving (Sanders, 2009).

- Observation of infants crying during aircraft descent demonstrated that non-nutritive sucking reduced crying (Byers, 1986).

- Radiologists who review CT scan results seldom have the opportunity to know or even to see the patient. Turner and colleagues (2008) added patient photos (with the patient's consent) to CT scan results and compared these reports to those without photos. They found that the ones with photos attached had longer reports written and more often had incidental (additional) findings noted.

In this chapter, we will consider the many types of interventions that may be evaluated in nursing research studies and then discuss the actual implementation of an intervention.

INTERVENTIONS

Drawing upon the Nursing Interventions Classification taxonomy, Tripp-Reimer and colleagues (1996) examined the way in which the 27 classes of nursing interventions in the taxonomy (357 at the time) were structured. They found three dimensions:

1. *Intensity of care:* This dimension reflects the acuity level of the patient/client and whether the intervention is typical (routine) or novel (infrequent).

2. *Focus of care:* This dimension reflects several characteristics of the intervention, whether it is directed toward an individual, group, or entire community or population; if the action taken is on behalf of the target "patient" or provided directly; and if it is done by nurses independently or in collaboration with others.

3. *Complexity of care:* This dimension reflects the amount of knowledge and skill needed to carry out the intervention and the degree of urgency in doing so (p.15).

You can see that nursing interventions are not only many in number but also vary greatly in scope, intensity, duration, and target population.

The following discussion is not all-inclusive, but it will introduce you to the many types of interventions that may be examined for their ability to either improve health and well-being or reduce the negative effects of a health concern.

Educational interventions. Lobar and colleagues (2008) evaluated the experience of Asthma Amigos, individuals who were trained to provide community-based education about asthma in a Hispanic community. The Amigos participated in two 90-minute training sessions to prepare them to bring this information to neighbors, coworkers, friends, and acquaintances.

Self-care. Closely related to educational interventions, self-care interventions generally prepare individuals to manage their own chronic condition or implement behavior changes. Burke and colleagues (2009) interviewed 15 individuals who had completed a behavioral weight loss program that involved using a diary to self-monitor their diets. The researchers found that people's responses fell into three categories: the well-disciplined who closely followed the plan, those who followed it to some degree but really did not understand the link between the diary, self-monitoring, and weight loss, and those who had difficulty maintaining the self-monitoring behavior at all.

Lifestyle changes. Again, these are closely related to educational interventions and self-care interventions but focus primarily on primary prevention and risk reduction. Most common are changes in diet or activity, smoking cessation, and stress reduction.

Population-level interventions. A number of large community-based interventions have been evaluated, often focusing on lifestyle change at the community rather than the individual level. These may take the form of mass media campaigns, immunization pro-

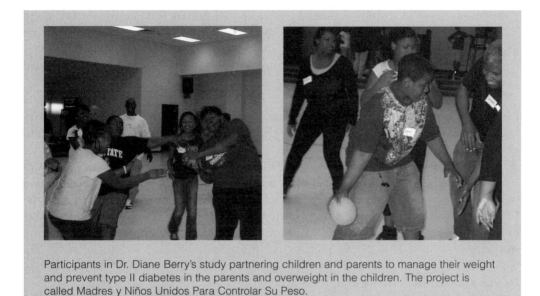

Participants in Dr. Diane Berry's study partnering children and parents to manage their weight and prevent type II diabetes in the parents and overweight in the children. The project is called Madres y Niños Unidos Para Controlar Su Peso.

Source: Courtesy of Diane Berry, PhD, ANP-BC.

grams, even changes in the laws meant to protect the citizenry, particularly but not limited to clean air, safe food, and clean water ordinances. For example, Alsever and colleagues (2009) studied the effects of a county smoke-free ordinance in Colorado. They compared hospitalization rates in the same county before and after the law went into effect and with a nearby county that did not have such an ordinance. They found a 27% drop in hospitalizations for acute myocardial infarction in the 18 months after the law went into effect, ascribing it to both the reduction in secondhand smoke and in smoking behavior.

Naturally occurring events. There are some human experiences that simply cannot be imposed upon humans but can be studied when they do occur. Many years ago, Goldfarb (1945) compared young children who were placed in foster care with those who were placed in institutions from infancy. Those in foster care had higher scores on intelligence, vocabulary, and language than did those in institutions. These differences in psychological development were ascribed to the richer environment of foster care compared with the stimulation deprivation of an institutional setting.

Physical care. A simple study by Adachi, Shimada, and Usui (2003) compared sitting and supine position effect on pain during labor. They found the sitting position superior in limiting pain in general and back pain specifically but no difference from the supine position in terms of abdominal pain.

Another pain-related study evaluated the effect of oral sucrose on behaviors indicating pain (crying, facial expression, heart rate, oxygen saturation) in sick infants undergoing heel sticks during prolonged (over 28 days) hospitalizations. Harrison and colleagues (2009) concluded that sucrose maintains its effectiveness over the course of a prolonged hospitalization.

Biofeedback. Tryon and colleagues (2006) tested the effect of feedback on the activity levels of 8- and 9-year-old boys diagnosed with attention deficit hyperactivity disorder and already on stimulant medication. Feedback was provided through an actigraphic device worn by the boys. The devices flashed green if the activity level during the quiet period of a 30-minute science class was under their baseline, red if they were over baseline, and yellow if close to the baseline. Edible rewards of moderate level were given if they kept the LED yellow, greater if they kept it at green, none if on red. Seven of the nine boys were able to keep their activity level 20% to 47% below their own baseline under the experimental condition.

Use of animal models. Although not a large proportion of nursing research studies, animal models are also used to answer health-related questions. For example, Choe and colleagues (2004) used adult male rats given surgically induced ischemic strokes to evaluate the effect on limb muscles. Their results suggested that the resultant muscle atrophy is due to disuse and undernutrition rather than to denervation.

Over-the-counter medications, herbals and supplements. There is great interest in the safety and efficacy of the various over-the-counter medications, herbal preparations, and nutritional supplements that are available without prescription. Paul and colleagues (2007) compared the effect of honey, honey-flavored dextromethorphan, and no treatment on nighttime coughing in children (not infants) aged 2 to 18 who had upper respiratory infections in a double blind, randomized study. They found honey to be most favorably rated by the parents of the children in the study.

Psychotherapeutic interventions. Counseling is often a portion or focus of psychoeducational intervention studies. For example, Schachman and colleagues (2004) created an intervention they called Baby Boot Camp as an adjunct to traditional childbirth education programs for military wives. Using resilience as their underlying framework, they helped pregnant military wives see how they could use the resources and coping strategies developed during life in the military to deal with the stresses of new motherhood. They also included use of the informal networks of military wives, especially those that formed within their spouses' military units.

Care management, care coordination, and follow-up care. Rush and colleagues (2008) report the use of Recovery Management Checkups (RMCs) for individuals with co-occurring substance use and mental health disorders. An RMC included locating the individuals for follow-up, assessing their current state of mental health, identifying need for further treatment, linking them to that treatment if needed, and following through to be sure it has been initiated.

Multicomponent interventions. Often it is clear that the synergy between multiple interventions is likely to make a combination of interventions more effective than a single facet of the intervention cluster would be on its own. For example, Schneider and colleagues (2009) described the multiple facets of the HEALTHY project intervention instituted in 42 middle schools in the United States:

1. Modification of the quantity and quality of food available within the participating schools

2. Increasing student physical activity through changes in the physical education curriculum

3. Behavioral education intervention to improve lifestyle choices, both within and outside of school

4. Promotional materials to support the program

5. Student peer communicators, also to support the program

You can see that this could be classified as a lifestyle change intervention as well.

Administrative and managerial changes in care processes. The way in which care is delivered often has a profound effect on the outcomes, either directly or through increased staff retention and satisfaction. Ferlise and Baggot (2009) reported piloting a closed-unit staffing model that included the following:

1. Staff would not be asked to float to other units.

2. Staff were sometimes asked to work extra hours.

3. Sick call and other unplanned missed days would be covered by unit staff.

4. Splitting or sharing shifts with colleagues to fill gaps was encouraged.

Staff turnover decreased and staff satisfaction increased as a result of the implementation of this staffing model.

Alternative and complementary interventions. Seskavich and colleagues (2004) compared the effect of stress management, imagery, touch therapy, and remote intercessory prayer with standard care provided in 30-minute sessions in patients undergoing percutaneous coronary intervention for acute coronary syndrome. Stress management, touch therapy, and imagery significantly reduced self-reported worry scores but not other mood indicators. Neither the remote prayer nor standard care reduced the worry scores.

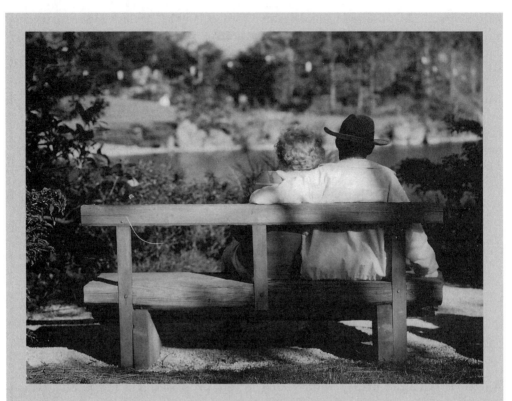

Dr. Ruth McCaffrey studied the effect of walking in gardens (a couple is shown here in the Morikami Japanese Gardens in Delray Beach, Florida) on depressive symptomatology in older adults.

Source: Courtesy of Ruth McCaffrey, DNP, ARNP-BC.

PREPARING TO IMPLEMENT THE INTERVENTION

Selecting and Training Interventionists

Selection

If you are not providing the intervention yourself, look for the following characteristics in the people who will be implementing the intervention:

- *Knowledge and skill related to the intervention:* Skill in providing a particular intervention often can be taught, but a broad base of knowledge related to the target problem is not so easy to obtain and so is important to look for in candidates.

- *Dependability:* It is critical that the intervention be provided not only correctly but as scheduled: as frequently as proposed and within the time frame proposed. Some people, for whatever reason they may have, simply cannot follow these rules and should not be selected.

- *Good judgment:* Interventionists will encounter unanticipated situations: refusals to participate, ill participants, expressions of suicide intent, and so forth. It is important that they be able to handle these situations wisely.

- *Objectivity:* This means providing *only* what the protocol calls for, nothing more and nothing less. This may be very difficult for caring people to do since they want to be helpful to people. Of course, if a serious problem is encountered, the interventionist should report it to staff if in a healthcare facility or provide a referral if working in the community. If an emergency arises, this takes priority over protocol and must be handled by the interventionist. Also, if the interventionist has an idea to improve the intervention, this should be discussed with the investigator, not tested independently.

Training

It is difficult to generalize since treatment protocols vary from very simple to highly technical and complex. An example of a moderately complex training program is in the study reported by Budin and colleagues (2008) who used a protocol guide developed by one of the investigators titled *Standardized psycho-educational and telephone counseling training manual* to conduct training before working with individuals with breast cancer (Haber, 2002, in Budin et al., 2008). The training included assigned readings, didactic sessions, role play, simulation exercises, and discussion.

Following is a general guide to providing a thorough training program for interventionists when an active intervention is planned:

1. *Purpose of the study:* Begin any training with a summary of the purpose and significance of the study in which the interventionists will be involved.

2. *Background information:* It is usually better to risk including already known information than to assume knowledge that may not have been retained. For example, if your target population has diabetes, you might include factors related to the development of diabetes, signs and symptoms, generally accepted treatment, common problems and sequelae associated with diabetes, self-care, adaptation to this chronic health concern, family responses, diabetic emergencies, and so forth as a review.

3. *Importance of maintaining the protocol:* Reasons why maintenance of protocol procedures and schedules are important should be explained thoroughly. Be sure to include circumstances that change this, such as the need for referrals if a problem arises, to whom a problem should be reported, and what to do if an emergency arises. Contingency plans should be worked out ahead of time to handle unforeseen situations and issues that may arise (Chow & Liu, 2004).

4. *Human subjects considerations:* Include the right to refuse all or part of the treatment or to withdraw from the study altogether and the right to know if new information arises that may affect a decision to continue with the study. Interventionists usually do not obtain consents but do need to know that they cannot proceed until a consent is signed and properly witnessed.

5. *The protocol itself:* A research protocol is the guidebook for the people carrying out the study. It is a working document that often is shared in the form of a notebook with sections for the raters (examiners) who will conduct the testing portion of the study, a detailed description of the treatment for the interventionists, IRB considerations for protection of the subjects (participants), schedules, lists of participating institutions, contact lists if questions arise, and other information and materials that the project team need to have readily accessible (see Figure 17-1). Raters and interventionists should carry these notebooks with them to research sites.

6. *Study design:* A brief description of the study design will help interventionists appreciate their pivotal role in the study.

7. *Rationale:* Given the study design and background information already provided, the rationale for selecting the proposed interventions should now be easier to understand.

8. *An outline of the treatment(s) that will be given:* Begin with a description of the entire treatment from beginning to end and provide an outline that interventionists can follow (for examples, see Tables 17-1 and 17-2). If several interventions are being compared, it is also a good idea to make the distinction between them clear and to be sure the interventionists appreciate the importance of keeping them distinct, not allowing the lines between them to become blurred in actual practice.

- Title page including title of the study, names of the investigators, IRB approval number, and funder if relevant
- Table of contents with page numbers for each major section
- Study team contact list
- Study abstract: a summary of the study
- Aims of the study written as objectives, with hypotheses if appropriate
- Recruitment procedures
- Participant flow chart from first contact with participant through screening, consent, testing, treatment assignment, intervention, posttesting, and follow-up testing, if any
- Inclusion and exclusion criteria including procedure for determining eligibility
- Consent procedures including explaining study, obtaining consent
- Test schedule
- Testing procedures including all tests and guidelines for administration
- Treatment schedule
- Treatments (interventions) including detailed procedures and record keeping
- Data safety monitoring board and procedures

Figure 17-1 Outline of a compete protocol for a clinical trial.

Source: Adapted from Piantadosi, 1997.

TABLE 17-1 Example of a Therapeutic Conversation Intervention

Peplau's Overlapping Phases of a Relationship	Therapeutic Strategies
Orientation: Participant gains trust, begins to engage in the relationship. The intervener introduces self and briefly explains the purpose of the visit. If the participant agrees to meet, phase-specific strategies are used as appropriate.	Protecting from distractions, conveying availability, consistency and interest, using a caring and respectful tone of voice and calm approach, adapting communication to the participant's cognitive ability, accepting some misunderstandings, focusing on the present, asking general questions, using nonverbal gestures and verbal encouragers, and allowing sufficient time to respond.
Identification: Participant begins to participate in the intimate interpersonal relationship. In addition to the orientation strategies used previously, the intervener uses phase-specific strategies as tolerated by the resident.	Sharing self, supportive touch, verbal support, paraphrasing, acknowledging emotions and concerns, and acknowledging autonomy. The intervener refrains from dishonest communication, demonstrations of impatience or frustration, correcting or pointing out errors, using diminutives or collective pronouns, and talking about the participant in his or her presence. Confrontational statements or questions such as those beginning with "Why?" are avoided.
Exploitation: Participant is engaged in and derives value from the relationship. In addition to the previous strategies, the intervener uses phase-specific strategies as appropriate.	Speaking as equals, establishing commonalities, giving recognition, expressing affection and positive regard, acknowledging and respecting the participant's individuality, clarifying vague communication, using open-ended as well as close-ended questions, listening for themes, and encouraging talk about feelings and concerns.
Resolution: Participant and intervener discuss termination. In addition to the previous strategies, the intervener uses phase-specific strategies as appropriate.	Encouraging talk about this relationship and other significant relationships, summarizing and reminiscing about relationship, facilitating the participant's relationships with peers and center staff, and saying good-bye.

Source: Tappen and Williams, 2009.

TABLE 17-2 Example of a Scheduled Progression of Exercise Program

Time Period	Motor Control & Strength Exercises	Balance Exercises	Endurance Walking
Weeks 1 & 2	3 shallow knee bends 3 toe rises 3 push & pulls with assistance	Side step 3 steps right & left, step backward 3 steps, and 2 circles, assist as needed	10 minutes increase pace
Weeks 3 & 4	5 shallow knee bends 5 toe rises 3 push & pulls no assistance	Side step 5 steps right & left, step backward 5 steps, and 4 circles, assist as needed	10 minutes increase pace
Weeks 5 & 6	7 shallow knee bends 7 toe rises 5 push & pulls no assistance	Side step 7 steps right & left, step backward 5 steps, and 4 circles, assist as needed	10 minutes increase pace
Weeks 7 & 8	5 deeper knee bends 5 toe rises 7 push & pulls no assistance	Side step 5 steps right & left, step backward 5 steps, and 4 circles, less assistance	15 minutes
Weeks 9 & 10	7 deeper knee bends 7 toe rises 5 push & pulls light resistance	Side step 7 steps right & left, step backward 7 steps, and 6 circles, less assistance	15 minutes increase pace
Weeks 11 & 12	9 deeper knee bends 9 toe rises 7 push & pulls light resistance	Side step 9 steps right & left, step backward 9 steps, and 8 circles, same resistance	15 minutes increase pace
Weeks 13 & 14	7 deep knee bends 7 toe rises 5 push & pulls moderate resistance	Side step 5 steps right & left, step backward 5 steps, and 4 circles, minimal possible support	20 minutes
Weeks 15 & 16	9 deep knee bends 9 toe rises 7 push & pulls moderate resistance	Side step 7 steps right & left, step backward 7 steps, and 6 circles, minimal possible support	20 minutes increase to maximal pace

Source: Courtesy of Ruth M. Tappen, EdD, RN, FAAN.

9. *Fill in the detail:* Now go back and provide all of the detail needed to actually carry out the intervention. This portion should be both didactic (providing information) and skill based (providing opportunity to practice). You may want to acknowledge that the interventionists are probably quite familiar with the procedures involved but that doing them as part of a research study differs from doing them as a part of customary nursing practice.

10. *Approach to the participant:* Interventionists also need to know how to introduce themselves, explain the study, and explain how the participants will be involved. This should have been done during consenting but needs to be repeated during the treatment phase. Expectations of the participant and responsibilities of the interventionist need to be explained as well.

    If the participant is unable to respond for himself or herself (if you are working with infants, for example, or with people who are comatose or otherwise unable to speak), it is especially important that interventionists check with staff each time about their current condition before proceeding with the treatment.

11. *Relationship to staff:* If the study is being conducted in a healthcare facility or through the cooperation of another institution (school, place of employment, and so forth), it is important that study team members know how to relate to the staff of the cooperating organization. Good leadership skills can be very useful in this regard.

12. *Recording responses to the treatment:* The detail in which this is done will vary from one study to another, but it is important that interventionists record provision of treatment or a missed treatment and reason why it was missed. In some cases, the amount of treatment that was received (whole, partial or number of minutes, dose, and so forth) needs to be recorded at each session. Interventionists' observations should also be recorded as they may be helpful in reporting an adverse event if it should occur and in interpretation of the results at the end of the study.

13. *Expectations:* Here you describe the roles and responsibilities of interventionists, what they are allowed to decide independently, and what needs to be reported to the investigators, either immediately or shortly after it happens. Hours and pay may be explained if this hasn't been done already. The importance of consistency and dependability should also be addressed.

14. *Authorship:* This is a topic that should be discussed at the beginning of the study. Inexperienced members of the team may not understand (1) the need to check with the investigator before writing about or speaking to the public about a research study, or (2) the basis upon which authorship and the order of authors on a paper will be decided.

15. *Communication with other members of the team and with the investigator:* Interventionists are on the "front line" and often see, hear or become involved in situations that the investigator needs to know about. For example, in one long-term care facility, a new interventionist observed what appeared to be abuse of a resident. This was brought to the attention of the investigator. The nurse manager was informed and action was taken to prevent further instances of this type of treatment of a vulnerable resident.

    Interventionists are often very interested in the topic of the study underway. As they work with participants, they may have creative ideas for improving the intervention or for further study. Keeping lines of communication open will encourage team members to share these ideas and perhaps become involved in pilot studies of the new ideas.

Chow and Liu (2004) reported the most common deficiencies found during Food and Drug Administration (FDA) inspections of research sites. Protocol nonadherence was the most common, closely followed by inadequate or inaccurate records. Consent form deficiencies and drug accountability problems were also found. Adverse events were the other type of problem found on these inspections. Nesbitt (2004) calls for *perfect adherence to the study protocol* as the standard to which we should aspire. Any deviation or violation of the protocol should be reported immediately.

Informing Facility Staff

There is another group of stakeholders involved in making the implementation of the planned intervention a success. These are the staff of the facility you are conducting the study in, both administrative and staff level personnel. Permission to conduct the study in the facility should have been obtained during the planning of the study and should have been reported to the IRB. This, however, is only the beginning of the relationship with a cooperating institution. All staff members need to know what is expected of them and how they can help to make the study a successful one.

Now that implementation is about to begin, the staff and management of the facility need to know what to expect of the research team and how they themselves will be involved. In some instances, staff of the institution will make the initial approach to a potential participant. This will require training of the staff member similar to what is described in the chapter on human subjects as well as training specific to the study being conducted. In other instances, staff will actually become part of the research team, implementing the intervention to be tested. In this case, they will need far more training, including information about the conduct of research, the rights of participants in the study and guidance in distinguishing research protocol from regular care.

A different scenario occurs when research team members become ancillary members of the caregiving team. Staff still need to understand the study's purposes and procedures but not in such great detail. Without this understanding, they may inadvertently interfere with study procedures, even in rare instances compete with the intervention or sabotage it. An example:

> A small pilot study of the effect of participation in a reminiscence group on depressive symptomatology and quality of life was being conducted in an assisted living facility. Residents of the facility were invited to join the group which met two mornings a week, at the same time as the recreational therapist conducted the daily news report and discussion group. The recreation therapist perceived the reminiscence group as competition and began to both vigorously recruit new members to the news group and to reenergize the conduct of the group, making it far more therapeutic in nature than it had been in the past. With these activities underway, the news group was no longer the "usual care" comparison it had been intended to be when the reminiscence group study was initiated.

Another caveat related to working with caregiving staff is to be respectful of their time and regular responsibilities. Investigators cannot expect that their studies are the primary concern of caregiving staff. It is reasonable to expect some assistance and support for the study but, without compensation, staff cannot be expected to do the majority of the work of the study unless the study belongs to them as it would in the case of an action research design.

It is also important to check with nursing management about the type of documentation of patient or client participation in a study they require. In some instances, a considerable amount of information needs to be added to the medical record. In other instances, a record of the patient or client's participation in the study and evidence of consent is all that is needed.

Patients and families often look to their regular care providers for assurance that participation in a clinical study is a good idea. Physicians, therapists, nurses, and nursing assistants often influence this decision. Information about the study and its purposes will help staff make informed responses to the people in their care.

IMPLEMENTATION

No matter how well prepared you are, there will likely be some surprises and some adjustments to be made once you begin implementation. It is hard to predict what these might be but here are just a few examples to illustrate what might be encountered.

- Post hip fracture patients that had traditionally been transferred to the long-term care facility research site for rehabilitation were being retained by hospitals in their own step-down rehabilitation units.

- The director of nursing who had enthusiastically approved the facility's participation in the study resigned just before the study was scheduled to begin.

- A tornado damaged the school building and knocked out power, putting staff, families, and students into crisis mode, leaving no time or energy for participation in the study for several months.

- The FDA found some deficits in record keeping and shut down all research studies conducted in the institution that was to be the research site until these problems were remedied.

- The sixth graders who had agreed to participate and whose families had consented to their participation in a fitness study found the active games that were planned to be "only for little kids" and the incentives for staying in the study uninteresting.

The last "surprise" could have been prevented through pilot work, by the way.

Just a reminder as you are responding to these and other surprises: major adjustments such as a new research site or changes in the intervention need approval by the IRB before proceeding.

Monitoring Adherence to Protocol

It is not enough to teach people how to implement the intervention. Regular monitoring through onsite visits, e-mail communications, telephone conferences, and submitted reports is essential to maintaining the protocol and preventing drift. At a minimum, the investigator needs to have biweekly contact with all interventionists not only to monitor them but also to troubleshoot as questions and concerns arise.

If facility staff are providing the intervention, regular monitoring of actual implementation and of their record keeping also needs to be done.

Monitoring Participant Safety

Investigators are responsible for assuring the safety of participants in every study. When an intervention is provided, this responsibility becomes a continuous task throughout every aspect of the study.

The amount of risk varies from one study to another and is the basis upon which the extent of the monitoring is determined. In small studies with minimal risk, the monitoring may be done by the investigator. In more complex studies, safety may also be reviewed by a single monitor. If the study is very complex and poses a higher level of risk, a data safety monitoring board (DSMB) is needed. The National Institutes of Health require a DSMB for multiple-site clinical trials that might pose a risk to the participant (NIH, 1998). Members of the DSMB should have expertise related to the conduct of research and the topic under study but not be members of the study team; they must be independent or external to the study. The DSMB is expected to meet regularly (quarterly, for example) to review interim data from the study and reports of any adverse events that may have occurred. Serious adverse events (SAEs) are expected to be reported immediately to the DSMB and the IRB. These may include the following:

- Death
- Life-threatening event
- Hospitalization
- Disability
- Congenital anomaly
- Treatment is required to prevent permanent damage (Cook & DeMets, 2008, p. 176).

The IRB usually requires a written plan for data and safety monitoring. This plan may include the following:

- Level of risk to participants
- Identification of the monitor: the investigator, a single monitor, or a DSMB
- How often data and reports will be reviewed

- The specific data and reports that will be reviewed
- To whom the results of the reviews will be submitted (NIH-OHSR, 2006; NIH, 2000).

All of this is done in addition to the usual reports to an IRB and the usual oversight done by the investigator and the IRB.

CONCLUSION

The intervention phase of research requires active involvement of the investigator and members of the research team. A carefully designed intervention based upon previous research and an underlying theoretical framework are the basis for undertaking this phase of the study. Those providing the intervention need to be well trained, the provision of the intervention needs to be monitored and recorded meticulously, and safety of participants needs to be assured throughout the study.

REFERENCES

Adachi, K., Shimada, M., & Usui, A. (2003). The relationship between the parturient's positions and perceptions of labor pain intensity. *Nursing Research, 52*(1), 47–51.

Alsever, R. N., Thomas, W. M., Nevin-Woods, C., Beauvais, R., Dennison, S., Bueno, R., et al. (2009). Reduced hospitalizations for acute myocardial infarction after implementation of a smoke-free ordinance—City of Pueblo, Colorado 2002-2006. *Journal of the American Medication Association, 301*(5), 480–483.

Budin, W. C., Hoskins, C. N., Haber, J., Sherman, D. W., Maislin, G., Cater, J. R., et al. (2008). Breast cancer: Education, counseling and adjustment among patients and partners in a randomized trial. *Nursing Research, 57*(3), 199–213.

Burke, L. E., Swigart, V., Turk, M. W., Derro, N., & Ewing, L. J. (2009). Experiences of self-monitoring: Successes and struggles during treatment for weight loss. *Qualitative Health Research, 19*(6), 815–825.

Byers, P. H. (1986). Infant crying during aircraft descent. *Nursing Research, 35*(5), 260–262.

Choe, M-A., An, G. J., Lee, Y-K., In, J. H., Choi-Kwon, S., & Heitkemper, M. (2004). Effect of inactivity and undernutrition after acute ischemic stroke in a rat hindlimb muscle model. *Nursing Research, 53*(5), 283–292.

Chow, S-C., & Liu, J-P. (2004). *Design and analysis of clinical trials: Concepts and methodologies.* New York, NY: Wiley-Interscience.

Cook, T. D., & DeMets, D. L. (2008). *Introduction to statistical methods for clinical trials.* Boca Raton, FL: Chapman & Hall/CRC.

Ferlise, P., & Baggot, D. (2009). Improving staff nurse satisfaction and nurse turnover: Use of a closed-unit staffing model. *Journal of Nursing Administration, 39*(7/8), 318–323.

Goldfarb, W. (1945). Effects of psychological deprivation in infancy and subsequent stimulation. *American Journal of Psychiatry, 102*, 18–33.

Harrison, D., Loughnan, P., Manias, E., Gordon, I., & Johnston, L. (2009). Repeated doses of sucrose in infants continue to reduce procedural pain during prolonged hospitalizations. *Nursing Research, 58*(6), 427–434.

Lobar, S., Brooten, D., Youngblut, J. M., Hernandez, L., Herrera-Perdigon, J., Royal, S., et al. (2008). The experience of being an Asthma Amigo in a program to decrease asthma episodes in Hispanic children. *Journal of Pediatric Nursing, 23*(5), 364–371.

Moore, E. A. (2009, November 11). The fun theory: Treadmill race track, piano stairs, and more. *Health Tech.* Retrieved April 30, 2010, from http://news.cnet.com/8301-27083_3-10395335-247.html

National Institutes of Health. (1998). *NIH policy for data and safety monitoring.* Retrieved April 30, 2010, from http://grants.nih.gov/grants/guide/notice-files/NOT98-084.html
   ◇ NIH policy on data and safety monitoring that is worth reading if you need to set up a data and safety monitoring board for your study.

National Institutes of Health. (2000). *NIH Guide: further guidance on a data and safety monitoring for phase I and phase II trials.* Retrieved April 30, 2010, from http://grants.nih.gov/grants/guide/notice-files/NOT-OD-00-038.html

National Institutes of Health, Office of Human Subjects Research. (2006). *Sheet 18: Guidelines for NIH intramural investigators and institutions review boards on data and safety monitoring.* Retrieved April 30, 2010, from http://ohsr.od.nih.gov/info/pdf/InfoSheet18.pdf

Nesbitt, L. A. (2004). *Clinical research: What it is and how it works.* Boston: Jones and Bartlett.

Paul, I. M., Beiler, J., McMonagle, A., Shaffer, M. L., Duda, L., & Berlin, C. M. (2007). Effect of honey, dextromethorphan, and no treatment on nocturnal cough and sleep quality for coughing children and their parents. *Archives of Pediatric and Adolescent Medicine, 161*(12), 1140–1146.

Piantadosi, S. (1997). *Clinical trials: A methodological perspective.* New York, NY: John Wiley & Sons.

Sanders, L. (2009, November 21). Junk food turns rats into addicts. *Science News, 176*(11), 8.

Schachman, K. A., Lee, R. K., & Lederma, R. P. (2004). Baby boot camp: Facilitating maternal role adaptation among military wives. *Nursing Research, 53*(2), 107–115.

Schneider, M., Hall, W. J., Hernandez, A. E., Hindes, K., Monty, G., Pham, T., et al. (2009). Rationale, design and methods for process evaluation in the HEALTHY study. *International Journal of Obesity, 33,* S60–S67.

Seskavich, J. E., Crater, S. W., Lane, J. D., & Krucoff, M. W. (2004). Beneficial effects of Noetic therapies in mood before percutaneous intervention for unstable coronary syndromes. *Nursing Research, 53*(2), 116–121.

Tappen, R. M., & Williams, C. (2009). Therapeutic conversation to improve mood in nursing home residents with Alzheimer's disease. *Research in Gerontological Nursing, 2*(4), 267–275.

Tripp-Reimer, T., Woodworth, G., McClosky, J. C., & Bulechek, G. (1996). The dimensional structure of nursing interventions. *Nursing Research, 45*(1), 10–17.

Tryon, W. W., Tryon, G. S., Kazlousky, T., Gruen, W., & Swanson, J. M. (2006). Reducing hyperactivity with a feedback actigraph: Initial findings. *Clinical Child Psychology and Psychiatry, 11*(4), 607–617.

Turner, Y., Silberman, S., Jaffe, S., & Hadas-Halpern, I. (2008). *The effect of adding a patient's photograph to the radiographic examination.* Paper presentation at Radiological Society of North America 2008 annual meeting, Chicago, IL.

Varon, J., & Acosta, P. (2008). Therapeutic hypothermia. *Chest, 133*(5), 1267–1274.

PART 4

Analysis and Interpretation Phase

CHAPTER 18

Quantitative Data Management

As soon as you begin collecting data, it is time to consider what to do with it as it comes in. You could just allow the data to accumulate and deal with it later, but there are several reasons not to do this. The first reason is probably obvious: if you do not begin to manage the data right away, you will have a huge job awaiting you later. More important, however, you may not know that problems are also accumulating. Following are some examples of common problems in the data to be alert for:

- Signatures on consents are not witnessed; copies of the consent have not been given to every participant.

- Duplicate identification (ID) numbers have been inadvertently assigned to participants (this can happen, for example, if you use the last four digits of the Social Security number which has been a common practice).

- Rating scales are scored incorrectly. This is most likely to happen with scales that have complicated scoring rules.

- Scale scores are not correctly totaled (mathematical errors).

- The wrong version of a test was used, the short form of the CES-D (a depression scale) or STAI (an anxiety scale), for example, instead of the long form.

- A page is missing from the test packet, so items are missing.

- An important variable such as age or gender has been left out by mistake.

- Items are missed or left blank.

- Responses to open-ended questions are difficult to read or too abbreviated to be useful.

Most of these errors are more likely to occur if you have someone else collecting or entering data for you or if participants are completing the forms themselves either on paper or electronically. Failure to correct these problems as quickly as possible may lead to serious problems later, particularly when you try to analyze the results of the study.

A third reason to begin data management as soon as data collection begins is to make it possible to conduct preliminary analyses of the results at several points during the study. If the study is funded, the funder may require interim reports including some preliminary results. Also, if your study involves an intervention, the preliminary analysis may indicate some concerns about the intervention that would otherwise not be known until the end of the study. A series of periodic preliminary or interim analyses are essential if the intervention requires a data and safety monitoring plan (Cook & DeMets, 2008). Finally, if you are using multiple data collectors you will also need to check interrater reliability periodically. Even if you have only one data collector, you still need to be alert to the possibility of rater drift over time, which can be detected through preliminary analysis.

The remainder of this chapter discusses a series of actions that will help you to manage your data. These actions are critical in a large, complex study, but they are useful in smaller quantitative studies as well. Some guidance on setting up a database for analysis completes this chapter.

MANAGING THE DATA

The more data you collect, the more important it is that you manage it well. In this section, a number of tasks related to data management are described. Some are one-time actions; others are done continuously, throughout the data collection phase of your study. Some may seem a little tedious, such as maintaining a tracking system, but keeping your data organized prevents many problems.

Set Up a Tracking System

As soon as you enroll your first participant, you should set up a paper or electronic tracking system. This allows you to monitor the success of your recruitment strategies, your randomization to treatment groups, characteristics of the sample that might be critical (for example, have you been able to recruit as many men as women?), and whether or not you have been able to keep up with your time frame for the study (a time frame is illustrated in Chapter 22).

For most studies, the tracking system does not have to be elaborate. In fact, keeping it as simple as possible is probably a good idea. The tracking system may be a simple table listing each participant by name or ID number, date the consent was signed, date of pretesting, date the intervention (if any) began, dates of posttest and follow-up testing, and a comment column that allows the addition of critical information such as reason for withdrawal from the study, a problem that has arisen, or loss of the participant due to having moved, become ill, or died. The table can be created in a word-processing program or spreadsheet. It is most important to keep the table or spreadsheet up to date and to check it regularly to monitor progress and identify possible problems that need to be corrected. There are commercial software products available to track complex clinical trials, but they are expensive and unnecessary unless you are conducting several clinical trials at one time.

Table 18-1 illustrates a very simple tracking system for a community-based study without an intervention that may be used in hard copy or electronically. Note that one ID number is missing, which may occur inadvertently or may indicate it had been assigned to someone who changed his or her mind about participation before enrolling. Any who withdraw after having given their consent need to be listed and reasons for the withdrawal added to the comment column. In some studies, the order in which different tests are administered may affect responses. This is reflected in the column marked Test Version. Each of the four versions has the tests in a different order. You'll also notice that the date of data entry and completion of the transcriptions are also included.

TABLE 18-1   Sample Tracking System

ID	Test Version	Date	Name	Age	Gender	Housing Unit	Diagnostic Group	Consent	Examiner	Audio	Video	Database Entry Completed	Transcription Done	Comments
1024	4	4-7-09	DX	23	M	Roman Gdns	1	Yes	RA	Yes	No	12-3-09	1-7-10	Decl video
1025	3	11-8-09	RS	35	F	Sunny Isles	2	Yes	CL	No	Yes	12-3-09	1-7-10	
1027	3	11-10-09	WA	21	F	Griffin Estates	1	Yes	RA	Yes	Yes	12-3-09	1-7-10	
1028	2	11-10-09	BE	27	M	Roman Gdns	1	Yes	WA	Yes	No	12-3-09	1-7-10	Decl video
1029	2	11-11-09	SD	31	M	Griffin Estates	2	Yes	CL	Yes	No	12-5-09	1-8-10	Decl video
1030	1	11-12-09	CD	33	F	Sunny Isles	1	Yes	WA	Yes	Yes	12-5-09	1-8-10	

Notes: 1 = diagnosed diabetes; 2 = no diabetes; decl = declined; with = withdrew; inc = incomplete.

Assure the Security of the Data

It is very likely that you have assured all participants both verbally and in a written consent form that all the information they provide will be kept confidential. In some studies when the information sought is especially sensitive, anonymity is assured. It is your responsibility to ensure that participants' confidence in these assurances is not violated, that their personal health information is not shared with unauthorized individuals, and that it cannot be inadvertently exposed. Following are some suggestions for maintaining the security of your data:

- Allow access only to those who have had training regarding the protection of human subjects.

- Store all paper files in locked file cabinets, preferably within a locked storage area.

- Use password protection to guard all electronic data files.

- Separate participants' names from the remaining data. Keep participant name and Social Security numbers (if needed) in a separate secure file.

- In some large studies, the data files are kept on a secure computer that is designated for this purpose only.

- Create backup copies of all electronic data files and store them in a separate secure location.

- If you are working on networked files, talk with the network administrator about your data security needs.

Develop a Filing System for Your Data

Whether paper, electronic, or a combination of both, the data you have collected is not only personal and confidential (if not anonymous) but also very valuable. A well-organized filing system for the original data, whether field notes, audiotapes, videos or test packets, will prevent having misplaced or lost information. Consents may be filed with test information or separately, but it is important to be able to connect them with the data if a problem arises or an audit is conducted.

Review Each Packet/Response

As indicated at the beginning of the chapter, a number of errors and omissions may occur during data collection. The sooner these are caught and corrected, the better. With some, it may only be possible to correct for future data collection. In other cases, scoring may be corrected and blanks filled in on collected data.

Create Codes for Open-Ended Questions

This is a task that cannot be completed until a substantial amount of data has been collected. There are several different ways to create these codes. The first is to anticipate participants' answers and create the codes (categories) before data collection begins. This can be done if you are relatively certain of the range of answers that will be obtained. The number of participants who select "other" will be one indication of how successful your prediction of their responses was.

A second approach is to create the codes after the data have been collected. You can list all of the responses, tabulate any that were used multiple times to reduce the list, and then cluster responses that are similar. Ideally, you want to reduce the categories to a manageable number (no more than 5 or 6, say) for analysis but this is not always possible. For example:

> A study of 160 individuals discharged from a rehabilitation unit yielded 93 different admitting diagnoses and 106 different discharge diagnoses. Some individuals had as many as 7 or 8 diagnoses. Use of ICD-9 diagnostic codes reduced the number but not enough to produce manageable categories. Instead, the diagnoses were clustered (cardiovascular, cancer, fracture) into broad diagnostic categories that yielded a more manageable set of 8 categories.
>
> The same study included a list of medications commonly prescribed to manage urinary incontinence (Box 18-1). The original list is the left column; the categorization by pharmacotherapeutic action is on the right.

Box 18-1   Bladder Medications

Original List	Categorized List
1. Oxybutynin	1. Bladder relaxants
2. Tolterodine	Oxybutynin
3. Duloxetine	Tolterodine
4. Terazosin hydrochloride	Solifenacin
5. Doxazosin mesylate	Trospium
6. Tamsulosin hydrochloride	Darifenacin
7. Solifenacin	2. Alpha blockers
8. Trospium	Terazosin hydrochloride
9. Darifenacin	Tamsulosin hydrochloride
10 Alfuzosin	Alfuzosin
11. Other (list) _____	3. Duloxetine
_____	4. Other

In some studies, the coding may become quite complex. In this case you may decide that calculation of intercoder agreement or reconciliation of any coding disagreements is necessary.

SELECTING THE SOFTWARE FOR THE DATABASE

There are a few questions to ask yourself before sitting down at your keyboard to create the database. Answers to these questions will affect your choice of software and how you design your database:

- Are your data entirely quantitative? This includes nominal data, such as gender, marital status, type of residence, or any other item that can be neatly divided into a small number of categories that numbers can be assigned to. Another common type of nominal data are the yes-no questions such as "Have you ever been told by a healthcare provider that you have asthma?" The responses can be 0 = no, 1 = yes. If a person is genuinely uncertain, you may need to add a third category or decide to treat it as unknown or missing, but to the extent possible, you want to encourage people to answer "yes" or "no," not "maybe." Gray (2009) goes one step further, suggesting that any missing value be coded for the reason it is missing:
  - Not applicable
  - Refused
  - Did not know
  - Forgot to answer

  Knowing the reason why data are missing will help you decide how to handle it during the analysis.

- Are there substantial amounts of open-ended responses that you may want to analyze qualitatively? If so, you probably want to create a second, qualitative, database using qualitative data analysis software if the data are extensive or a word-processing program if they are not.

- Will the data analysis be very simple, involving just descriptive data such as means, percents, totals, and subtotals by various groupings? If so, you may use very simple software such as Excel, Minitab, or a similar program. However, most research studies require data analysis that goes beyond this very basic information, in which case you will want to use more sophisticated data analysis software such as SPSS, SAS, STATA, EcStatic, SYSTAT or STATISTIX (Salkind, 2008).

- Will you want to present your results graphically? Sometimes a picture really is worth a thousand words, and a few well-designed graphs, charts, or tables may enliven your written report or presentation. If this is the case, you will want to select data analysis software that produces attractive graphs, charts, and other visual displays. JMP is an example, but other programs also do this well.

- Is there better support available for one software package versus another? If you encounter a problem you cannot resolve on your own, is there somewhere or someone you can turn to for help? Quantitative data analysis software is complex. You do not have to be a novice researcher to encounter problems that you cannot resolve on your own. Online help guides are not always sufficient; in some cases, they are more difficult to understand than the software itself, although the software producers have made considerable progress in improving their online support. Salkind (2008) suggests you call the tech support number to see how long you are on hold before someone responds to your call. Some software producers offer only online help—you can test this the same way.

- What is the cost of the software? The cost of some quantitative data analysis packages to a private individual is astronomical. However, many universities and other research-intensive organizations purchase multiuser licenses so that an individual may pay a very reasonable amount for access to the software. In other cases, there are discount prices for students and for faculty doing research. It is worthwhile to inquire about these. There are also free programs available online, but be sure they will meet your needs before adopting them. Many are very limited in scope.

- Is the software compatible with your system? As operating systems change, the data analysis software may temporarily be incompatible with the newest version. Further, the memory capacity (RAM) of your desktop or laptop may need to be increased to accommodate a very large program. Check these requirements before making your selection.

DATABASE CREATION

Test the Program

Before launching the effort to create a complete database, it is a good idea to practice with the software you have selected. You can do a trial run on a "mini" database with just a few (3 or 4) variables and a few (less than 10) hypothetical responses. Use a name for this database that will make it clear it is just a trial run. Call it "Mini," "Trial," or "Junk," and remember to delete it when you are done.

Tutorials are available for many software packages. These are usually worthwhile, but they are not a substitute for trying to set up a mini database on your own.

Once you have mastered creation of a trial database, you are ready to create the real one.

Develop a Codebook

A codebook is a working document that provides all the detailed information needed to transfer information from the test packet into the database. The codebook assures consistency in data input. For example, you do not want to use no = 0 and yes = 1 in some instances but no = 1 and yes = 2 in others. Imagine the confusion this would create!

The codebook may simply be a copy of the test packet with coding information added (in some studies, the codes are built into the test packets). You may also put some of this information into the database so that it comes up automatically when you enter the data.

Create the Database

There are several ways to build a database. You may create it either within the analysis program such as SPSS or SAS, or you may create an external file and import it into the analysis program. In either case, it is important to structure the database so that the programs run smoothly and the analyses are done correctly.

SPSS Databases

When you open SPSS and select *Type in Data*, SPSS Data Editor offers two tabs, Data View and Variable View. Using Variable View, you can list variables and define them (Figure 18-1). Gaur and Gaur (2009) provide a very simple description of database set up within SPSS.

1. *Name the variable:* Use names that tell you what the variable represents (*ID*, *age*, *gender*, and so forth) instead of symbols names (Var1, Var2, or QuesA, QuesB) which are hard to remember.

2. *Define the type of variable* you have named, whether it is numeric (a number), string (text), or a date.

3. Then you can *label* the variable, explaining what the short name stands for. For example, MMSE stands for Mini-Mental State Examination, BNT for the Boston Naming Test.

4. If you anticipate having any missing data, you can also specify how *missing* values will be designated, such as 88 or 99. If not designated, SPSS will assume the number is real and include it in any analysis.

5. Under the *Measure* column you can specify whether the variable is nominal, ordinal, or scale (interval or ratio).

Once the above steps are completed, you can switch to Data View and enter your data line by line (Figure 18-2), each line representing one participant or one testing/data collection session.

SAS Databases

The procedure for creating a SAS database is similar. Using *proc* (i.e., procedure) *FSEDIT*, you indicate that a new database is being created and give it a name using SAS conventions for naming files.

Data input is easier if you list the variables in the same order as they appear in the test packet. Variables are added by entering their name, indicating whether they are numeric

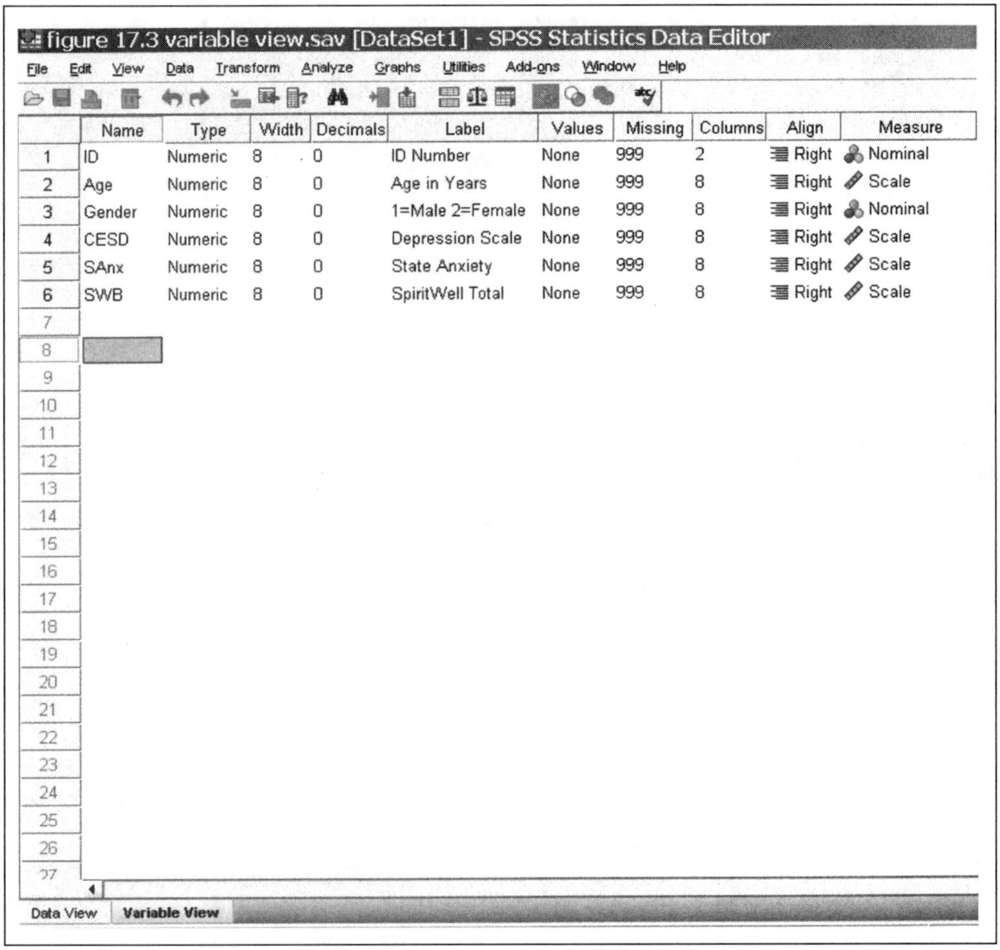

Figure 18-1 Example of SPSS dataset using variable view.

Source: SPSS for Windows, Rel. 17.0.0. (2008). Chicago: SPSS, Inc.

(N) or character ($) and the maximum length of the number or letter string for the variable and labels (which are optional). Missing data may be indicated by a dot (.) (Delwiche & Slaughter, 1995; Schlotzhauer, & Littell, 1997). An example of an SAS database may be found in Figure 18-3. If you look at the way the data are characterized and entered in Figures 18-1, 18-2, and 18-3, you can see that these systems lead you to create a *data matrix* (Gray, 2009). Usually, one line of data represents one participant. The line may contain all the data for the individual or for just one testing time. If you include several test times on one line, be sure to identify this in the variable names. For example, weights obtained at

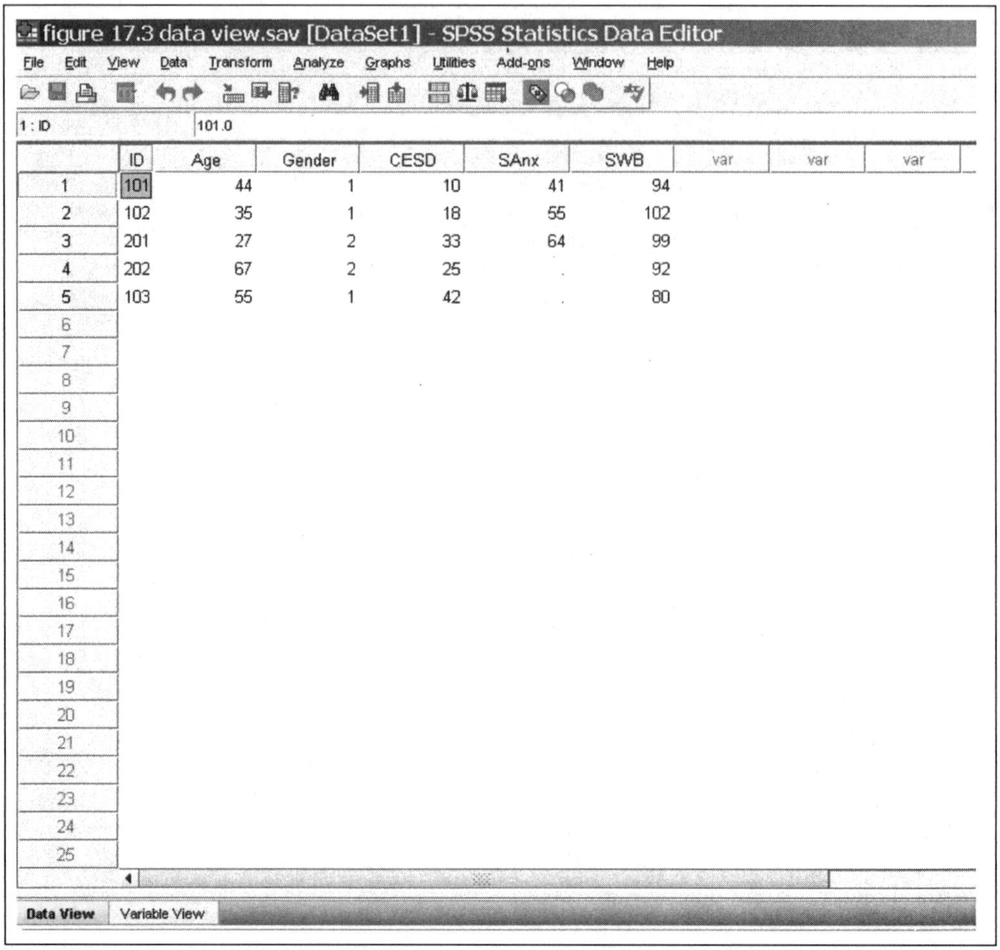

Figure 18-2 Example of SPSS dataset using data view.

Source: SPSS for Windows, Rel. 17.0.0. (2008). Chicago: SPSS, Inc.

pre-, post-, and follow-up testing times could be called *wt1*, *wt2*, and *wt3*, or *wta*, *wtb*, and *wtc*. It is best to use a consistent format to denote testing times. Alternatively, you may use one line per testing session and identify these using codes such as 1 = pretest, 2 = posttest, and 3 = 6-week follow-up for an additional variable called *datapt* (data point).

An alternative that can be used for smaller datasets is to use instream data input. The lines of data are simply entered within a SAS data statement and read when the statement is submitted.

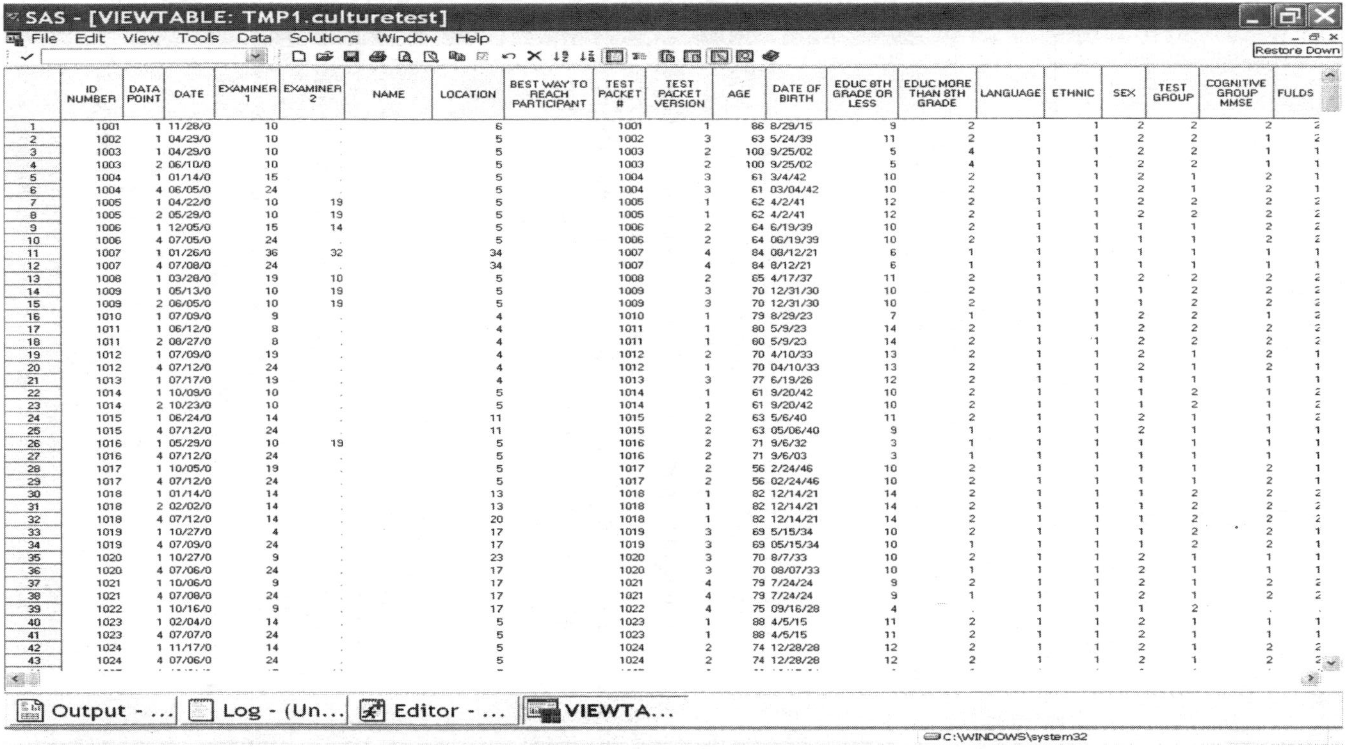

	ID NUMBER	DATA POINT	DATE	EXAMINER 1	EXAMINER 2	NAME	LOCATION	BEST WAY TO REACH PARTICIPANT	TEST PACKET #	TEST PACKET VERSION	AGE	DATE OF BIRTH	EDUC 8TH GRADE OR LESS	EDUC MORE THAN 8TH GRADE	LANGUAGE	ETHNIC	SEX	TEST GROUP	COGNITIVE GROUP MMSE	FULDS
1	1001	1	11/28/0	10	.		6		1001	1	86	8/29/15	9	2	1	1	2	2	2	2
2	1002	1	04/29/0	10	.		5		1002	3	63	5/24/39	11	2	1	1	2	2	1	2
3	1003	1	04/29/0	10	.		5		1003	2	100	9/25/02	5	4	1	1	2	2	1	1
4	1003	2	06/10/0	10	.		5		1003	2	100	9/25/02	5	4	1	1	2	2	1	1
5	1004	1	01/14/0	15	.		5		1004	3	61	3/4/42	10	2	1	1	2	1	2	1
6	1004	4	06/05/0	24	.		5		1004	3	61	03/04/42	10	2	1	1	2	1	2	1
7	1005	1	04/22/0	10	19		5		1005	1	62	4/2/41	12	2	1	1	2	2	2	2
8	1005	2	05/29/0	10	19		5		1005	1	62	4/2/41	12	2	1	1	2	2	2	2
9	1006	1	12/05/0	15	14		5		1006	2	64	6/19/39	10	2	1	1	1	1	2	2
10	1006	4	07/05/0	24	.		5		1006	2	64	06/19/39	10	2	1	1	1	1	2	2
11	1007	1	01/26/0	36	32		34		1007	4	84	08/12/21	6	1	1	1	1	1	1	1
12	1007	4	07/08/0	24	.		34		1007	4	84	8/12/21	6	1	1	1	1	1	1	1
13	1008	1	03/28/0	19	10		5		1008	2	65	4/17/37	11	2	1	1	2	2	2	2
14	1009	1	05/13/0	10	19		5		1009	3	70	12/31/30	10	2	1	1	1	2	2	2
15	1009	2	06/05/0	10	19		5		1009	3	70	12/31/30	10	2	1	1	1	2	2	2
16	1010	1	07/09/0	9	.		4		1010	1	79	8/29/23	7	1	1	1	2	2	1	2
17	1011	1	06/12/0	8	.		4		1011	1	80	5/9/23	14	2	1	1	2	2	2	2
18	1011	2	08/27/0	8	.		4		1011	1	80	5/9/23	14	2	1	1	2	2	2	2
19	1012	1	07/09/0	19	.		4		1012	2	70	4/10/33	13	2	1	1	2	1	2	1
20	1012	4	07/12/0	24	.		4		1012	1	70	04/10/33	13	2	1	1	2	1	2	1
21	1013	1	07/17/0	19	.		4		1013	3	77	6/19/26	12	2	1	1	1	1	1	1
22	1014	1	10/09/0	10	.		5		1014	1	61	9/20/42	10	2	1	1	1	2	1	2
23	1014	2	10/23/0	10	.		5		1014	1	61	9/20/42	10	2	1	1	1	2	1	2
24	1015	1	06/24/0	14	.		11		1015	2	63	5/6/40	11	2	1	1	2	1	1	2
25	1015	4	07/12/0	24	.		11		1015	2	63	05/06/40	9	1	1	1	2	1	1	1
26	1016	1	05/29/0	10	19		5		1016	2	71	9/6/32	3	1	1	1	1	1	1	1
27	1016	4	07/12/0	24	.		5		1016	2	71	9/6/03	3	1	1	1	1	1	1	1
28	1017	1	10/05/0	19	.		5		1017	2	56	2/24/46	10	2	1	1	1	1	2	1
29	1017	4	07/12/0	24	.		5		1017	2	56	02/24/46	10	2	1	1	1	1	2	1
30	1018	1	01/14/0	14	.		13		1018	1	82	12/14/21	14	2	1	1	1	2	2	2
31	1018	2	02/02/0	14	.		13		1018	1	82	12/14/21	14	2	1	1	1	2	2	2
32	1018	4	07/12/0	14	.		20		1018	1	82	12/14/21	14	2	1	1	1	2	2	2
33	1019	1	10/27/0	4	.		17		1019	3	69	5/15/34	10	2	1	1	1	2	2	1
34	1019	4	07/09/0	24	.		17		1019	3	69	05/15/34	10	1	1	1	1	2	2	1
35	1020	1	10/27/0	9	.		23		1020	3	70	8/7/33	10	2	1	1	2	1	1	1
36	1020	4	07/06/0	24	.		17		1020	3	70	08/07/33	10	1	1	1	2	1	1	1
37	1021	1	10/06/0	9	.		17		1021	4	79	7/24/24	9	2	1	1	2	1	2	2
38	1021	4	07/08/0	24	.		17		1021	4	79	7/24/24	9	1	1	1	2	1	2	2
39	1022	1	10/16/0	9	.		17		1022	4	75	09/16/28	4	.	1	1	1	2	.	.
40	1023	1	02/04/0	14	.		5		1023	1	88	4/5/15	11	2	1	1	2	1	1	1
41	1023	4	07/07/0	24	.		5		1023	1	88	4/5/15	11	2	1	1	2	1	1	1
42	1024	1	11/17/0	14	.		5		1024	2	74	12/28/28	12	2	1	1	2	1	2	2
43	1024	4	07/06/0	24	.		5		1024	2	74	12/28/28	12	2	1	1	2	1	2	2

Figure 18-3 Example of SAS database.

Source: The output for this figure was generated using SAS software, Version 9.2 of the SAS System for Windows. Copyright © 2007 SAS Institute Inc. SAS and all other SAS Institute Inc. product or service names are registered trademarks or trademarks of SAS Institute Inc., Cary, NC, USA.

Raw data in text or ASCII files that have only printable characters, tabs, blanks, and marks for the ends of lines may also be used. These files are created in word-processing, spreadsheet, or database programs and then imported into SAS, SPSS, or other analysis programs (Der & Everitt, 2002, p. 11).

External Files

SPSS, SAS, and other data analysis programs accept datasets created in other programs. When you use this approach, it is most important that you use conventions acceptable to the data analysis program. Variable names, for example, cannot begin with a number (MMSE5 is acceptable but 5MMSE is not) or contain blanks or certain symbols that have other functions such as an equal sign or parenthesis. Values can be entered using decimal points but not as fractions. Conventions for separating values and indicating ends of lines of data also need to be observed. Consult your software help facility, tech consultant, or a statistician for help setting up a database that can be imported into your statistical analysis program.

Data Input

You are ready now to enter your data. Accuracy is paramount, so try to do this at a time when distractions and interruptions can be kept to a minimum. There are several ways to check the accuracy of the data input. Entering the data twice and comparing the databases is an effective but time-consuming strategy. Random checks of accuracy require less time but pick up most problems. The range of possible scores can be specified when setting up the database so that you can be alerted if a value outside the range is entered. Values outside the expected range can also be found when you are reviewing the frequencies and ranges of each variable when data analysis begins.

CONCLUSION

Data management is an interim step between data collection and data analysis. Proactive data management can help you detect potential problems when they can still be corrected. It also allows for the preliminary analyses that are often required, either for reports or for data and safety monitoring. Beginning researchers are likely to need guidance from expert researchers, software tech support, tutorials, and manuals as well as their consultant statistician when setting up all but the simplest databases, but these tasks become much easier with practice.

REFERENCES

Cook, T. D., & DeMets, D. L. (2008). *Introduction to statistical methods for clinical trials*. Boca Raton, FL: Chapman & Hall/CRC.

Delwiche, L. D., & Slaughter, S. J. (1995). *The little SAS book*. Cary, NC: SAS Institute.

Der, G., & Everitt, B. S. (2002). *A handbook of statistical analysis using SAS*. Boca Raton, FL: Chapman, Hall/CRC.
    ◇ A helpful introduction to statistical analysis, this one uses examples and printouts from SAS.

Gaur, A. S., & Gaur, S. S. (2009). *Statistical methods for practice and research*. Los Angeles, CA: Response Books.

　◇ Easy to follow directions for entering data into an SPSS database can be found here.

Gray, D. E. (2009). *Doing research in the real world*. Los Angeles, CA: Sage.

　◇ Very basic but practical guidance on the practice of research.

Salkind, N. J. (2008). *Statistics for people who (think they) hate statistics*. Los Angeles, CA: Sage.

SAS for Windows, Version 9.2. (2007). Cary, NC: SAS Institute.

Schlotzhauer, S. D., & Littell, R. (1997). *SAS system for elementary statistical analysis*. Cary, NC: SAS Institute.

SPSS for Windows, Rel. 17.0.0. (2008). Chicago: SPSS, Inc.

CHAPTER 19

Basic Quantitative Data Analysis

If you are afraid of numeric data and feel (correctly or incorrectly) that your math skills are not up to par, you may face this phase of research with some trepidation. It may help to know that your clinical knowledge and experience are as vital to data analysis as are your mathematical skills.

On the other hand, if you enjoy working with numeric data and feel prepared to do so, this will be like any other phase of research except that this phase requires a basic knowledge of statistical analysis and some computer skills. For more complex analysis you need either your own or your consultant's expertise in statistics.

In either case, this phase is one of discovery. It is exciting to finally see the results of your study:

- Did the intervention work? Are participants who received it better off than they were before? How much better off? If they are not better off, why aren't they?

- Was your hypothesis about the relationship of interest correct? If not, are there any clues why not? How strong is the relationship?

- Were there any surprises? Unanticipated results that need explanation?

- Do the findings support existing theory? Do they suggest modification of the theory?

There are a few steps to take yet to obtain answers to these questions, but by the time you complete the data analysis, you will have some answers.

Beginning researchers usually need the guidance of an expert researcher or statistician to complete this phase adequately. Remember, however, that it is your study and that you have become the expert on your study topic. It is best to stay involved in the data analysis even if you cannot do it on your own. You need to understand what has been done and what the results mean. An analysis cannot be done mechanically: the theory and meaning that underlie each measure must always be kept in mind and are essential to the interpretation of the results. Reed (1995) reminds us that "Data alone do not yield up the theory any more than brushes will produce a painting" (p. 95).

A deliberate, thoughtful, step-by-step process for analyzing quantitative data is described in this chapter. The description is basic and does not require a high level of statistical skill.

DATA CLEANING

Now that all of the data have been entered into the database and the database has been imported into the analysis program if you were using an external file, it is time to review it once more for any errors that could affect the outcomes of the analysis. The following are a few things to consider:

- Look at the data matrix on screen or in the printout: are any lines too short ("truncated") or too long? Any symbols that should not be there? For example, review of a large (7500 subjects) data matrix that had been imported into SAS revealed #### has been entered as a value for the length of stay variable for several people. On another variable, gender, which was coded 1 = male and 2 = female, one value entered was *y*. In the first case, the ### probably means that the data were missing: a check of the original data confirmed this and a period (.) which is a SAS convention for missing data was used to replace the ###s. In the second case, the *y* was probably a typo: this was also confirmed, and a 2 for female was used to replace the *y*.

- Recheck the scoring of tests to be sure it was done correctly. You may do a random check to verify this. Do not just look at the first few lines of data, however, but in the middle and at the end of the database as well.

- Make sure the correct coding categories were used. For example, it is critical that each person receiving treatment #1 be coded as a member of treatment group 1. One way to double check this is to compare a randomly selected number of participants' treatment group membership codes with the treatment group assignment noted on the test packet and on your tracking sheet.

- Another way to double-check is to compare the value on one variable with the value on another. For example, you may use the assignment of ID numbers to indicate treatment group: all in treatment group 1 have a 1000–1999 ID number; all in treatment group 2 have a 2000–2999 ID number, and so forth. Another example would be to compare country of origin or language spoken with the indicated ethnic group membership. Each study will have different variables that can be cross-checked in this manner.

- Look for *outliers*, any number (value) that is outside the expected range for a variable. For example, an age of 101 is possible; an age of 201 is not. If the maximum score on a scale is 60, then any value over that indicates an error, whether in scoring or in data entry.

To find outliers, you can look at the frequencies for each variable on screen or in a printout. Every variable needs to be checked, even if you have put limits on their range within the data entry programs.

- While you are going through the steps above, watch for the frequency of missing data, especially for a pattern in the missing data. Handling missing data at this phase of the study presents some challenges discussed in the next section.

MISSING DATA

Sources

There are a number of reasons why data may still be missing despite efforts to fill in as much as possible during data collection:

- The participant may have refused to answer a question or take a particular test.
- The participant withdrew, moved, became ill, or died.
- An item or test was missed inadvertently.
- Participant fatigue, agitation, or other negative response made it necessary to omit all or part of the data collection.
- A participant deliberately omitted the test or item because he or she thought it was not applicable or did not understand the question.
- Poor directions or poorly worded questions elicited no response or the wrong response. Here is an example:

  > We asked long-term care facility staff to rate resident rehospitalizations as avoidable or unavoidable. To our astonishment, only 3.7% were rated avoidable. Conversation with nursing staff explained this extremely low rate: the ratings were focused on the time at which the decision to rehospitalize the resident was made. Later in the project, which was designed to reduce avoidable rehospitalization, staff began to recognize that events in the days prior to hospitalization (increasing dehydration, for example) or capability of staff (to start infusions or intervene with anxious families of dying patients, for example) should also be considered, they began to see more rehospitalizations as avoidable.

- The data were collected but missed during data entry. If the missing data can be retrieved from the original files, the problem is easy to resolve.

Once all of the above are done, however, the remaining missing data need to be evaluated (Cook & DeMets, 2008; Little & Rubin, 2007):

1. Are the missing data random in nature? If so, then loss of information is more of a concern than is bias in the results.

2. Is there a pattern to the missing data? Is it a systematic problem? If so, this may introduce a bias into the data and subsequent analysis (Hardy, Allure, & Studenski, 2009). Little and Rubin (1987) emphasize that these patterns cannot be ignored but must be evaluated.

It is important to identify the reasons why data are missing. Feedback from participants and the observations of data collectors may provide valuable information regarding the reasons for missing data. Analysis of the data may also provide information about the source of bias. An example of the type of bias that might be found through analysis of the data:

- Tests of function such as the independent activities of daily living (IADLs) often ask the participant if he or she can prepare a meal or balance a checkbook. Many older married men do not know how to cook and so will answer "no" or skip the question even though they could prepare a meal if they were taught how to cook. Likewise, many older married women have let their spouses balance the checkbook and will answer "no" or skip the question about balancing a checkbook although they could do it if taught.

- Another IADL function item asked participants if they played games of skill. Analysis of responses found a significant difference between ethnic groups (European Americans, African-Americans, Afro-Caribbeans and Hispanic Americans) in the number of participants who left this question unanswered. Here are the differences (Tappen, Rosselli, & Engstrom, 2010):

Ethnic Group	Percent Who Never Did This Activity
African-American	18%
Afro-Caribbean	23%
European American	15%
Hispanic American	9%

Items such as these need to be worded carefully to obtain the desired information: do you want to know if the person *actually does* this activity or if the person *could* do it or both?

These examples illustrate gender and ethnic group biases in the data that cannot be ignored. The participants with missing data were not necessarily *unable* to perform the task although they *did not perform* the task. Replacing the missing data with the code for "not done" could lead to the highly erroneous conclusion that more men than women were unable to function in the kitchen, more women than men were unable to do the simple math to balance a checkbook, and more African-American and Afro-Caribbean people were unable to play games of skill. Instead, a very simple replacement of the missing data with the participants' mean on the remaining activities that they did perform or a calculation of their individual means on a smaller number of items that they did perform would have been a more reasonable approach. Further analysis of the results of using the participant's mean on other items suggested that it was acceptable in this instance. However, in many cases a more complex approach is advisable.

Replacing Missing Values

There are several ways to address the problem of missing data after your initial evaluation has been completed. Replacement of missing data with a value derived from existing information is called *imputation*. Alternative approaches include *deletion with weighting of remaining cases* and *direct analysis of the incomplete data* (Rubin & Little, 2009). Missing data may be confined primarily to a single variable such as income—this is called a *univariate pattern*. Or it may be found in certain cases when participants have withdrawn from the study or refused to complete certain portions of it—this is called *unit nonresponse*. Missing data may be *systematic* in these and other ways, or it may be *missing completely at random*, abbreviated as MCAR (Little & Rubin, 2007).

Little and Rubin (1987, p. 44) quote an earlier comment by Dempster and Rubin that is worth repeating:

> The idea of imputation is both seductive and dangerous. It is seductive because it can lull the user into . . . believing that the data are complete . . . and it is dangerous because it lumps together situations where the problem . . . can be legitimately handled in this way and situations where standard estimators applied to the real and imputed data have substantial biases.

With this caution in mind, we will proceed to consider some basic principles in handling missing data:

1. Some missing data cannot be replaced. For example, if the participant's age is missing, there is no birth date from which to calculate it and age was not recorded at a previous data collection point, that information is permanently missing and imputation cannot be done.

2. Imputation uses existing information to estimate the missing values. With single item scales such as the powerful and ubiquitous self-rating of health "for your age would you say, in general, your health is excellent, good, fair, poor, or bad?" (Massey & Shapiro, 1982, p. 800), it is difficult to estimate the response that would have been selected by an individual participant. Missing items within a multi-item scale are more amenable to imputation.

3. The easiest (and most "seductive and dangerous") approach to replacing missing data is to use the group's mean (average) on the item. The problem is that there is little foundation for assuming that a particular participant's rating would be average. Further, if you replace too many missing values with the average, the variability among participants may be drastically reduced, an undesirable situation that may lead to erroneous conclusions.

4. A somewhat more targeted and justifiable approach is to use the average of the individual participant's scores or ratings on the remaining items of a multi-item scale. For example, if an IADL scale has 25 items and 2 are missing, the average score on the 23 items can be used to fill in the 2 missing scores. This assumes that scores on individual items are highly related, which needs to be established because it is not always the case. (In fact, very highly correlated items on a scale are considered *redundant* and often deleted during scale development).

5. Missing values may be estimated from values at previous time points. Again, this is based on the (often shaky) assumption that that particular score has not changed.

In fact, one of the primary reasons to employ multiple data collection points is to detect change over time. In some clinical trials, the *last observation carried forward* (LOCF) approach is used (Phillips & Haudiquet, 2003). In this instance, the data from the previous testing is used to replace the missing data. There are many problems associated with this approach. It is based upon the assumption that no outcomes of interest would have changed between testing times, a difficult assumption to support in many instances (Cook & DeMets, 2008). More complex approaches have been developed to avoid these problems.

6. Incomplete cases (participants) may be deleted, and the analysis may be done on those who completed the study. The problem with this approach is that the people who drop out are likely to differ from those who remain in important ways. Those who drop out may have had a disappointing response to the treatment being tested or they may be less persistent than those who completed. If, however, people were lost due to external circumstances unrelated to the study (a new job took them to another state, for example) then their loss may not affect the outcomes of the study. An alternative is to weight comparable complete cases to compensate for those that are lost (Little & Rubin, 2007).

7. There are several more complex calculations that may be made to estimate the values of the missing data. Instead of using the mean of others' scores, a regression analysis may be used to predict the values of the missing scores. This is called *regression imputation*. Other formulas for estimating the values of missing data include maximum likelihood and multiple imputations (Duffy & Jacobsen, 2005; Little & Rubin, 2007).

Expectation maximization (EM) is an algorithm that uses a formula designed for random missing information (Little & Rubin, 2007, p. 114). The first step involves computing expected values. In the second step, the effect of substituting these values is evaluated using maximum likelihood, a method of estimation used in factor analysis and structural equation modeling in a series of iterations until convergence is achieved (Munro, 2005, p. 439).

Multiple imputation avoids some of the disadvantages of using single imputation. Instead of using a single set of replacement values, somewhere between two and five different sets of replacement values (repetitions) can be contrasted and combined to obtain the best set of estimates for the missing values (Duffy & Jacobsen, 2005; Little & Rubin, 2007).

VISUAL REPRESENTATIONS

Now that all of the data have been entered into a database, the database has been cleaned, and missing data are filled in or replaced as much as possible, you are ready to initiate the actual analysis of the data. If your work has been careful and thorough up to now, this phase should go relatively smoothly and more quickly than you might at first imagine. Informally, this first stage of analysis is called "eyeballing" the data.

Many statisticians caution eager researchers not to skip this initial phase of analysis. Much of what is done here is not included in a final report or published article on your study but it is a valuable "first look" at characteristics of the sample (the participants), the outcomes of the study, and the relationship between the two. This first look may suggest relationships that were not anticipated and may cause you to use some additional analyses not anticipated when the study was designed. In other words, this may be a stage of discovery as well as evaluation.

Actually, you began eyeballing the data during the previous steps directed toward finding errors and dealing with missing data. Now you will eyeball the data once more to look at the characteristics of the results on each variable and how the variables are related one to another.

Graphics capabilities differ considerably from one data analysis package to another, but most should be able to generate the simple visual representations discussed here.

There are many ways to visually represent data. We will look at a few basic ones: stem and leaf, box plots, bar and pie charts, and plots. Data from a sample of 150 students at an urban university who were majoring in nursing and psychology will be used for illustrative purposes.

Stem and Leaf

You may have to use a little imagination to actually see these representations as a stem and leaf, but this is often the first graphic studied. An example can be seen in Figure 19-1. This is a stem and leaf representation of a sample of college students whose average age was 27 with a wide range of 18 to 61. The "stem" represents the number of years the students have lived in the United States, which ranged from 4 to 56 years. The "leaf" represents the number of students (frequency) in each category, from 4 to 56. You can see that the largest number had been in the United States for 22 years (this is the mode or most frequent value, by the way).

You can also see that the numbers seem to cluster in the 14 to 28 year range and that there are more at the lower end of the stem (fewer years in the United States) than at the higher end. Why this imbalance? Knowledge of the sample explains this imbalance. This is a diverse group of college students including European American, African-American, Hispanic American, and Afro-Caribbean students. A portion (not yet determined in this analysis) of the latter two groups were not born in the United States but came to the United States at various ages. This explains the imbalance to the lower end of the range of years in the United States. This is an important characteristic of this sample of college students.

Box Plots

A box plot is illustrated in Figure 19-1 to the right of the stem and leaf. The box plot also suggests an imbalance toward the lower end of the range. The horizontal line across the box indicates the median (middle value) or 50th percentile of this distribution. The top of the box is the 75th percentile (75% of the cases fall at or below this line), and the bottom

```
                        The UNIVARIATE Procedure
                           Variable: Years US

        Stem  Leaf                                          #        Boxplot
          56  0                                             1          0
          54  0                                             1          0
          52  0                                             1          0
          50  0                                             1          0
          48  00000                                         5          0
          46  0                                             1          0
          44  00                                            2          0
          42  0                                             1
          40
          38  000                                           3          |
          36  00                                            2          |
          34  0                                             1          |
          32  0                                             1          |
          30  000                                           3          |
          28  000000000                                     9          |
          26  00000000000                                  11      +------+
          24  0000000000                                   10      |      |
          22  000000000000000000000000000                 27      *--+--*
          20  00000000000000000000                        22      |      |
          18  0000000                                      7       |      |
          16  000000                                       6      +------+
          14  000000                                       6          |
          12  0000                                         4          |
          10  00000                                        5          |
           8  000000                                       6          |
           6  0000000                                      7          |
           4  000                                          3          |
              ----·----·----·----·----·--+-·
```

Figure 19-1 Stem and leaf and box plot for years in the United States in a sample of college students.

Source: The output for this figure was generated using SAS/STAT software, Version 9.2 of the SAS System for Windows. Copyright © 2007 SAS Institute Inc. SAS and all other SAS Institute Inc. product or service names are registered trademarks or trademarks of SAS Institute Inc., Cary, NC, USA.

is the 25th percentile (25% of the cases fall at or below this line). The dashed vertical line above and below indicate values that are not outliers. The zeros above this line from 44 to 56 years in the United States indicate outliers that lie outside (above or below) most of the distribution. The full length of the box represents the interquartile range (IQR), from the 25th to the 75th percentile, which constitutes the middle half of the distribution (Duffy & Jacobsen, 2005). A series of box plots (not shown) may be done to show differences in distribution among several groups. For example, they could be used to show the differences in years in the United States by ethnic group membership.

Bar Charts and Pie Charts

These charts are especially helpful in visualizing differences between several groups within a sample. The simplest bar and pie charts show the frequency (total number) within each group. For example, Figure 19-2 is a very simple pie chart that illustrates the proportion of the college student sample that is European American (26.75%), African-American (17.20%), Hispanic American (28.03%), and Afro-Caribbean (28.03%). It is quickly apparent that the African-American group is a little smaller than the other three groups, and there are a few less European Americans than there are Hispanic American and Afro-Caribbean students.

The bar chart in Figure 19-3 illustrates a slightly more complex relationship between nominal data (ethnic group) and interval data (depression scores): the mean scores on the CES-D depression scale (Radloff, 1977). In this instance, you can see that the Hispanic American students have higher CES-D scores than the others. The European American and Afro-Caribbean students have similar mean scores; the African-American students fall in between.

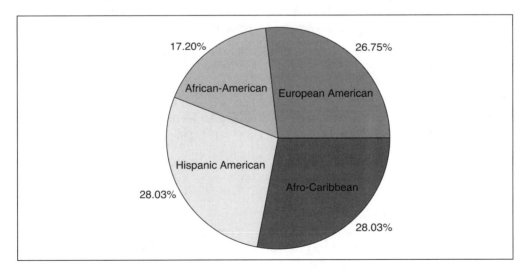

Figure 19-2 Pie chart showing proportion of each ethnic group within the sample.

Source: The output for this figure was generated using SAS/STAT software, Version 9.2 of the SAS System for Windows. Copyright © 2007 SAS Institute Inc. SAS and all other SAS Institute Inc. product or service names are registered trademarks or trademarks of SAS Institute Inc., Cary, NC, USA.

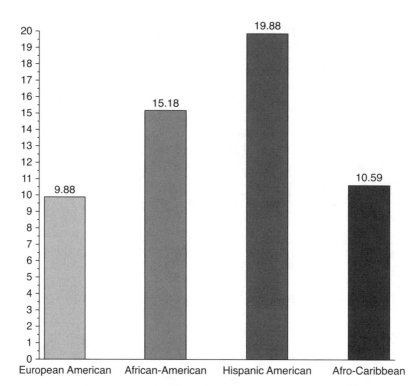

Figure 19-3 Bar chart: Mean depression scores of nursing and psychology students by ethnic group membership.

Source: The output for this figure was generated using SAS/STAT software, Version 9.2 of the SAS System for Windows. Copyright © 2007 SAS Institute Inc. SAS and all other SAS Institute Inc. product or service names are registered trademarks or trademarks of SAS Institute Inc., Cary, NC, USA.

Plots

The relationship between interval data on two or more variables can be visually represented in plots. Figure 19-4 is a plot of age by years in the United States for the European American and African-American students. Compare this plot with Figure 19-5 of the same variables for the Hispanic American and Afro-Caribbean students.

Neither plot has the straight line that would represent a perfect correlation between age and years in the United States. However, a close look at them shows that the Figure 19-4 plot is closer to a straight line. There are fewer asterisks a distance from the diagonal line than in the plot in Figure 19-5. Why the difference? Fewer Hispanic American and Afro-Caribbean students were born in the United States. Consequently, the relationship

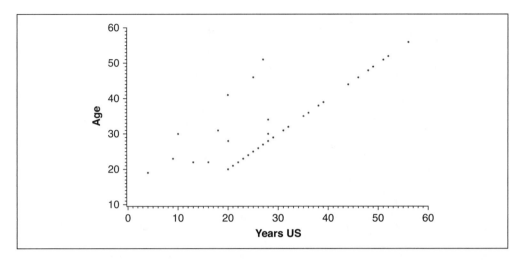

Figure 19-4 Plot of age by years in the United States: European American and African-American college students.

Source: The output for this figure was generated using SAS/STAT software, Version 9.2 of the SAS System for Windows. Copyright © 2007 SAS Institute Inc. SAS and all other SAS Institute Inc. product or service names are registered trademarks or trademarks of SAS Institute Inc., Cary, NC, USA.

between their age and years in the United States is not as strong as it is for the European American and African-American students.

BASIC DESCRIPTIVE STATISTICS

It is time now to begin describing the characteristics of your sample numerically. There are some basic characteristics that are almost always reported: sample size, age, gender, ethnicity, income, health status, and location (place of residence, type of facility, and so forth).

Basic descriptive statistics are essential to virtually every quantitative data analysis. They are used to (1) continue examination of the distribution of values within the dataset, and (2) to describe the characteristics of the sample.

Normality

We look more formally now at the distribution of the values or scores in the dataset to evaluate the extent to which the data are normally distributed.

Skew

You may recall from your basic statistics course that a normal distribution of the values of a specific variable is bell-shaped and symmetrical (O'Rourke, Hatcher, & Stepanski,

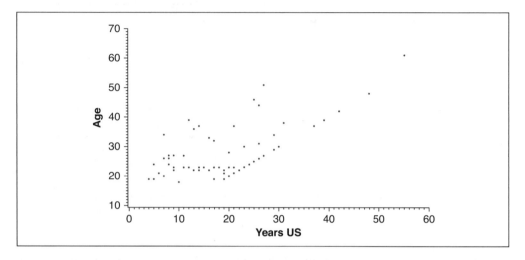

Figure 19-5 Plot of age by years in the United States: Hispanic American and Afro-Caribbean college students.

Source: The output for this figure was generated using SAS/STAT software, Version 9.2 of the SAS System for Windows. Copyright © 2007 SAS Institute Inc. SAS and all other SAS Institute Inc. product or service names are registered trademarks or trademarks of SAS Institute Inc., Cary, NC, USA.

2005) (see Figure 19-6). If you turn the stem and leaf on its side, you can see the extent to which the shape of the "leaf" does or does not resemble the bell-shaped curve. In Figures 19-7 and 19-8, you can see that the distribution of values for years in the United States is not normal: there are too many values in the lower range and too few in the higher range. This is a *positive skew*. The distribution of age has even more cases near the lower end of the range and fewer at the high end of the range, also a positive skew.

A *negative skew* would be a "pile up" of scores in the high values (Evans, 1996, p. 57), which are on the right hand side of the graph. Both positive and negatively skewed data are less symmetrical than the normal, bell-shaped curve. The basic descriptive statistics for these two variables can be found in Figures 19-9 and 19-10. You can see at a glance that the skewness for age is greater than the skewness of years in the United States.

Central Tendency

The mean, median, and mode are technically *measures of central tendency*. They are important and relatively easy to understand statistics. The *mode* is the value that occurs most often. The *median* is the middle score in the distribution, with 50% of the values or scores above it and 50% below. The *mean* is the average of all the scores. You can see in Figures 19-9 and 19-10 that the means, medians and modes of both variables differ from each

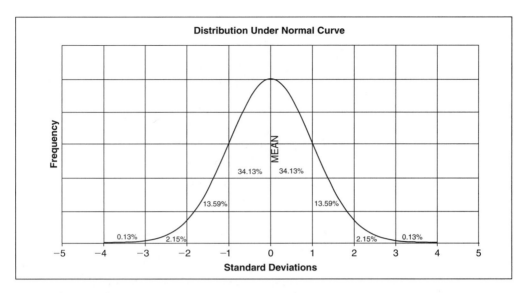

Figure 19-6 Example of normal curve and standard deviations above and below 0 (the mean). Percentages are the area under the curve, the proportion of subjects that fall within each standard deviation.

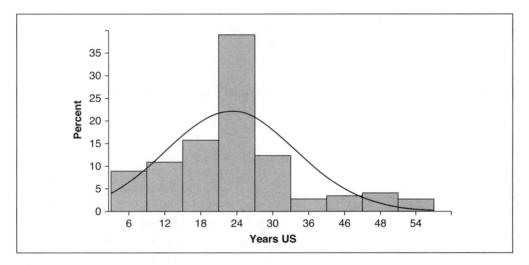

Figure 19-7 Histogram and normal distribution curve for years in the United States of college student sample.

Source: The output for this figure was generated using SAS/STAT software, Version 9.2 of the SAS System for Windows. Copyright © 2007 SAS Institute Inc. SAS and all other SAS Institute Inc. product or service names are registered trademarks or trademarks of SAS Institute Inc., Cary, NC, USA.

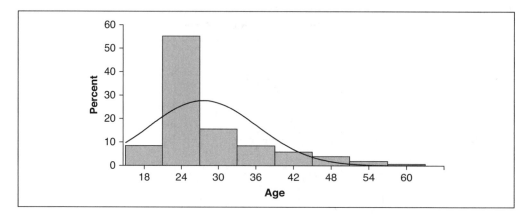

Figure 19-8 Histogram and normal distribution curve for age of college student sample.

Source: The output for this figure was generated using SAS/STAT software, Version 9.2 of the SAS System for Windows. Copyright © 2007 SAS Institute Inc. SAS and all other SAS Institute Inc. product or service names are registered trademarks or trademarks of SAS Institute Inc., Cary, NC, USA.

other somewhat, but the difference is greater for age, the more highly skewed distribution (Evans, 1996). In a perfect bell-shaped normal distribution, the mean, median, and mode would be the same. This is often not the case in research studies, especially those with small samples or samples selected to emphasize a specific characteristic such as poor functional status or severe pain where you would expect data to be skewed to the low side for function and high side for pain.

Dispersion
The range, variance, and standard deviation, also found in Figures 19-9 and 19-10, are measures of *dispersion* or the extent to which they differ from the average or mean. The *range* is also easy to understand: it is simply the distance between the highest and lowest values. For example, the lowest age in the college student sample is 18 and the highest is 61 so the difference is 43. The range or distance between these endpoints can be divided into various portions. Quartiles are the portions created when the range is divided into fourths or quarters, with 25% of the sample in each quartile. The interquartile range (IQR) was defined earlier and is illustrated in the box plot section. *Variance* is a much more complex but important statistic. It is defined as the *average of the squared deviations from the mean* (Evans, 1996, p. 85). You can see in Figures 19-9 and 19-10 that the variance of years in the United States (116.78) is greater than the variance of age (74.59).

The *standard deviation* is a related statistic that is frequently reported. Technically, the standard deviation is the square root of the variance. More important, the standard deviation is

N	154
Mean	27.5714286
Std Deviation	8.63709672
Skewness	1.61466762

Central Tendency

Mean	27.57143
Median	24.00000
Mode	23.00000

Dispersion

Std Deviation	8.63710
Variance	74.59944
Range	43.00000
Interquartile Range	8.00000

100% Maximum	61
99%	56
95%	48
90%	41
75% (Third Quartile)	30
50% Median	24
25% (First Quartile)	22
10%	21
5%	20
1%	18
0% Minimum	18

Figure 19-9   Basic descriptive statistics for the variable age.

Source: The output for this figure was generated using SAS/STAT software, Version 9.2 of the SAS System for Windows. Copyright © 2007 SAS Institute Inc. SAS and all other SAS Institute Inc. product or service names are registered trademarks or trademarks of SAS Institute Inc., Cary, NC, USA.

related to actual values of a variable and can be interpreted directly in terms of distance from the mean (Evans, 1996). An example will help illustrate this. The average (mean) number of years in the United States was 23 and the standard deviation was 10.80. One standard deviation below the mean would be 12.26 years in the United States and one standard deviation above would be 33.86 years in the United States. If you look back to the normal distribution

N	146
Mean	23.0684932
Std Deviation	10.8065482
Skewness	0.92314299

Central Tendency

Mean	23.06849
Median	22.00000
Mode	23.00000

Dispersion

Std Deviation	10.80655
Variance	116.78148
Range	51.00000
Interquartile Range	10.00000

100% Maximum	56
99%	55
95%	48
90%	39
75% (Third Quartile)	27
50% Median	22
25% (First Quartile)	17
10%	9
5%	7
1%	5
0% Minimum	5

Figure 19-10 Descriptive statistics for variable years in the United States.

Source: The output for this figure was generated using SAS/STAT software, Version 9.2 of the SAS System for Windows. Copyright © 2007 SAS Institute Inc. SAS and all other SAS Institute Inc. product or service names are registered trademarks or trademarks of SAS Institute Inc., Cary, NC, USA.

curve, you will remember that, given a normal distribution, 34.13% of the sample will be within 1 standard deviation below the mean, and another 34.13% will be within 1 standard deviation above the mean, altogether 68.26% of the whole sample (Salkind, 2008).

Why are these measures of central tendencies and dispersion so important? They provide a numerical "snapshot" of your data to you and to people reading the reports of your studies. Why is comparison with a normal curve done so often? Data distributions that are markedly different from the normal curve distribution may affect the results of your analyses. In particular, using nonnormal data can bias correlation results and cause misleading results when calculating inferential statistics. Major departures from the normal distributions may call for some statistical intervention (O'Rourke, Hatcher, & Stepanski, 2005).

BIVARIATE ASSOCIATION

The term *bivariate* refers to relationships between two variables (O'Rourke, Hatcher, & Stepanski, 2005). The Pearson product moment correlation coefficient represented symbolically as *r* is the most commonly used bivariate measure of association. Uses of the Pearson *r* and cautions about its interpretation can be found in the chapter on reliability, but there are several other points relevant to analysis of study outcomes, as opposed to use in evaluation of reliability, that need to be mentioned.

You can create a *correlation matrix* by entering several variables at one time as a set of variables to be analyzed (see Figure 19-11). This helps you see the differences in the strengths of relationships between various pairs of variables. For example, in Figure 19-11, you can see that the relationship of age to years in the United States is $r = .74, p < .0001$, a strong and statistically significant (that is, not by chance) relationship. It is also in the positive direction, as age goes up, years in the United States also rise. There are also some negative relationships such as the relationship of depression scores to degree of immersion in the dominant (mainstream American) society as measured by the Stephenson Multigroup Acculturation Scale (SMAS) $r = .44$ (rounded) (Stephenson, 2000). This moderately strong association suggests that depressive symptomatology is less when acculturation is higher and higher when the person is less acculturated. Such a relationship calls for further investigation: Is this true of everyone in the sample? Or of people in just one of the ethnic groups? Is it due to the type of questions asked (i.e., would this relationship hold if other measures of depression and acculturation were used)? Note also that some of the very weak correlations such as the number of years in the United States and the depression score are not significant (the *p* value for significance is found under each correlation value).

Interpretation of the strength of a correlation is often done. Even in the preceding paragraphs, correlations were described in terms of their strength. The following is a common way to interpret the strength of a correlation:

.90 to 1.00	Very strong
.70 to .90	Strong
.40 to .70	Moderate to strong
.20 to .40	Low to moderate
.10 to .20	Very low or weak
.00 to .10	Little or no relationship

	Age	Years in U.S.	Depression Score	Stephenson ESI Score	Stephenson DSI Score
Age	1.00000				
Years in U.S.	0.741453 < .0001	1.00000			
Depression Score	0.00474 0.9623	−0.08936 0.3917	1.00000		
Stephenson ESI Score[1]	−0.14365 0.1477	−0.22111 0.0313	−0.05234 0.6014	1.00000	
Stephenson DSI Score[2]	0.26859 0.0061	0.36840 0.0002	−0.43777 < .0001	−0.05512 0.5802	1.00000

Notes: [1]Ethnic Society Immersion Subscale; [2]Dominant Society Immersion Subscale.

Figure 19-11   Pearson correlation coefficients: Correlation matrix.

Source: The output for this figure was generated using SAS/STAT software, Version 9.2 of the SAS System for Windows. Copyright © 2007 SAS Institute Inc. SAS and all other SAS Institute Inc. product or service names are registered trademarks or trademarks of SAS Institute Inc., Cary, NC, USA.

Remember the size or strength of a correlation is not affected by the sign, positive or negative. You can have a strong positive (.80) or strong negative (−.80) correlation between two variables (Munro, 2005; Salkind, 2008).

There is one more step in an interpretation of a correlation. You can square the correlation, for example .80 multiplied by .80, to calculate the *coefficient of determination* or proportion of the variance accounted for by the correlation (Evans, 1996). A strong correlation such as .80 accounts for 64% of the variance (.80 × .80 = .64 or 64%). This may help to interpret the relationships found in the correlation matrix in Figure 19-11. The correlation of $r = .74$ between age and years in the United States accounts for 55% of the variance ($R^2 = .5471$). For the relationship between depression and acculturation, $r = −.44$ or $R^2 = .19$, accounting for 19% of the variance between depression and acculturation, which is far less but still of interest theoretically.

ADDITIONAL MEASURES OF ASSOCIATION

There are times when another measure of association is more appropriately used (O'Rourke, Hatcher, & Stepanski, 2005). The *Spearman rank-order correlation coefficient* (r_s) should be used, as its name implies, when ordinal (i.e., ranked or ordered) data is analyzed.

It may also be used if the data distribution is seriously skewed (i.e., not normally distributed) (O'Rourke, Hatcher, & Stepanski, 2005).

The *chi-square statistic* (χ^2) is useful when both variables are nominal level data (i.e., simple counts of people within a category such as gender or ethnic group membership). A frequently used statistic, chi-square compares the *observed* (actual) frequencies in each cell to the *expected* frequencies.

Figure 19-12 shows a contingency table for the association between gender and ethnic group membership. The question we are asking in this case when calculating the statistic is whether or not the differences in frequency of males and females across the four ethnic groups are greater than what we would expect by chance. In other words, if males constitute about one-third of the sample as a whole, do we find that same or similar distribution of males and females in each ethnic group? Or is the difference greater than that? If the percents were added to this table, you would see the following:

	Males	Females
European Americans	24%	76%
African-Americans	33%	66%
Hispanic Americans	32%	68%
Afro-Caribbean	45%	55%

If you add the percentages *across* (i.e., the rows, not the column) you would see that the distribution of males and females is one third to two thirds almost exactly in the African-American and Hispanic American students. The Afro-Caribbean group has a higher pro-

	Gender	
Ethnic Group	Male	Female
European American	10	32
African-American	9	18
Hispanic American	14	30
Afro-Caribbean	19	23

Note:	df	value	probability
Chi-square	3	4.42	.21

Figure 19-12   Chi-square table for gender and ethnicity of college student sample.

Source: The output for this figure was generated using SAS/STAT software, Version 9.2 of the SAS System for Windows. Copyright © 2007 SAS Institute Inc. SAS and all other SAS Institute Inc. product or service names are registered trademarks or trademarks of SAS Institute Inc., Cary, NC, USA.

portion of males; the European American group has a lower proportion. The resulting chi-square is 4.42 with 3 degrees of freedom (see Figure 19-12). The resulting probability is $p = .22$ or a 22% probability that such a distribution could occur by chance. Using the .05 level of significance (5% probability of occurrence by chance), we conclude that the distribution of males and females across ethnic groups is not significant.

There are only a few cautions in using the chi-square statistic (Evans, 1996). First, it requires at least five cases per cell (a cell is each square in Figure 19-12). This assumption was not violated in the analysis of gender and ethnicity. Second, the observations must be independent of each other. In other words, the results from one person (one case) must appear only one time in one cell. This assumption was not violated either. However, it is easy to encounter a situation in which you might violate it if you were not aware of the rule. For example, you could ask people why they came to a community health fair. Some participants might give you two or three reasons: "I saw a flyer at the mall," "My friend was coming," and "I'd like to have my cholesterol level checked." You cannot evaluate all three answers at once by gender, age group, or income group with a chi-square analysis.

Fisher's Exact Test may be used instead of the chi-square if the sample is small with less than five cases per cell. The *Mann-Whitney U Test* is used instead of chi-square if the data are ordinal in nature. It is useful, for example, when you compare two groups in an ordinal or ranked outcome from poor to excellent. For example, you could compare an active ingredient (acetaminophen) with a placebo in the treatment of pain from an ankle sprain and ask participants to rank the degree of pain control as poor, fair, good, and excellent, which are ordinal in nature (unlike a chi-square analysis that assumes no order to the various groupings) (Stokes, Davis, & Koch, 2000).

CONCLUSION

The basic data cleanup, replacement of missing data, visual representations, descriptive statistics, and bivariate association statistics described in this chapter are useful in the analysis of virtually every nursing research study. For some studies, the analysis is complete after accomplishing these basic steps. For other, more complex studies, it is necessary to continue with the more advanced analytic techniques described in the next chapter. Whether the analysis is basic or advanced, you will want to have a good statistics textbook, a guide to whatever statistical analysis software you are using, and guidance from an expert researcher and/or statistician to help you complete your quantitative data analysis correctly.

REFERENCES

Cook, T. D., & DeMets, D. L. (2008). *Introduction to statistical methods for clinical trials.* Boca Raton, FL: Chapman Hall/CRC.

Duffy, M. E., & Jacobsen, B. S. (2005). Univariate descriptive statistics. In B. H. Munro (Ed.), *Statistical methods for health care research* (pp. 33–72). Philadelphia, PA: Lippincott, Williams & Wilkins.

Evans, J. D. (1996). *Straightforward statistics.* Pacific Grove, CA: Brooks/Cole.

Hardy, S. E., Allure, H., & Studenski, S. A. (2009). Missing data: A special challenge in aging research. *Journal of the American Geriatrics Society, 57*, 722–729.

Little, R. J. A., & Rubin, D. B. (1987). *Statistical analysis with missing data*. New York, NY: John Wiley & Sons.

Little, R. J. A., & Rubin, D. B. (2007). The analysis of social science data with missing values. In S. Sarantakos (Ed.), *Data analysis* (pp. 99–128). Los Angeles, CA: Sage.

Massey, J. M., & Shapiro, E. (1982). Self-rated health: A predictor of mortality among the elderly. *American Journal of Public Health, 72*(6), 800–808.

Munro, B. H. (2005). *Statistical methods for health care research*. Philadelphia, PA: Lippincott, Williams & Wilkins.
  ◇ A readable textbook written for the healthcare professional.

O'Rourke, N., Hatcher, L., & Stepanski, E. J. (2005). *A step-by-step approach to using SAS for univariate and multivariate statistics*. Cary, NC: SAS Institute.

Phillips, A., & Haudiquet, V. (2003). TCH E9 guideline statistical principles for clinical trials: A case study. *Statistics in Medicine, 22*(1), 1–11.

Radloff, L. S. (1977). The CES-D Scale: A self-report depression scale for research in the general population. *Applied Psychological Measurement, 19*(3), 385–401.

Reed, P. G. (1995). A treatise on nursing knowledge development for the 21st century: Beyond post modernism. *Advances in Nursing Science, 17*(3), 70–84.

Salkind, N. J. (2008). *Statistics for people who (think they) hate statistics*. Los Angeles, CA: Sage.
  ◇ If you are really having difficulty understanding basic statistical concepts, this textbook may be of help to you.

Stephenson, M. (2000). Development and validation of the Stephenson Multigroup Acculturation Scale (SMAS). *Psychological Assessment, 12*(1), 77–88.

Stokes, M. E., Davis, C. S., & Koch, G. G. (2000). *Categorical data analysis using the SAS system*. Cary, NC: SAS Institute.

Tappen, R., Rosselli, M., & Engstrom, G. (2010). Evaluation of the functional activities questionnaire (FAQ) in cognitive screening across four American ethnic groups. *Clinical Neuropsychologist*. (In press).

CHAPTER 20

Inferential Analysis

In the previous chapter, the strategies for becoming familiar with your dataset and calculating some very basic statistics were explained. In this chapter, we will advance this discussion to some of the most common statistical measures used to draw conclusions about the data. Specifically, we will discuss *analysis of variance and regression,* which are technically part of the same family of statistics known as the general linear method but are used to achieve different analytical goals. For the most part, analysis of variance is used to test hypotheses concerning the existence of differences between the means of two samples, subsets of the same sample, or between two or more data points from the same sample. Regression, on the other hand, is used to predict relationships among a set of variables including at least one outcome (dependent) variable. A few of the more common variations of each of these statistical techniques will also be discussed, including *t* tests and logistic regression.

ANALYSIS OF VARIANCE

ANalysis Of VAriance is often abbreviated as ANOVA. Iversen and Norpoth said they once had a student who thought this was the name of an Italian statistician (1987). We can think of analysis of variance as a whole family of procedures beginning with the simple and frequently used *t* test and becoming quite complicated with the use of multiple dependent variables (MANOVA, to be explained later) and covariates (ANCOVA, also to be explained later). Although the simpler varieties of these statistics can actually be calculated by hand, it is assumed that you will use a statistical software package for your calculations. If you want to see how these calculations are done, you could try to compute a correlation, chi-square, *t* test, or ANOVA yourself (see Yuker, 1958), but in general it is too time consuming and too subject to human error to do these by hand.

Important Terminology

There are a number of terms that are used in these analyses that you need to be familiar with to understand the analyses themselves and the results. Many will already be familiar to you.

Statistical significance. Indicates the probability that the differences found are a result of error, not the treatment. Stated in terms of the P value, the convention is to accept either a 1% ($P \leq .01$) or 1 out of 100, or 5% ($P \leq .05$) or 5 out of 100, possibility that any differences seen could have been due to error (Cortina & Dunlap, 2007).

Research hypothesis. A research hypothesis is a declarative statement of the expected relationship between the dependent and independent variable(s).

Null hypothesis. The null hypothesis, based upon the research hypothesis, states that the predicted relationships will not be found or that those found could have occurred by chance, meaning the difference will not be statistically significant.

Effect size. Defined by Cortina and Dunlap as "the amount of variance in one variable accounted for by another in the sample at hand" (2007, p. 231). Effect size estimates are helpful adjuncts to significance testing. An important limitation, however, is that they are heavily influenced by the type of treatment or manipulation that occurred and the measures that are used.

Confidence intervals. Although sometimes suggested as an adjunct or replacement for the significance level, confidence intervals are actually determined in part by the alpha (significance level) (Cortina & Dunlap, 2007). Likened to a margin of error, the confidence intervals indicate the range within which the true difference between means may lie. A narrow confidence interval implies high precision; we can specify believable values within a narrow range. A wide interval implies poor precision; we can only specify believable values within broad and generally uninformative range.

Degrees of freedom. In their most simple form, degrees of freedom are 1 less than the total number of observations. This sometimes confusing term refers to the smallest number of values (terms) that one must know to determine the remaining values (terms). For example, if you know the weights of 12 out of a sample of 13 people and also the sum (grand total) of the weights of these 13 people, you can easily calculate the weight of the 13th person. In this case, the degrees of freedom would be 12 or 13 minus 1 degree of freedom. If you had a second sample of 13 people and again needed to know the weights of 12 to calculate the 13th, the degrees of freedom for these two subsamples together would be 12 + 12 = 24. Not all calculations of degrees of freedom are this simple, but they are based upon this principle (Iversen & Norpoth, 1987; Keppel, 2004).

Variance. A measure of the dispersion of scores around the mean, or how much they are spread out around the mean. Statistically, it equals the square of the standard deviation (Iversen & Norpoth, 1987; Munro, 2005).

Mean. The arithmetic average of a set of numbers, usually the scores or other results for a sample or subsample. Simple to calculate by hand unless you have a very large sample.

Variable. A characteristic or phenomenon that can vary from one subject to another or from one time to another (O'Rourke, Hatcher, & Stepanski, 2005).

Independent variable. In experimental research, the independent variable is the *treatment or manipulation* that occurs. In nonexperimental research, it is the theoretical causative factor that affects the dependent or outcome variable; in other words, it is the *explanatory* variable, also called the *predictor* variable.

Dependent variable. In experimental research, the dependent variable is the measured outcome of the treatment (in the broadest sense of the term treatment). In nonexperimental research, the dependent variable is the theoretical result of the effects of the independent variable(s). It is also called the *criterion* variable.

t Tests

The cardinal feature of *t* tests and ANOVAs also provides an important clue to their usage: these statistical procedures analyze the means of at least one continuous (interval or ratio) response variable in terms of the levels of a categorical variable, which has the role of predictor or independent variable (Der & Everitt, 2006).

The simplest of these statistics are *t* tests. They may be used when:

1. There is just *one predictor* or independent variable that has *just two values* such as male/female, treated/not treated, or hospital #1 patients/hospital #2 patients.

2. There is a *single criterion or dependent variable* measured at the interval or ratio level.

You can see that the applicability of the *t* test is limited by these criteria. In most cases that do not fit these criteria, ANOVA becomes the procedure of choice.

There are two common types of *t* tests (O'Rourke, Hatcher, & Stepanski, 2005):

1. *Independent samples:* This type of *t* test is appropriate when there are two subsamples being compared on an outcome measure. For example, you might randomly assign severe asthma patients to an environmental control education program or a general asthma education program and compare the number of times they used their rescue inhalers in the 3 months following intervention. (Note that this is a posttest-only design; there is no pretest.)

2. *Paired sample:* This type of *t* test is appropriate when the same subjects constitute each sample being compared under two different sets of conditions. Because they are the same people, the results are obviously not independent of one another and are said to be paired or correlated. For example, you could compare severe asthma patients' use of rescue inhalers before and after they attend an educational program on environmental control. (Note that this is a one group pretest-posttest design.)

T-tests may be used in nonexperimental situations as well. Most common is a comparison of naturally occurring groups or events such as the difference between male and female students' mathematical abilities (an example of independent samples), or a comparison of marital discord scores before and after the birth of the first child (an example of paired samples). An example of each of these *t* tests will help to clarify terms and demonstrate their use.

Independent Samples

Graduate nurse practitioner students and first year medical students were invited to participate in a special clinical practicum. Because the experience was optional, the project leaders knew that the volunteers might not be representative of their classes. However, they were still struck by apparent differences between the two groups and looked at the sociodemographic data to see if the differences were statistically significant. For the purposes of demonstrating the use of *t* tests, we will look at the analysis of just one variable, their age. The project coordinators looked at the descriptive data first. One aspect was the mean and standard deviation of the students' ages by college (see Table 20-1). The mean age of nurse practitioner students ($M = 37.58$, $SD = 8.54$), certainly looked different from the mean age of the medical students ($M = 24.84$, $SD = 2.81$). Note also that the standard deviations are quite different suggesting more variability in the ages of the practitioner students than in the ages of the medical students, evidenced also by the differences in the range, 23 to 60 versus 21 to 36, respectively.

The next step was to subject the results to *t* test analysis (see Table 20-2) using the *t* test for independent samples since the two sets of means and standard deviations come from two different (independent) subsamples.

First, look at the lower line of results in Table 20-2 to find what is called the folded *F* result. This is a particular type of *F* test of the variances of the two samples (remember how different the standard deviations were?). The folded *F* indicates that the differences are significant, so the *t* test result for samples with unequal variances (Satterthwaite method) is the appropriate statistic. The *t* value of 14.20 and *P* value of $< .0001$ indicate a statistically significant difference between the ages of the graduate nursing students and the medical students. The observed difference between the means of the two samples is 12.75. Clearly, the nurse practitioner students are significantly older than the medical students as a group. The printout also includes confidence intervals. The 95% confidence interval is reported because the .05 significance level was selected. The confidence intervals are of less than usual interest in this instance because there is little doubt that the ages reported are relatively accurate and of little interest in generalizing this result to the larger population of medical students and nurse practitioner students. They would be much more important if we were analyzing the means on a confidence scale or a cultural competency measure for both groups of students.

TABLE 20-1   **Age of Nurse Practitioner and Medical Students: Means, Standard Deviations, and Ranges**

	N[a]	Mean	SD[b]	Range
Nurse practitioner students	99	37.60	8.54	23–60
Medical students	113	24.84	2.81	21–36

Note: [a]N = number in sample; [b]SD = standard deviation.

TABLE 20-2 Comparison of the Ages of Nurse Practitioner and Medical Students: Independent *t*-Test Results

	N	Mean	95% CI[a]	(Mean)	SD	95% CI	(SD)
1. Nurse practitioner students	99	37.59	35.89	39.30	8.54	7.49	9.93
2. Medical students	113	24.84	24.32	25.37	2.82	2.49	3.24
Diff 1-2 pooled method		12.75	11.08	14.43	(6.18)	5.65	6.84
Diff 1-2 Satterthwaite method		12.75	10.98	14.53			

Method	Variances	*df*[b]	*t*	*p*
Pooled	Equal	210.00	14.98	<.0001
Satterthwaite	Unequal	116.65	14.20	<.0001

Equality of Variances

Method	Num *df*	*df*	*F*	*p*
Folded *F*	98	112	9.19	<.0001

Notes: [a]CI = confidence interval; [b]*df* = degrees of freedom.

There is one more calculation that should be made, the effect size. The effect size statistic answers the question: Is this a relatively large difference? As a reminder, the effect size is the degree (extent) to which the mean of one sample differs from the mean of another sample. The calculation is related to standard deviation units (O'Rourke, Hatcher, & Stepanski, 2005, p. 180). The formula for calculating the effect size in this example is relatively simple:

$$\text{effect size} = \frac{\text{First Sample Mean} - \text{Second Sample Mean}}{\text{Pooled Estimate of the Population Standard Deviation}}$$

$$d = \frac{(M_1 - M_2)}{Sp}$$

The difference between the two means in our example is 12.75 (37.59 mean for the practitioners minus the 24.84 mean for the medical students).

The pooled standard deviation is 6.18, which you can find circled in the table in Table 20-2.

Our calculation is 12.75 ÷ 6.18 which equals 2.06. Filling in all these numbers in the formula, we have

$$\frac{(37.59 - 24.84)}{6.18} = 2.06 \qquad d = 2.06$$

Our effect size is 2.06 which, if you check the tables provided by Cohen (1988) is a large effect size (small = .20, medium = .50, and large = .80 or greater) (O'Rourke, Hatcher, & Stepanski, 2005, p. 182).

If you can understand this very simple example in all its detail, then you are ready to consider the more complex variations to follow.

Paired Samples

The groups to be compared in paired sample *t* tests are matched or correlated. In other words, they are related, not independent of one another. To illustrate the use of *t* tests in paired samples, we will look at the responses of some of those students who participated in that special clinical experience. Since the nurse practitioners and medical students were assigned to interdisciplinary teams for this experience, the project coordinators were interested in whether or not the experience changed their perspectives on physician-nurse collaboration. A measure of collaboration (Sterchi, 2007) was administered before and after this experience and the pretest-posttest results were first compared using simple paired-sample *t* tests. Table 20-3 shows the differences in means for just the medical students from pretest to posttest.

Table 20-4 shows the results of a paired *t* test comparing the pretest scores to the posttest scores of the medical students. You can see that the difference in mean scores from pretest ($M = 51.48$, $SD = 6.53$) to posttest ($M = 52.70$, $SD = 6.16$) is only 1.22 points on the scale. A higher score indicates a more positive attitude toward physician-nurse collaboration (Sterchi, 2007). The 95% confidence limits are .20 and 2.243, indicating that the *actual difference* in the pretest and posttest means has a 95% probability of lying between .20 and 2.23. Since zero does not lie within this range, you can reject the null hypothesis (O'Rourke, Hatcher, & Stepanski, 2005) of no difference between pretest and

TABLE 20-3 Mean Collaboration Scores for Medical Students at Pretest and Posttest

	N	Mean	SD	Range
Pretest Score	86	51.48	6.53	29–60
Posttest Score	86	52.70	6.16	29–60

posttest scores. However, the lower bound of the confidence interval is almost zero suggesting that the mean gain of the studied population could be as little as 0.2. With this result, the researcher needs to wonder about the practical utility of the interdisciplinary experience in regard to changing perspective on physician-nurse collaboration.

We turn now to the test of significance and see that the *t* value is 2.40 and the *P* value (probability) is .0186, which is significant because it is at or below the conventional cutoff of .05. We can tentatively conclude, then, that the experience had an effect on perceived collaboration.

The effect size should also be calculated, especially since the change in score was relatively small. Using the same formula as before:

$$d = \frac{(M_1 - M_2)}{Sp} = \frac{51.48 - 52.70}{4.71} = \frac{1.22}{4.71} = .2591 \qquad d = .2591$$

Rounding the result, we can say that $d = .26$, a small effect size, confirming our impression of its size.

There are limitations to the *t* test. It accommodates only two levels of the predictor variable, which is nominal or categorical in nature, and just one outcome variable, which is at the interval or ratio level of measurement. To accommodate more levels of the predictor variable and more complex analyses, we turn now to the analysis of variance or ANOVA.

ANOVA

Analysis of variance extends the *t* test to three or more groups. It is especially useful in examining the impact of different treatments (Muller & Fetterman, 2002). If you had

TABLE 20-4 **Collaboration Ratings in Medical Students: Comparison of Pretest and Posttest Mean Scores Using Paired Samples *t*-Tests**

		Statistics			
N	Mean	SD	Std Error	Minimum	Maximum
86	1.22	4.71	.50	-11.00	13.00

95% Confidence Interval	(Mean)	SD	95% Confidence Interval (Std Dev)	
.20	2.23	4.71	4.10	5.55

	t-Test		
Difference	df	t	p
Posttest Score-Pretest Score	85	2.40	.0186

three subsamples to compare on one outcome measure, you could do this with a set of three *t* tests. But this approach is inefficient and increases the risk of type I error. Instead, analysis of variance performs these comparisons simultaneously and produces a significant result if any of the sample means differ significantly from any other sample mean (Evans, 1996, p. 339). ANOVA compares the variation or difference *between* the means of the subsamples or groups with how much variation there is *within* each group or subsample (Iversen & Norpoth, 1987, p. 25).

F Ratio

Analysis of variance computations produce an *F* ratio. There is usually variation within the groups as well as between the groups. An *F* ratio is the ratio of between-treatment group variations to within-treatment group variation (Evans, 1996, p. 345). *F* ratios close to 1 indicate the differences are random or chance differences. *F* ratios much larger than 1 indicate that the difference is greater than would be expected by chance (Iversen & Norpoth, 1987, p. 31).

In an experiment, for example, we would look first at the standing of the groups (subsamples) before treatment is given. At this point, the groups should be equivalent on the outcome variable of interest although there will be some variation across subjects within the group. After the treatment or treatments are completed, the groups are compared to see if there is evidence of an effect from the treatment.

The resulting *F* ratio is a relatively robust statistic, but if your data departs too much from normality, you may need to use nonparametric alternatives, which you will find described in statistics textbooks (Der & Everitt, 2006).

One-Way ANOVA

One-way ANOVA is the basic analysis of variance. It involves (1) a single predictor or independent variable that is categorical in nature but may have two or more values, and (2) a single criterion or dependent variable at the interval or ratio level of measurement (O'Rourke, Hatcher, & Stepanski, 2005, p. 210).

One-way ANOVA involves only one predictor variable. As with *t* tests, there are two basic types, a *between-subjects* model, which is similar to the independent sample *t* test, and a *repeated-measures* model, which is similar to the paired *t* test (O'Rourke, Hatcher, & Stepanski, 2005). We will look at examples of each model.

Between subjects. A group of community-dwelling older adults who volunteered for memory screening were matched across ethnic groups on income and years of education to produce a sample of 225 African-Americans, European Americans, and Hispanic Americans. Because there were exactly 75 participants in each ethnic group, this was a *balanced* design. A between-subjects one-way analysis of variance was done comparing the three ethnic groups on their mean depression score (Sheikh & Yesavage, 1986).

As you can see from the results of the ANOVA in Table 20-5, there are significant differences across the three ethnic groups given the *F* ratio of 3.78 and probability of $P = .02$.

TABLE 20-5   Comparison of Depression Scores by Ethnic Group: One-Way Between Subjects Analysis of Variance

Source of Variation	df	Type I SS	Mean Square	F	p
Ethnic Group	2	15.055	7.527	3.78	.0243
	df	Type III SS	Mean Square	F	p
Ethnic Group	2	15.055	7.527	3.78	.0243

Means and Standard Deviations

	N	Geriatric Depression Scale Mean	SD
African-American	75	5.41	1.20
European American	75	5.97	1.45
Hispanic American	75	5.97	1.55

Tukey's Studentized Range (HSD) Test

Ethnic Group Comparison	Difference Between Means	Simultaneous 95% Confidence Intervals	
Hispanic to European American	0.0008	−0.5504	0.5519
Hispanic to African-American	0.5541	0.0067	1.1014*
European American to Hispanic	−0.0008	−0.5519	0.5504
European American to African-American	0.5533	0.002	1.1044*
African-American to Hispanic	−0.5541	−1.1014	−0.0067*
African-American to European American	−0.5533	−1.1044	−0.0022*

Note: *Significant at .05 level.

Note there are results for both type I and type III sums of squares. The type III sum of squares results is appropriate for unbalanced designs, but in this case, with a balanced design, you can see that the results for type I and type III are the same. If you were reporting these results, you would use this statement:

$$F(2,223) = 3.78, P = .02$$

Although the *F* test is significant, it does not tell us what comparisons across the three ethnic groups were the source of the significance. In other words, it tells us that an effect occurred but not what effect(s) occurred (Evans, 1996). To answer the question, "Which means are different?," there are several calculations that can be done. If these comparisons are planned in advance (before analyzing the data) they are called *a priori* or planned comparisons. Another term for these calculations is *contrasts* (Muller & Fetterman, 2002). The most common comparisons or contrasts following one-way ANOVA are a group of pairwise comparisons of the means. To obtain this important information, a Tukey test (a post-hoc test) was performed. You can see at the bottom of Table 20-5 that pairwise comparisons of the means were done for the three ethnic groups. Although there are six comparisons listed, actually there are only three unique sets of information. The asterisks indicate the pairs of comparisons that are significant at the $P = .05$ or better level. Inspection of the results provides the answer to the question of which means are different. In this example, the depression score mean for the African-American group was significantly different (lower) than the means for the Hispanic and European American groups.

These calculations for pairwise comparisons include an adjustment factor for the number of comparisons that will be made. Remember that too many comparisons may lead to rejection of the null hypothesis when the null hypothesis is true (Type 1 error). There are a number of these multiple comparisons procedures available. This includes the Bonferroni or Dunnett for planned comparisons and the Tukey and Scheffé for unplanned comparisons (Muller & Fetterman, 2002). The Tukey's HSD (honestly significant differences) produces a conservative estimate. The Scheffé test can be used with both balanced and unbalanced designs (Munro, 2005).

Again, there is one more calculation needed to complete this analysis, the R^2 for the predictor variable, which in this example is ethnic group membership. The R^2 will tell you the percent of the variance in the scores on the Geriatric Depression Scale that is accounted for by the predictor variable—the ethnic group. It is relatively easy to calculate the R^2 if you do not find it on your ANOVA printout:

$$R^2 = \frac{\text{Type III SS}}{\text{Corrected Total SS}}$$

$$R^2 = \frac{15.005}{446.959} = .033 \quad R^2 = .03$$

This is a relatively small R^2. It indicates that ethnic group membership accounts for 3% of the variation in the depression scores, a significant but small effect.

Repeated Measures Designs. These designs are also called *within-subjects* designs because more than one measurement is obtained on each participant. The simplest of these designs is the testing of the same participants under two or more different treatment conditions. For example, you could first engage participants with mild hypertension in a series of yoga relaxation classes to reduce blood pressure. After a washout period, the second treatment, adherence to the DASH diet (DHHS, NIH, 2006), would be instituted, and a second set of measurements would be taken. A third or even fourth treatment could be added to this experiment.

Advantages of this design, which uses participants as their own controls, is that fewer participants are needed and the treatment groups do not differ (Munro, 2005). These advantages, however, are often outweighed by the disadvantages:

- High attrition rate (the number of participants lost from the study between the two treatment conditions).
- Order effect: Participants may not be as enthusiastic about trying the second or third treatment option, reducing adherence.
- Carryover effect: Participants may continue to experience or benefit from the effects of the first treatment (O'Rourke, Hatcher, & Stepanski, 2005).

Counterbalancing helps to overcome the last two disadvantages; this involves providing the treatments in different orders. For example, one half of the sample would follow the DASH diet first, while the other half would attend the yoga sessions first. The washout period, a separation of a week or more between treatments, is also helpful.

Mixed Designs. A second repeated measures design uses different participants in each treatment group. This eliminates order and carryover effects, but it does mean that the participants in each treatment group will not be identical. Even with random assignment to treatment group, there will probably be some variation between groups at baseline. This second repeated measures design is called a *mixed design* because it will generate both between-group (the different treatment groups) and within-group (change or lack of change from one time to another) measures. The analysis of the results will provide three types of information:

- Change over time
- Differences between the groups
- The interaction of time and group effects (Munro, 2005).

In the case of a study with one experimental group and one control group, both of whom are tested prior to treatment and at the end of treatment, it is the interaction of time and treatment group that is of greatest interest.

An example will help clarify the use of mixed design and interpretation of the results. An experimental study comparing the effects of exercise and social conversation on the mood of nursing home residents with Alzheimer's disease was conducted. Enrolled participants (consent was provided by next of kin, guardian, or proxy healthcare surrogate and assent obtained from the participant) were randomly assigned to one of three treatment groups:

- An exercise program that combined simple strength and endurance exercises. Done with minimal conversation.
- Social conversation designed to engage the person in discussion of everyday activities and interests but not to address the person's concerns or emotional

needs, a "friendly visitor" level of conversation. Designed to provide an attention control group.

- Combined exercise and conversation

To illustrate use of mixed designs, we will look at the results on just one outcome measure, the Sad subscale of the AD-RD Mood Scale (Tappen & Williams, 2008). (See Table 20-6 for means, standard deviations, and ranges of the Sad subscale scores by treatment group.) A diagram of the study design might help make it clear what model was used (see Figure 20-1). Data from this study will also be used to illustrate the use of ANCOVA.

The interaction effect of treatment group over time is the result that addresses the primary study hypotheses that exercise alone or in combination with conversation will improve mood but that social conversation alone will not (see Table 20-7). Unfortunately, neither the univariate nor multivariate tests for interaction effects are significant given an F value of 1.21 and P value of .3029. The *main* effects of group and time can also be inspected. There is no group (between-subjects) effect with an F value of .28 and P value of .7544. The time (within-subjects) effect is also not significant with an F value of .63 and P value of .4292.

Given the nonsignificant results, neither inspection nor reporting of the planned contrasts are done in this instance. During the study, however, the investigators noted that involving participants in the intended treatment was a challenge for the interventionists. When participants were tired, irritable, or not feeling well, they were likely to refuse treatment. Interventionists kept records of the number of minutes per session each participant engaged in the assigned treatment. If the difference in the amount of treatment provided were controlled, would there be a significant difference in the outcomes for the three treatment groups? To answer this question, an analysis of covariance (ANCOVA) was done using the measure of treatment intensity (total minutes of treatment over the entire 16 weeks of the treatment phase of the study) as a covariate.

ANCOVA

Analysis of covariance is a procedure in which the effects of factors called covariates are extracted or controlled before the analysis of variance is done (Der & Everitt, 2006). The

TABLE 20-6   Sad Mood Scores of Individuals with Alzheimer's Disease: Pretest and Posttest Means, Standard Deviations, and Range by Treatment Group

	Pretest			Posttest		
	M	SD	Range	M	SD	Range
Exercise	7.379	(2.55)	4–13	6.482	(2.64)	4–14
Conversation	7.357	(3.10)	4–15	7.285	(2.87)	4–15
Combined	6.800	(1.90)	4–11	7.033	(3.07)	0–17

Treatment Groups	Testing Times	
	Pretest	Posttest
Exercise		
Conversation		
Combined Exercise and Conversation		

Figure 20-1   Diagrammatic representation of the Exercise vs. Conversation Study of nursing home residents with Alzheimer's disease.

covariates are usually *confounding variables* or *extraneous variables* that contribute to the variation and reduce the magnitude of the differences between the groups being compared. Controlling for these extraneous or confounding variables can reduce the error variance and increase the power of the analysis (Munro, 2005).

There are two main instances when ANCOVA is used:

1. When a variable is known to have an effect on the dependent (outcome) variable in an analysis of variance

TABLE 20-7   Mixed Design (Repeated Measures ANOVA) Comparison of Sad Mood Following Treatment in Nursing Home Resident with Alzheimer's Disease

Source	*df*	Type III Sums of Squares	Mean Square	*F*	*p*
Between Subjects	86	901.033			
Treatment group	2	6.012	3.006	0.28	.7544
Residual between	84	895.021	10.655		
Within Subjects	87	359.570			
Time (pretest-posttest)		2.606	2.606	0.63	.4292
Group X Time Interaction	2	10.008	5.004	1.21	.3029
Residual within	84	346.956	4.130		
Total	173	1260.603			

Note: N = 87.

2. When the groups being compared are not equivalent on one or more variables, either because they were not randomized or in spite of randomization (Munro, 2005, p. 200)

The second use of ANCOVA is controversial because it is impossible to identify with any certainty all of the ways in which nonrandomized groups might differ. Another concern is that the use of ANCOVA is based upon the assumption that the covariate is not related to the experimental treatment (Keppel, 2004).

Returning to the exercise and conversation treatment example, an analysis of covariance controlling for baseline level of sadness and treatment intensity (the number of minutes of treatment received over the entire course of treatment, which was 4 months) is shown in Table 20-8. The resulting F value for the effect of the treatment is 4.02 and level of significance is .0215. The adjusted means (least squares means) show the greatest amount of sadness in the conversation group, the least in the exercise group. Preplanned pairwise comparisons show a significant difference between the group receiving conversation treatment and the group receiving the exercise treatment. The other comparisons are not significant.

By controlling for any baseline difference in sad mood or difference in the amount of treatment received, the effect of the exercise treatment becomes evident. However, this use of ANCOVA is the second, more controversial use—to equalize groups that are, despite

TABLE 20-8   Comparison of Sad Mood in Nursing Home Residents with Alzheimer's Disease Using Analysis of Covariance Controlling for Baseline Mood and Treatment Intensity

Source	df	Type III SS	Mean Square	F	p
Baseline Sad Mood	1	153.895	153.895	25.08	< .0001
Treatment Intensity	1	53.733	53.788	8.76	.0040
Treatment	2	49.384	24.692	4.02	.0215

Least Squares (Adjusted) Means	
Exercise	5.823
Conversation	8.191
Combine	6.825

Preplanned Comparisons: pr > t

	Exercise	Conversation	Combined
Exercise		.0061	.1272
Conversation	.0061		.0937
Combined	.1272	.0737	

random assignment, not equal on all possible factors that might affect the outcome of treatment. Interpretation of the results needs to be done with extreme caution.

Two-Way ANOVA

The ANOVA-based analyses discussed so far have employed a single independent variable at the nominal or categorical level of measurement (the independent variable is the treatment variable in experimental research or explanatory variable in nonexperimental research). Two-way analysis of variance allows you to examine the effects of two between-subjects independent variables at once, including the interaction between the two independent variables (Munro, 2005; O'Rourke, Hatcher, & Stepanski, 2005).

Let's return to the fictional yoga versus DASH diet example to illustrate two-way analysis of variance. The mode of delivery of the intervention is a second important independent variable that could also be tested. This model is illustrated in Figure 20-2: two modes of delivery, electronic via an online program and a live group that meets twice weekly to learn yoga or the DASH diet. Further, combining yoga and diet is of interest and will add another level of treatment to produce what is called a *3 × 2 factorial design:* three treatments by two modes of intervention delivery. Each of the six squares in the diagram is referred to as a *cell*.

Reporting of the results of a two-way analysis of variance follows a similar pattern to other analysis of variance models. Begin with the *main effects*, which in this study would be mode of delivery and type of treatment. If either is significant, you can proceed to examination and reporting of the planned comparisons such as the difference in outcome between yoga, the diet, and the combination of yoga and diet. Finally, you can examine and report the *interaction effect* between the two independent variables. A significant interaction means that the differences in treatment depend on the mode of delivery.

MANOVA

One additional procedure from the analysis of variance family, often a very useful one, is the multivariate analysis of variance or MANOVA. You have encountered mention of

Intervention	Mode of Delivery	
Yoga	Electronic	Group
DASH Diet	Electronic	Group
Yoga + Diet	Electronic	Group

Figure 20-2 Diagrammatic representation of a two-way analysis of variance study.

avoiding type I error (rejecting the null hypothesis when it is true) several times already in this chapter. When you have a number of criteria or outcome variables that are conceptually related, instead of analyzing each one separately using ANOVA, you can begin the analysis with a MANOVA.

For example, in a research study that compared two types of cognitive stimulation, one that used a specific cognitive retraining protocol and the other that used life review to provide general cognitive stimulation, there were several outcome measures related to face-name association (ability to remember names of people). These four face-name associated variables were entered into a MANOVA that produced a significant effect (see Table 20-9).

Examination of the results of a MANOVA should begin with multivariate F value derived from Wilks lambda or any of the other statistical tests (e.g., Hotelling-Lawley's trace). If this is not significant, your analysis ends here because you cannot reject the null hypothesis that the groups have equal means on the outcome variables. If the multivariate F value is significant, however, you may proceed to examine the univariate ANOVAs generated for each of the outcome variables. If the univariate F statistic is significant, then

TABLE 20-9 Comparison of Cognitive Retraining and Life Review Interventions in Individuals with Mild Cognitive Impairment: MANOVA of Face-Name Association Outcomes

MANOVA Test for Effect of Treatment		
Statistic	F	p
Wilks' lambda	0.860	.0573
Pillai's trace	0.133	.0573
Hotelling-Lawley trace	0.153	.0573
Ray's greatest root	0.153	.0573

Univariate Tests for Effect of Treatment Adjusted Means						
	Cognitive Retraining	Life Review	df	Type III SS	Mean Square	F	p
Face-Name Trial 1	2.972	1.774	1	24.240	24.240	5.71	.0198
Face-Name Trial 2	2.972	2.354	1	58.441	58.441	7.63	.0074
Face-Name Trial 3	4.459	2.870	1	42.562	42.562	4.53	.0371
Face-Name Recognition	16.783	14.225	1	110.369	110.369	7.70	.0072

you can proceed down one more level of specificity to the pairwise comparisons (O'Rourke, Hatcher, & Stepanski, 2005).

Most of these steps, the examination of the univariate *F* and the pairwise comparisons, are already familiar. The multivariate *F*, however, is new to this procedure. To return to the results in Table 20-10, you can see that the multivariate *F* derived from Wilks' lambda is .866 and the *P* value is .0573, just barely significant at the *P* = .05 level. Proceeding to the univariate *F* statistics, you find that all four have *F* values significant at the *P* = .05 or better level. Because there were only two treatment groups involved in each of these comparisons, there is no need for additional pairwise comparisons in this instance.

Interpretation of this one-way, between-subjects design MANOVA is relatively straightforward. If the results are significant, you can say that the treatment groups were compared simultaneously on the four outcome variables related to face-name association and that the analysis revealed a significant multivariate effect (O'Rourke, Hatcher, & Stepanski, 2005, pp. 293–294). The univariate *F* tests indicate significant effects of treatment on each of the four outcome variables. Inspection of the adjusted means indicates higher achievement on each of these tests of face-name association for the group that received the specific cognitive retraining when compared to the group that received the general stimulation (life review) intervention. Effect size statistics such as the partial eta squared (η^2) may also be generated and reported as part of the results of your analysis.

TABLE 20-10   **Simple Linear Regression**

Source	df	Sum of Squares	Mean Square	*F* e	*p*
Model	1	922.52940	922.52940	40.95	< .0001
Error	689	15523	22.52999		
Corrected Total	690	16446			
	Root MSE	4.74658	R-Square	0.0561	
	Dependent Mean	13.29799	Adj R-Sq	0.0547	
	Coeff Var	35.72080			

Parameter Estimates

		Unstandardized Coefficients		Standardized Coefficients		
Variable	df	B	Standard Error	Beta	t	p
Intercept	1	23.48576	1.60386	−.23684	14.64	< .0001
Age	1	−0.14023	0.02192		−6.40	< .0001

Note: Dependent Variable: Animal Category Fluency Test Score; Independent Variable: Respondent Age; Number of Observations Used: 691.

There are some drawbacks to the use of MANOVA. Technically, if the MANOVA is not significant, you have to ignore a statistically significant result for one or more of the sets of outcome variables analyzed. Due to the effects of intercorrelation within groups, MANOVA can sometimes be significant when the ANOVAs are not and vice versa (Bray & Maxwell, 1985).

REGRESSION ANALYSIS

In this second half of the chapter, we will focus on prediction of the dependent variable based on knowledge of the independent variable rather than on comparison of means. The discussion will be limited to the most basic and commonly used linear regression analyses. Regression analyses can become very complex in some of their iterations. You will find these discussed in advanced statistics textbooks.

The primary assumption behind linear regression analysis is clearly described by Evans (1996):

> Its most essential assumption is that variables *x* and *y* have a straight-line relationship with each other. . . . If that assumption is true for a set of pairs of scores, then *y* values can be predicted from *x* values. The stronger the correlation between *x* and *y*, the more accurate the predictions. (p. 160)

The *x* variable, by the way, is the predictor (independent) variable, and the *y* variable is the criterion (dependent) variable. We can do much more than this with regression, but this is the fundamental basis of regression: to predict values of *y* from values of *x*.

Simple Linear Regression

There is an interesting and deceptively simple set of cognitive function tests called the category fluency tests. To administer the test, the examiner asks the person being tested to name as many animals, fruits, vegetables, words beginning with *F*, modes of transportation, items of clothing, or other categories in 1 minute. The answers are recorded and the score is simply the number of relevant, nonredundant items or words generated in one minute. The simplicity of the test makes it easy to understand. The number of factors that might influence the total score makes it an interesting example to illustrate linear regression analysis.

We will begin with the simplest linear regression: one independent variable and one dependent variable. To do this, we will regress respondent age on the animal category fluency test (see Table 20-10)[1]. As you can see in the modified SAS printout in Table 20-10, the dependent variable is the animal fluency test score (number of nonduplicate animals named in 1 minute), and the independent variable is the age of the respondent. Details of the derivation and interpretation of the many statistics found in a simple linear regression result are provided in Box 20-1.

---

[1]This research was supported by funds from the Johnnie B. Byrd Sr. Alzheimer's Center and Research Institute, Inc., Huntington Potter, PhD, principal investigator, John Schinka, PhD, project director.

Box 20-1 Explanation of Table 20-10: Details of a Simple Linear Regression Output

Regarding Table 20-10, you can see that the total degrees of freedom (690) are one less than the responses that were analyzed (691). The model sum of squares plus the error sum of squares should equal the total sum of squares, and it does. The mean square is the sum of squares divided by the related number of degrees of freedom. The *F* value of 40.95 is the result of testing the overall model. It is calculated by dividing the model mean square (922.529) by the error mean square (22.529). The size of this *F* value and *P* value of < .0001 indicate a significant model. Root MSE is then obtained by finding the square root of the mean square and estimates the standard deviation of the error. The coefficient of variation is the ratio of the root MSE to the size of the dependent mean. It tells us that the error standard deviation is 35.7% of the mean value of the dependent variable (animal category fluency) mean. The *R* square, or R^2, is the correlation of the dependent and independent variables squared. It tells us the percentage of the variation in values of animal category fluency scores explained by age (definitions from Freund & Littell, 2000).

The parameter estimates are found at the bottom of the table. To understand them, we have to consider the basic equation that underlies regression analyses:

$Y = a + bX$ Y = the dependent variable
            X = the independent variable
            a = the intercept
            b = the slope of the line, called the *regression coefficient* (Polit, 2009).

The independent and dependent variables are already familiar, but *a* and *b* need further explanation. The regression coefficient *b* is the rate of change in *Y* per unit change in *X*. If *X* and *Y* values were plotted on a graph such as those shown below, *b* would be the slope of the regression line. The regression coefficient *b* is calculated from what are called deviation scores (the differences between the values for *X* (age) and *Y* (test scores) and the means of *X* and *Y* which are summed and divided by the sum of the squared deviations of *X*. Similarly, the intercept constant is calculated from the mean of *Y* from which the mean of *X* times the regression coefficient is subtracted (definitions from Munro, 2005, p. 265).

When two or more independent variables are involved, as is the case in multiple regression, they usually employ different units of measurement making it difficult to compare them. To allow for comparison, these values can be standardized. To do this, the original (raw) values of the independent variables are converted into *Z* scores with a mean of 0 and standard deviation of 1.0, and the estimates are calculated on the *Z* scores. This produces standardized regression coefficients called *beta weights* (βs). The nonstandardized coefficients are *b* weights. The standardized beta weights can be compared to see the relative importance of each of the independent variables in a multiple regression analysis (Freund & Littell, 2000; Polit, 2009).

continues

Box 20-1 Continued

The lower portion of the table provides parameter estimates that may be used to estimate (predict) values of the animal category scores given the age of the respondent. The predicted animal category score is the intercept value (23.48576) minus the dependent variable parameter estimate (−.14028) times the age of the respondent. It is unlikely that we would actually try to predict the scores on the basis of age alone because the amount of variance explained by age, the R^2, is only 5%. Confidence intervals may also be calculated using the standard errors of the parameter estimate or they may be generated by the statistical software program. The last column provides the t value. The t value of −6.40 is calculated by dividing the parameter estimate by the standard error. The P value is significant.

It is not necessary to memorize all of this information, but it is helpful to understand how each of the statistics is derived and how they are related one to the other.

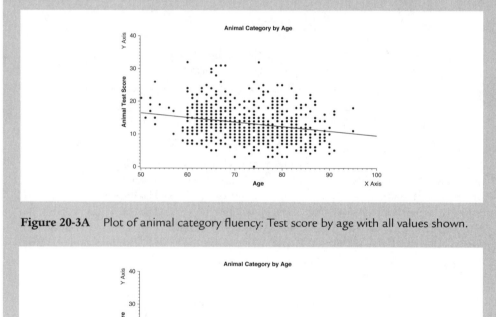

Figure 20-3A Plot of animal category fluency: Test score by age with all values shown.

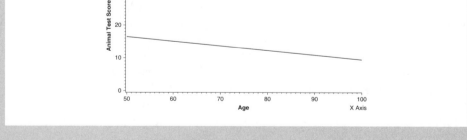

Figure 20-3B Plot of animal category: Fluency by age illustrating the slope line of X by Y.

The information gained from this simplest form of linear regression is somewhat limited and not often reported. The addition of other independent variables usually generates more informative results and, often, an explanation of a greater proportion of the variance of the dependent variable.

Multiple Regression with Two or More Independent Variables

Multiple regression is used to examine the "collective and separate effects of two or more independent variables on a dependent variable" (Pedhazur, 1982, p. 6). The discussion will begin with the use of continuous-level (interval or ratio) independent variables and then address the use of nominal-level (categorical) independent variables through what is called dummy or effect coding.

We will continue to use the animal category fluency test score as an example to explain multiple regression analysis. You may have felt that some fundamental information about the variables was missing from the discussion in the previous section. If so, you were correct. To remedy this, Table 20-11 provides basic statistics about the two variables, animal category fluency and age, and two additional variables that will be added to the next analysis, years of education and cognitive function as measured by the Mini-Mental State Examination (MMSE) (Folstein, Folstein, & McHugh, 1975).

Most of the information provided in Table 20-11 should be easy to understand now. Altogether, there were 692 respondents, but there is information missing on the Animal Category Fluency test for one respondent, so the N for that variable is only 691. The mean number of animals named in one minute was 13.287 ($SD = 4.88$), but the range was very wide, 0 to 32. The age range was also wide, from 50 to 95 with a mean of 72.708 ($SD = 8.24$). Years of formal schooling also had a wide range from 1 to 21 with a mean of 12 (equivalent to finishing high school) ($SD = 4.13$). Cognitive scores need a little more explanation. The range of possible scores on the MMSE is 0 to 30. The lower scores indicate some degree of cognitive impairment: mild if between 18 and 23, moderate at about 10 to 18 and advanced or severe if below 10. Just these few numbers provide a much clearer idea of who the respondents were. You may have noticed that neither gender nor ethnic group membership was mentioned. These are nominal (categorical) variables that will be addressed later. The regression analyses discussed so far include only continuous (interval or ratio-level) data.

One more section of Table 20-11 needs to be examined. Below the simple statistics, you will find the Pearson correlation coefficients for all possible combinations of the four continuous variables of interest. The first number under each variable combination is the correlation (r), the second number is the probability of r (the significance level of the correlation); the third number is the N or sample size. Note that all the correlations are significant at the $P < .0001$ level. Several combinations have a lower N because of the missing data on one animal category fluency score. The lowest correlation is between years of education and age, $r = -.15$, a negative correlation. This indicates that, as age rises, the years of education declines. The highest correlation is between years of education

TABLE 20-11   Correlation Matrix for Variables of Interest for Regression Analysis

Four Variables: Animal Category Fluency, Age, Years of Education, Cognition

Simple Statistics

Variable	N	Mean	Std Dev	Sum	Minimum	Maximum
Animal Category Fluency	691	13.28799	4.88204	9182	0.0000	32.00000
Age	692	72.70809	8.24420	50314	50.00000	95.00000
Years of Education	692	12.00145	4.13642	8305	1.00000	21.00000
Cognition	692	26.13295	3.66541	18084	9.00000	30.00000

Pearson Correlation Coefficients

	Animal Category Fluency	Age	Years of Education	Cognition
Animal Category Fluency	1.00000	−0.23684	0.35790	0.42749
		< .0001	< .0001	< .0001
	691	691	691	691
Age	−0.23684	1.00000	−0.15998	−0.23161
	< .0001		< .0001	< .0001
	691	692	692	692
Years of Education	0.35790	−0.15998	1.00000	0.47962
	< .0001	< .0001		< .0001
	691	692	692	692
Cognition	0.42749	−0.23161	0.47962	1.00000
	< .0001	< .0001	< .0001	
	691	692	692	692

and MMSE score, $r = .47$. As years of education increase, the MMSE score tends to increase also. That the MMSE score is so sensitive to education has been a concern for many years for clinicians using the test because it is meant to measure cognitive ability, not educational achievement.

We turn our attention now to Table 20-12, which provides the results of a linear regression with two or more independent variables. The F value of 68.72 and $P < .0001$ indicate that we can reject the null hypothesis. The R square of .23 indicates that this model explains 23% of the variance in animal category fluency. The adjusted R^2, often a little lower than the R^2, is useful in keeping us from adding too many independent variables simply to raise the resulting R^2 (Munro, 2005). Interpretation of the *t* values is not as straightforward as it is in a simple *t* test. In this case the *t* value and related probability tell you whether or not there is an effect for age, for example, over and above the effect of the other two independent variables (education and cognition) (Freund & Littell, 2000). The null hypothesis for this *t* value would be that there is no effect due to age. The *P* value of < .0001 indicates that there is an effect and that the null hypothesis should be rejected.

Upper and lower confidence intervals may also be generated for the regression analysis. Remember that prediction of the values of the dependent variable *y* from values of the independent variable *x* is the fundamental purpose of regression. Prediction values of the dependent variable can be generated for each value of the independent variable along with 95% confidence intervals for each value. Because this may become a very long list of values (in this example *N* = 691, so there are 691 listed) only a sample of 15 of these predicted

TABLE 20-12   Regression with Two or More Independent Variables (Multiple Regression)

Source	df	Sum of Squares	Mean Square	F	p
Model	3	3796.08986	1265.36329	68.72	< .0001
Error	687	12650	18.41281		
Corrected Total	690	16446			

Root MSE		4.29102	R-Square	0.2308	
Dependent Mean		13.28799	Adj R-Sq	0.2275	
Coeff Var		32.29244			

Parameter Estimates

Variable	df	Unstandardized Coefficients		Standardized Coefficients		
		B	Standard Error	Beta Weight	t	p
Intercept	1	5.847	2.11378		2.77	0.0058
Age	1	−0.081	0.02040	−.137	−3.96	< .0001
Years of Education	1	0.225	0.04506	.190	4.99	< .0001
Cognition	1	0.40629	0.05159	.305	7.88	< .0001

Notes: Dependent Variable: Animal Category Fluency; Independent Variables: Age, Years of Education, Cognition; Number of Observations Used: 691

values and some useful statistics are included. As you can see in Table 20-13, values are provided for each observation. We are looking only at the first 15 that were entered into the database, observations 1 through 15. The actual value of the dependent variable, animal category fluency is next, followed by the value predicted by the regression equation and standard error. Then you can see the 95% confidence intervals for the expected (predicted) value (not the actual value) listed. Most of these seem to be relatively close to the predicted value. However, the difference between the actual and predicted value of the dependent variable (animal category fluency) are quite different in some cases. The residuals column provides specific information on this. These residuals are the difference between the actual and predicted values. For example, the difference (residual) between actual and predictive values for observation #2 is −7.698, and for observation #10 it is 9.6482, which are quite large. Others are not so large, but they do suggest that the regression equation is not entirely accurate in predicting animal category fluency scores. At the end of this long list of observations are some helpful statistics. The first one, sum of residuals, should be zero, and it is in this case. The second one, sum of squared residuals, should be equal to the error sum of squares in the analysis of variance reported in the top portion of the output (not shown in this table), and inspection shows that they are identical. The last statistic, PRESS, indicates the presence of outliers if it is much larger than the previous statistic, which it is not (Freund & Littell, 2000). None of these three statistics indicate a problem with the data used in this analysis.

Multicollinearity

The choice of independent variables to include in a regression equation is often a challenge for the researcher. Theory underlying the study, results of prior studies and the study hypothesis should guide the selection. It is tempting to include as many variables as possible to boost the R^2 and improve the predictive power of the equation, but this approach increases the risk of multicollinearity among the independent variables.

Collinearity may be defined as redundancy among the variables. In other words, some of the independent variables added to a regression equation may contribute little to the information that has already been contributed by other variables. Muller and Fetterman (2002) call these "extremely unimportant predictors" as opposed to those that do contribute, which can be extremely important sources of information (p. 164). Uncontrolled collinearity, they note, creates difficulties in the analysis of the regression equation and makes interpretation of the results problematic.

If the correlation matrix, illustrated in Table 20-11, provided all the information we needed to identify collinearity, this would be relatively easy to evaluate. Certainly, highly correlated variables are likely to contribute to collinearity. However, there are other statistics that provide better diagnostic information. The first is the variance inflation factor (VIF) (see Table 20-14), which illustrates the results of these diagnostics applied to the regression of age, education, and cognition on animal category fluency scores. As you can see, all three variance inflation factors are relatively similar in size, ranging from 1.06 to 1.34 (rounded). One rule of thumb for interpreting the VIF is that values under 10 are not

TABLE 20-13   Dependent Variable: Animal Category Fluency Scores

Output Statistics

Observation	Dependent Variable	Predicted Value	Standard Error Mean Predicted	95% Confidence Intervals	Mean	Residual
1	11.0000	15.9337	0.2881	15.3681	16.4993	−4.9337
2	3.0000	10.6988	0.2957	10.1182	11.2793	−7.6988
3	20.0000	15.2869	0.3345	14.6302	15.9436	4.7131
4	8.0000	9.4304	0.3986	8.6478	10.2129	−1.4304
5	11.0000	8.9914	0.4017	8.2028	9.7800	2.0086
6	15.0000	15.6912	0.2959	15.1101	16.2722	−0.6912
7	12.0000	13.4673	0.1805	13.1129	13.8218	−1.4673
8	18.0000	15.9694	0.2637	15.4516	18.4875	2.0306
9	12.0000	15.3509	0.3654	14.6334	16.0684	−3.3509
10	26.0000	16.3518	0.4635	15.4417	17.2619	9.6482
11	19.0000	13.6563	0.2180	13.2283	14.0844	5.3437
12	7.0000	10.5212	0.2630	10.0049	11.0376	−3.5212
13	7.0000	10.5232	0.3180	9.8988	11.1476	−3.5232
14	6.0000	11.0104	0.3108	10.4001	11.6207	−5.0104
15	12.0000	12.8889	0.3409	12.2195	13.5583	−0.8889

Sum of Residuals	0
Sum of Squared Residuals	12650
Predicted Residual SS (PRESS)	12798

an indicator of concern. Another approach is to look at any values that are greater than $1/(1 - R^2)$ (Freund & Littell, 2000, p. 98). Since the R^2 for this regression is .23, the result would be 1.29870 or 1.30. Only the VIF for cognition is higher than this and only by a very small amount. SPSS also generates a Tolerance statistic which is based upon VIF (Tolerance = 1/VIF). If it is low, there may be a problem with collinearity.

The second diagnostic is a little more complex because it analyzes the structure of the relationships among the variables and produces a set of statistics that have not been addressed before. Only a summary of this approach will be provided. Find the last condition index number in the lower portion of the table (it is circled to help you find it). Compare this figure with the variance proportions of the independent variables (age,

TABLE 20-14   Statistics to Evaluate Multicollinearity

| | | Parameter Estimates | | | | | |
| | | Unstandardized Coefficients | | Standardized Coefficients | | | |
Variable	df	B	Standard Error	Beta	t	p	Variance Inflation (VIF)
Intercept	1	4.84723	2.11378		2.77	0.0058	
Age	1	−0.081	0.02040	−.137	−3.96	< .0001	1.05931
Education	1	0.225	0.04506	.190	4.99	< .0001	1.30124
Cognition	1	0.406	0.05159	.305	7.88	< .0001	1.33960

Collinearity Diagnostics (Intercept Adjusted)

| | | | Proportion of Variation | | |
Number	Eigenvalue	Condition Index	Age	Education	Cognition
1	1.60403	1.00000	0.10149	0.18975	0.20081
2	0.88092	1.34939	0.87035	0.12796	0.03486
3	0.51505	(1.76474)	0.02816	0.68229	0.76433

Notes: Dependent Variable: Animal Category Fluency; Number of Observations Used: 691.

education, and cognition). This condition number is 1.76474, which is not especially large. Compare this with the proportion of variance in the same row for each of the independent variables. None of these is larger than the condition number indicating again that multicollinearity is not a serious concern in this example (Freund & Littell, 2000).

Dummy Coding
After encountering all those difficult technical terms, this next one, *dummy coding*, might provide some comic relief. Despite its odd name, however, dummy coding extends the reach of multiple regression in some very useful ways. Up to this point, all of the variables entered into the regression analyses have been continuous variables, measured at the interval or higher level. (In some cases, ordinal variables can also be used). Dummy coding allows us to include nominal- or categorical-level variables (called "qualitative" in some texts) as well.

If the categorical variable has only two values, such as male and female for gender, died or survived for mortality data, or controlled and not controlled for diabetic management, then these dichotomous independent variables can be entered into the equation without recoding. If the variable is *polytomous* (having more than two levels), however, then you must recode it before entering it into the equation (Hardy, 1993).

There are two categorical variables not yet included that were of interest in the analysis of influences on animal category fluency test scores: gender and ethnic group membership. Gender is a dichotomous variable and can be entered without recoding. However, since this study included members of four distinct ethnic groups, African-American, Afro-Caribbean, Hispanic American, and European American, ethnicity is polytomous and needs to be recoded.

Recoding involves conversion into a set of dichotomous variables. The number of dichotomous variables created should be one less than the total number of levels of this variable. In the case of ethnic group membership, this would be 4 minus 1 = 3, as follows:

Ethnic 1	African-American = 1	Not African-American = 0
Ethnic 3	Hispanic American = 1	Not Hispanic American = 0
Ethnic 4	Afro-Caribbean = 1	Not Afro-Caribbean = 0

The European Americans were designated the *reference group* because they are the group on which most of these cognitive measures were first tested, but technically this choice is an arbitrary one, and any ethnic group could have been selected as the reference group (Hardy, 1993).

To illustrate the use of dummy coding, we first consider the regression equation with the addition of gender alone (Table 20-15). If you compare the results in Table 20-15 with those in Table 20-12 you will see the following:

- Degrees of freedom are increased from 3 to 4.
- The R^2 and adjusted R^2 are only minimally increased.
- Gender has a significant t value, but it is smaller (less significant) than the t values of the other independent variables.
- The beta weight for gender is small relative to the others.
- The VIF for gender is smaller than the VIF of the other independent variables. The condition number also suggests that multicollinearity is not a problem.

Adding ethnic group membership increases the complexity of the output and changes the status of the variable gender (see Table 20-16). Comparing this result with the previous one in which only gender had been added, you can see the following differences:

- The degrees of freedom have increased again, from 4 to 7, reflecting the increased number of independent variables.
- The R^2 and adjusted R^2 have increased.
- Gender is no longer significant at $t = 1.47$, $P = .1412$.
- The beta coefficient (beta weight) for gender is clearly smaller than the beta weights for the other independent variables.

TABLE 20-15 Dummy Coding Example: Addition of a Dichotomous Variable Gender

Analysis of Variance

Source	df	Sum of Squares	Mean Square	F	p
Model	4	3881.57536	970.39384	52.98	< .0001
Error	686	12564	18.31504		
Corrected Total	690	16446			

Root MSE	4.27961	R-Square	0.2360
Dependent Mean	13.28799	Adj R-Sq	0.2316
Coeff Var	32.20658		

Parameter Estimates

Variable	df	Unstandardized Coefficients B	Standard Error	Standardized Coefficients Beta	t	p	Variance Inflation (VIF)
Intercept	1	7.04511	2.17985		3.23	0.0013	
Age	1	−0.08111	0.02034	−0.13694	−3.99	< .0001	1.30238
Education	1	0.4496	0.04496	0.18788	4.93	< .0001	1.30238
Cognition	1	0.41828	0.05175	0.31398	8.08	< .001	1.35517
Gender	1	0.82861	0.38354	−0.07256	−2.16	0.0311	1.01298

Collinearity Diagnostics (Intercept Adjusted)

Number	Eigenvalue	Condition Index	Proportion of Variation Age	Education	Cognition	Gender
1	1.62041	1.00000	0.09679	0.17977	0.19519	0.01574
2	0.99086	1.27881	0.01623	0.01991	0.00004914	0.95365
3	0.88059	1.35652	0.86009	0.13454	0.03394	0.00321
4	0.50815	1.78573	0.02688	0.66578	0.77082	0.02740

Notes: Dependent Variable: Animal Category Fluency; Independent Variable: Age, Years of Education, Cognition, Gender; Number of Observations Used: 691.

TABLE 20-16 Dummy Coding Example: Addition of a Polytomous Variable Ethnic Group Membership

Source	df	Sum of Squares	Mean Square	F	p
Model	7	4418.70868	631.24410	35.85	< .0001
Error	683	12027	17.60905		
Corrected Total	690	16446			

Root MSE	4.19631	R-Square	0.2687
Dependent Mean	13.28799	Adj R-Sq	0.2612
Coeff Var	31.57975		

Parameter Estimates

Variable	df	Unstandardized Coefficients B	Standard Error	Standardized Coefficients Beta	t	p	Variance Inflation (VIF)
Intercept	1	10.77027	2.24819		4.79	< .0001	
Age	1	−0.09652	0.02032	−0.16296	−4.75	< .0001	1.09879
Education	1	0.18086	0.04500	0.15319	4.02	< .0001	1.35654
Cognition	1	0.39677	0.05127	0.29784	7.74	< .0001	1.38332
Gender	1	−0.56442	0.38319	−0.04943	−1.47	0.1412	1.05166
Ethnic 1	1	−2.24510	0.48017	−0.23005	−4.68	< .0001	2.26084
Ethnic 3	1	−2.85321	0.53372	−0.25239	−5.35	< .0001	2.08168
Ethnic 4	1	−1.99900	0.65674	−0.12595	−3.04	0.0024	1.59912

Collinearity Diagnostics (Intercept Adjusted)

Number	Eigenvalue	Condition Index	Proportion of Variation Age	Education	Cognition	Gender
1	1.73395	1.00000	0.08417	0.04878	0.08709	0.00002112
2	1.54109	1.06073	0.01207	0.14111	0.10266	0.03370
3	1.18801	1.20811	0.00097364	0.00137	0.00042200	0.06802
4	0.97168	1.33584	0.01435	0.05472	0.00209	0.77717
5	0.84811	1.42985	0.84726	0.05218	0.03704	0.04133
6	0.49711	1.86763	0.01015	0.665555	0.74844	0.03729
7	0.22003	2.80721	0.03103	0.04629	0.01225	0.04247

(continues)

TABLE 20-16   Dummy Coding Example: Addition of a Polytomous Variable Ethnic Group Membership (continued)

| | Collinearity Diagnostics (Intercept Adjusted) Proportion of Variation | | |
Number	Ethnic 1	Ethnic 3	Ethnic 4
1	0.07634	0.05730	0.00356
2	0.05581	0.5647	0.01427
3	0.01048	0.06649	0.37795
4	0.00238	0.03927	0.01988
5	0.03049	0.00640	0.00025332
6	0.00687	0.00317	0.00041588
7	0.81764	0.77070	0.58367

Notes: Ethnic 1 African-American–Not African-American; Ethnic 3 Hispanic American–Not Hispanic American; Ethnic 4 Afro-Caribbean–Not Afro-Caribbean; Dependent Variable: Animal Category Fluency; Independent Variables: Age, Education, Cognition, Gender, Ethnic Group; Number of Observations Used: 691.

- The variance inflation factors (VIF) for Ethnic 1 and Ethnic 3 are higher than the VIF of the other variables. However, the condition number of 2.807 is higher than any of the proportion of variance figures for the independent variables, which range from .012 for cognition to .817 for Ethnic 1, suggesting that multicollinearity is not a serious problem.

- The beta weights and significance levels for the ethnic group variables suggest that they do influence the animal category fluency test scores, especially for the African-American and Hispanic American to other ethnic groups' comparisons. This is not a desirable outcome for this test, the results of which should not be influenced by age, education, or ethnic group membership, only by cognitive functionality.

Selection

You could see in the previous section on dummy coding that entering additional independent variables can have an effect on both the weight of other variables and on the overall results of the regression. As mentioned earlier, selecting the variables to enter into the regression equation and deciding which ones should be retained is often a challenge. Theory and prior research results should be your primary guides, but they do not always provide enough guidance. Another approach is to use the results of the analysis to make these decisions.

There are a number of different selections you can make to conduct this exploratory regression analysis:

- *Maximum* R^2: This analysis begins by selecting one or two variables that produce the highest R^2, interchanges them until those with maximum improvement in R^2 are identified, and then brings in additional variables and interchanges them until the optimum combination is found.

- *Forward selection:* This analysis begins with the simple (one variable) model that produces the largest R^2 and adds variables until no further increase is found. Selected variables are not deleted later in this approach.

- *Backward elimination:* This analysis begins with all of the variables in the regression and then deletes those with the least significance, one at a time, until all remaining variables are at the prespecified level of significance.

- *Stepwise:* Begins with the one variable model that produces the largest R^2, then adds and deletes variables until no further improvement can be made.

The automatic, atheoretical process involved in these selection-based regression analyses is a source of some concern. Der and Everitt (2006) caution that a variable that is eliminated might contribute to a different solution if retained for a theory-based reason. They also quote Agresti (1996) who noted that when all effects are weak, the largest of the weak effects might be overestimated and that some variables should be included due to theoretically based interest in them. Most important, if you include a large enough number of variables, one or more that really are not important may appear to be important due to chance.

Hierarchical Linear Regression

Instead of putting all the variables into the analysis at once as is done in multiple regressions or entering them in an order determined by preset limits such as significance level, hierarchical linear regression employs a series of steps or blocks of variables determined in advance on a theoretical basis.

This is an advanced technique that will not be described in detail but summarized so the reader will have a general idea of when it is an appropriate choice and how it works.

Newlin and colleagues (2008) examined the relationship of religion and spirituality to glycemic control in black women who had type 2 diabetes. They used a four-step block entry hierarchical regression to conduct the analysis. At step 1, sociodemographic variables including age, income, and education, were entered as a block. At step 2, BMI (body mass index) and the number of diabetes-related medications were entered. The religion and spirituality subscale scores of the Spiritual Well-Being Scale were entered at step 3. Finally, at step 4, diabetes-specific emotional distress and social support scores were entered. Glycemic control, the dependent variable, was measured using the (Hb)A1c test. Religion and spirituality were found to be significantly related to glycemic control, holding the sociodemographic and clinical factors (BMI and diabetes medications) constant.

Sample Size

The temptation to include (some would say "throw in") as many variables as possible in the regression equation and the problems associated with doing this have already been mentioned but are emphasized once more when considering the sample size needed to conduct these analyses. A common rule of thumb is to have at least 10 subjects per variable in the analysis (Munro, 2005). Any less than that will result in unstable outcomes and appreciable shrinkage of the adjusted R^2. You can also conduct a power analysis to determine the sample size needed. You can find the formulas to do this in Cohen (1988) or generate a power analysis from your statistical analysis program.

Logistic Regression

Up to this point, we have addressed regression of independent variables on a continuous dependent variable. Logistic regression addresses the use of a *categorical* dependent variable in the equation. If this variable is dichotomous (having only two different values), then logistic regression is done. If the dependent variable has three or more values, then a polytomous regression is done. These analyses may also be done with dependent variables that can be ordered such as:

Mild-1		Independent-1
Moderate-2	OR	Needs Assistance-2
Severe-3		Dependent-3

To illustrate the use of logistic regression with a dichotomous categorical variable, we will return to the 692 individuals who volunteered for cognitive screening. This time we will focus on a question related to ethnic group membership and primary language. Inspection of the data indicates that only one person for whom Spanish was the primary language was not Hispanic American but Afro-Caribbean. Given this situation, an analysis of factors predicting Spanish as primary language is only appropriate for the Hispanic American subsample. Of these 171 individuals in the dataset, data are missing on 9 of them so 162 responses are used in the analysis. Experience with this group and information from the literature suggests that those for whom Spanish is their primary language are likely to be older, have fewer years of education, be less actively involved in activities outside of their ethnic enclave, more likely to suffer from depression, and born outside the United States. To test these ideas (which could be restated as formal hypotheses), we will run a logistic regression of six independent variables: age, gender, education, born in the United States, depression, and function to predict the dependent categorical measure (Spanish as primary language vs. Spanish not the primary language). The results may be seen in Table 20-17.

We look now at the results in Table 20-17 to find out if the hypothesized independent variables predicted whether or not participants had Spanish as a primary language and what that effect was. The number of missing values was already discussed. We see next that Spanish was the primary language of 93 individuals; English was the primary language for 69. The modeling is based upon those whose primary language was Spanish (Spanish = 1), but it could have been based upon those whose primary langue was English—this choice should be based on the relationship of interest. Next we note that the convergence criterion is satisfied. Then we see the model fit statistics. Lower levels of these statistics are considered favorable (Allison, 1999). The three chi-squares for the model are similar although the Wald, which is the focus of our attention, is somewhat lower but still significant.

The Wald chi-squares and their significance levels for each independent variable are of particular interest. You can see that gender (a dichotomous variable), age, and function are not significant predictors of Spanish as a primary language. The Wald chi-square (similar to a *t* value although squared) is largest for those born in the United States and small for gender and function. Similarly, the beta weights for gender and function are small while the largest ones are for being born in the United States.

Logistic regression analyses produce *odds ratios* for the independent variables. The odds of an event or condition are the ratio of the probability of occurrence to the probability of nonoccurrence (Munro, 2005, p. 305). We can use the born in the United States variable as an example of the calculation of the odds ratio using information found in Tables 20-18 and 20-19. The relationship of primary language (English or Spanish) to country of origin (the United States or other) is diagrammed in Table 20-18. You can quickly see that only one (5%) of the individuals born in the United States reported that Spanish was their primary language. In contrast, only 48 (32%) of the 148 who were not born in the United States reported that English was their primary language.

To obtain the odds ratio just for this variable, we can generate a new logistic regression with born in the United States as the only independent variable, or we can calculate it from the cells in Table 20-18. Calculating the odds from the cells allows us to see how an odds ratio is generated. Table 20-19 shows the calculations that we will review. As you can see, four *probabilities* may be calculated first, addressing four possible conditions that reflect the relationships in the four cells of the contingency table. From these results, two odds are calculated, the odds that the individual was born in the United States if English is his or her primary language (.4375) and the very small odds (.0100) that Spanish would be the primary language of an individual born in the United States in this sample. The odds ratio of 43.75 is calculated from these last two results and is the same as the odds (43.75) reported in the logistic regression of born in the United States in Spanish as a primary language. This is a high odds ratio suggesting that country of origin is a powerful predictor of Spanish as a primary language in older Hispanic Americans.

TABLE 20-17   Logistic Regression

Response Profile

Ordered Value	Spanish	Total Frequency
1	1	93
2	0	69

Probability modeled is Spanish = 1 (Spanish as primary language)

Model Convergence Status
Convergence Criterion (GCONV = 1E-8) Satisfied

Model Fit Statistics

Criterion	Intercept Only	Intercept and Covariates
Akaike's information criterion	223.011	182.085
Schwartz criterion	226.099	206.786
−2 Log L	221.011	166.085

Testing Global Null Hypothesis: BETA = 0

Test	Chi-Square	df	Pr > Chi-Square
Likelihood ratio	54.9257	7	< .0001
Score	46.7125	7	< .0001
Wald	27.8544	7	0.0002

Analysis of Maximum Likelihood Estimates

Parameter	df	Unstandardized Coefficients B	Standard Error	Wald Chi-Square	Pr > ChiSq	Standardized Estimate Beta
Intercept	1	−8.2773	3.8875	4.5336	0.0332	
Gender	1	−0.1603	0.4258	0.1418	0.7065	−0.0394
Age	1	−0.0448	0.0281	2.5374	0.1112	−0.1824
Born in the US	1	3.8794	0.0639	13.2961	0.0003	0.7350
Education	1	−0.1132	0.0508	4.9551	0.0260	−0.2852
Depression	1	0.1863	0.1093	2.9076	0.0882	0.2087
Function	1	−0.0176	0.0280	0.3935	0.5305	−0.0758

(continues)

TABLE 20-17   Logistic Regression (continued)

Odds Ratio Estimates

Effect	Point Estimate	95% Wald Confidence	Limits
Gender	0.852	0.370	1.963
Age	0.956	0.905	1.010
Born in the US	43.75	6.015	389.420
Education	0.893	0.808	0.987
Depression	1.205	0.973	1.493
Function	0.983	0.930	1.038

Notes: Response (Dependent) Variable: Spanish; Number of Response Levels: 2
Number of Observations Read: 171; Number of Observations Used: 162.

TABLE 20-18   Frequency Table and Chi-Square Analysis

Primary Language and Country of Origin: Older Hispanic Americans

Primary Language	Country of Origin US	Other	Total
Spanish is primary language	1	100	101
English is primary language	21	48	69
Total	22	148	170

Chi-Square Analysis

Statistic	df	Value	Prob
Chi-square	1	31.5463	< .0001
Likelihood ratio chi-square	1	34.9690	< .0001
Continuity ad. chi-square	1	28.9870	< .0001
Mantel-Haenszel chi-square	1	31.3608	< .0001
Phi coefficient		0.4308	
Contingency coefficient		0.3956	
Cramer's V		0.4308	

TABLE 20-19 Calculation of Probabilities, Odds, and Odds Ratios: Primary Language and Country of Origin

Probabilities	
21/69 = .3043	Probability was born in US if English primary language
48/69 = .6956	Probability was not born in US if Spanish primary language
1/101 = .0101	Probability of Spanish primary language if born in US
100/101 = .99	Probability of Spanish primary language if not born in US

Odds	
.3043/.6956 = .4375	Odds born in US if English is primary language
.0101/.9909 = .0100	Odds Spanish primary language if born in US

Odds Ratio	
.4375/.0100 = 43.75	

Source: Based upon procedures described by Munro, 2005, p. 317 (data are original).

Remembering the definition of odds as the ratio of occurrence to nonoccurrence, we can diagram it as:

$$\frac{\text{Occurrence}}{\text{Nonoccurrence}}$$

If you are not interested in the individual probabilities, you can calculate the odds directly by dividing the occurrence cell value by the nonoccurrence cell in each column and then dividing the result for those not born in the United States column by the result for those born in the United States column (see Table 20-20).

	First Column	Second Column
Occurrence (Of Spanish as primary language) Nonoccurrence (Of Spanish as primary language)	$\dfrac{1}{21} = .0476$	$\dfrac{100}{48} = 2.083$

2.083/.0476 = 43.75

This is just a shorter, more direct way to calculate the odds ratio.

There is more that you can do with logistic regression analyses. As with multiple regression, you can select a method for addition and deletion of variables to achieve the optimum combination, but the same cautions apply to use of this procedure as applied to multiple

TABLE 20-20   Contingency Table: Occurrence vs. Nonoccurrence of Spanish as Primary Language by Country of Origin

	Country of Origin	
	U.S. (Born in US)	Other (Not born in US)
Occurrence (Spanish as primary language)	1	100
vs.		
Nonoccurrence (English as primary language)	21	48

Occurrence/Nonoccurrence

Odds	$1/21 = .0476$
	$100/48 = 2.0833$
Odds Ratio	$2.0833/.0476 = 43.75$

regression. Logistic regression can be used in one-to-one matched samples, which are of considerable interest in health-related research (Der & Everitt, 2006). Confidence intervals may be generated, and multinomial analyses (more than two levels of the outcome variable) may be used. If the levels of the outcome variable can be ordered, you can take advantage of this higher level of measurement as well (Allison, 1999). You can also enter variables in blocks as in hierarchical linear regression and apply a variety of diagnostic statistics, such as the ones mentioned earlier, to the logistic regression (Munro, 2005).

The data and results used to demonstrate the use of logistic regression in this chapter are only one small example of the wide range of uses for logistic regression and its variants.

As we end this chapter, it is important to note that there are other increasingly complex strategies within the regression family of analyses. They address a variety of situations such as relationships that are nonlinear, more sophisticated modeling techniques such as LISREL, and use of multiple dependent variables such as canonical analysis. Their use and interpretation are addressed in intermediate and advanced statistics textbooks.

CONCLUSION

One of the best ways to gain an appreciation of the analytic procedures described in this chapter is to apply them to a dataset, your own if possible, or one of the demonstration datasets that accompany most software packages and statistical textbooks.

Each of these procedures has its uses but also its drawbacks. It is important to understand both when you apply them in your research. Obtaining guidance from an experienced researcher and/or statistician will not only help you select the most powerful procedures for your dataset but also avoid inappropriate applications of them.

REFERENCES

Agresti, A. (1996). *Introduction to categorical data analysis*. New York: Wiley.

Allison, P. D. (1999). *Logistic regression using SAS: Theory and application*. Cary, NC: SAS Institute.

Bray, J. H., & Maxwell, S. E. (1985). *Multivariate analysis of variance*. Beverly Hills, CA: Sage.

Cohen, J. (1988). *Statistical power analysis for the behavioral sciences*. Hillsdale, NJ: Lawrence Erlbaum Associates.

Cortina, J. M., & Dunlap, D. P. (2007). On the logic and purpose of significance testing. In S. Sarantakos (Ed.), *Data analysis* (pp. 215–234). Los Angeles, CA: Sage.

Department of Health & Human Services (DHHS), NIH. (2006). *Your guide to lowering your blood pressure with DASH* (Pub. H06-4082). Washington, DC: Government Printing Office.

Der, G., & Everitt, B. S. (2006). *Statistical analysis of medical data using SAS*. Boca Raton, FL: Chapman & Hall/CRC.

Evans, J. D. (1996). *Straightforward statistics*. Pacific Grove, CA: Brooks/Cole.

Folstein, M. F., Folstein, S. E., & McHugh, P. R. (1975). Mini-Mental State: A practical method of grading the cognitive state of patients for the clinician. *Journal of Psychiatric Research, 12*, 189–198.

Freund, R. J., & Littell, R. C. (2000). *SAS system for regression* (3rd ed.). Cary, NC: SAS Institute.
  ✧ Good explanation of the elements of simple and multiple regressions. Note that SAS uses the terms parameter estimate for the unstandardized coefficient β and standardized estimate for β weights (standardized regression coefficients).

Hardy, M. A. (1993). *Regression with dummy variables*. Newbury Park, NJ: Sage.
  ✧ There is more to the use of dummy coding than was covered in this chapter. This little book delves into the subject without being too difficult to understand.

Iversen, G. R., & Norpoth, H. (1987). *Analysis of variance*. Newbury Park, NJ: Sage.

Keppel, G. (2004). *Design and analysis: A researcher's handbook* (4th ed.). Englewood Cliffs, NJ: Prentice-Hall.

Muller, K. E., & Fetterman, B. A. (2002). *Regression and ANOVA: An integrated approach using SAS Software*. Cary, NC: SAS Institute, Inc.

Munro, B. H. (2005). *Statistical methods for healthcare research*. Philadelphia: Lippincott, Williams & Wilkins.
  ✧ A readable introduction to statistics.

Newlin, K., Melkus, G. D., Tappen, R., Chyun, D., & Koenig, H. G. (2008). Relationships of religion and spirituality to glycemic control in black women with type 2 diabetes. *Nursing Research, 57*(5), 331–339.
  ✧ Provides an example of hierarchical linear regression with a relatively clear explanation of mediational model testing.

O'Rourke, N., Hatcher, L., & Stepanski, S. (2005). *A step-by-step approach to using SAS for univariate and multivariate statistics*. Cary, NC: SAS Institute.
  ✧ Not only is this a very clear explanation of t-tests and ANOVAs but this book offers help with interpreting the results and provides sample paragraphs illustrating how you summarize the results in a report or paper to be submitted for publication.

Pedhazur, E. J. (1982). *Multiple regression in behavioral research*. New York: Holt, Rinehart & Winston.
  ✧ A classic text on multiple regression.

Polit, D. F. (2009). *Data analysis and statistics for nursing research* (2nd ed.). Upper Saddle River, NJ: Prentice Hall.
  ✧ Contains an especially clear explanation of multiple regression that may be helpful to the new researcher.

Sheikh, J. I., & Yesavage, J. A. (1986). Geriatric Depression Scale (GDS): Recent evidence and development of a shorter version. In T. L. Brink (Ed.), *Clinical gerontology: A guide to assessment and intervention* (pp. 165–175). New York: Haworth Press.

Smith, H., Gnanadesikan, R., & Hughes, J. B. (2007). Multivariate analysis of variance (MANCOVA). In S. Sarantakos (Ed.), *Data analysis* (Vol. 3, pp. 309–328). Los Angeles, CA: Sage.

Sterchi, L. S. (2007). Perceptions that affect physician-nurse collaboration in the perioperative setting. *Association of Perioperative Registered Nurses, 86*(1), 45–57.

Tappen, R., & Williams, C. (2008). Development & testing of the Alzheimer's Disease & Related Dementias (AD-RD) Mood Scale. *Nursing Research, 57*(6), 426–435.

Yuker, H. E. (1958). *A guide to statistical calculations.* New York: G. P. Putnam's Sons.
   ◇ If you want to calculate a chi-square or t-test by hand, this is the guide for you.

CHAPTER 21

Analysis of Qualitative Data

Once more, we consider the continuum from structured to unstructured, this time in the analysis of qualitative data. The most structured approach to the analysis of qualitative data uses coding and quantifying of the qualitative data. *Content analysis* is a specific case of the quantification of qualitative data. At the other end of the continuum are three of the great traditions in qualitative research: ethnography, grounded theory, and phenomenological analysis. In between lie a variety of coding and thematizing analyses that operate within a semistructured and unstructured framework. Each of these reflects a very different tradition (most are described in the theory and design chapters), which needs to be kept in mind as you match your data to the appropriate analytic framework.

Data collection and data analysis may occur virtually simultaneously in the most unstructured of these approaches, while the more structured analyses are done after the data has been collected and processed.

PROCESSING THE DATA

Faced with a mountain of observational notes and transcribed conversations, many qualitative researchers have thought to themselves "What do I do now?" Handling that mountain of qualitative data requires some organization. There are several activities you may need to complete during the data collection and analysis stages to manage the data and facilitate the final analysis:

1. *Keep notes organized with sources clearly identified.* It is common to think at the beginning of a study that we will never forget this participant and his or her story nor would we ever confuse our own ideas and interpretations with statements made by the participants. But our memories become consolidated over time, so the distinction between what we have thought and what we have heard from participants may blur.

   For these reasons, it is important to keep field notes separated by source: (1) transcribed quotes from participants, (2) observations of participants, (3) the researcher's feelings about the experience, and (4) researcher interpretations, preliminary constructions, and theme identification.

   The *language* of the notes is important as well. Recording the speech of the participant, the idioms, slang, jargon, phrases, and abbreviations characteristic of the people and the setting is important. Much cultural and personal meaning may be lost if this is not done. Exact quotes are preferable when possible. If you write in the language of the researcher or in a combination of researcher/participant language, be sure to make note of this (Spradley, 1979).

Spradley (1979) also distinguishes between *condensed* accounts that are made in the field and *expanded* accounts that include as much detail as you can, written as soon after exiting the field as possible. Be sure to put date, time, and place on each note.

2. *Prepare accurate transcriptions of notes and recordings.* This step is not an absolute necessity if you (1) plan to hand code (as opposed to using a software program), (2) will do all the analysis yourself, (3) write clearly, and (4) do not have a mountain of data. On the other hand, transcribing those condensed notes into an expanded account as soon as possible after the notes have been taken accomplishes two goals: readable notes and an opportunity to review what happened and plan the next data collection session.

Some types of analysis require transcriptions in electronic form, particularly if you plan to use qualitative analysis software. A transcriber with a foot pedal to stop and start a recorded session is worth the expense if you have a large number of audio recordings to transcribe. Or you can use a digital voice recorder designed for dictation or recording music and download the recordings into a transcription program. Eventually speech recognition may become accurate enough to do this for us (Gibbs, 2007).

For certain types of content, narrative, conversation, and discourse analysis, every emphasis, mispronunciation, and hesitation needs to be recorded. For an interpretive analysis, the tone of voice and emphasis need to be noted also. Listening to the recording should supplement reading the transcripts.

Accuracy of the transcription cannot be taken for granted. If you have someone typing your notes or recordings, it is very important to review the transcription for accuracy. Gibbs (2007) provides some examples of the types of errors a transcriptionist may make that can have a serious impact on the accuracy of your analysis (Gibbs, 2007, p. 19):

Transcribed: ever meant to   Actual: never meant to

Transcribed: denying neglect   Actual: benign neglect

3. *Upload the data into an analytic software program.* If you have a large amount of data or plan to conduct a very detailed or quantitatively based analysis, then qualitative data analysis software may be very helpful. The following is a brief list of the ways in which qualitative data analysis software can help you conduct your analysis:
   - Upload the texts.
   - Maintain lists of the codes you have created.
   - Mark text by code or theme.
   - Retrieve text that you have coded.
   - Support creation of a hierarchy of codes and themes.
   - Allow you to write memos and attach them to text.

Commonly used software packages include Ethnograph, NUD*IST, NVivo, Altas.ti, and MAX qda for most descriptive and interpretive analyses. VB Pro, Word Stat, and ZyINDEX can be used for content analysis (Krippendorff, 2004). Each has features that support qualitative data analysis. Gibbs (2007) warns that using these types of software leaves some researchers feeling that it has created a distance between them, their data, and the people the data represent. You may also want to remember that these programs are basically high-level sorters and organizers. They support your analytic work, they do not think for you.

WHY QUANTIFY?

Even in qualitative research, there are occasions where counting is useful. Some of these have been mentioned in earlier chapters:

- To describe the sample: Number of participants, their age, gender, years of education, income categories, stage of disease, and so forth

- To report the frequency of a response: Frequency of a response may indicate how general an opinion is or how common a particular experience has been. For example, you could report that 25% of the children interviewed had been hospitalized at least once due to an asthma attack. Or you could report that 75% of the adults interviewed mentioned difficulty explaining their problem with chronic fatigue to employers. Note that the frequency of mention is not equivalent to the intensity of the impact. This is better evaluated qualitatively ("This is what I fear most," "It has been the most difficult part of having chronic fatigue") or by asking people to rate the impact.

- To report the frequency of behaviors: This is often done with behaviors that have been recorded on video or on coding forms. This data lends itself to quantification and quantitative analysis. For example, you can report how often preschoolers with autism engage in solitary play versus interaction with classmates and teachers. The type of solitary play and of the interactions with others could be described qualitatively or coded and reported as frequencies.

- This coding and counting of observations can be done with either micro or macro units of analysis:

    Micro: At this level, every vocalization, even the hesitations, the hmms, and uhs are noted and counted. Incomplete sentences, unfinished thoughts, and word repetitions can also be counted.

    Macro: At this level, conversations may be coded as generally symmetrical (relatively equal exchanges) or asymmetrical (imbalanced, one speaks more often than the other). Even more macro would be a count of purposeful interactions among staff (reporting patient data or problem solving) versus social interactions (plans for the weekend or talk about the weather).

- Comparisons of frequencies across subgroups: This is just one step further into quantitative analysis. The number of observed expressions of sympathy or empathy from staff to patient may be compared in male and female staff. The number of instances and types of nurse–patient nonprocedural touch could also be compared in male nurses versus female nurses (Fisher, 2009).

- Combining quantified qualitative data with other quantitative data. This may be done in a mixed method study as a concurrent analysis of the data. While the emphasis here is on quantizing or quantifying qualitative data, the opposite can also be done: quantitative data may also *qualitized* (Tashakkori & Teddlie, 1998). For example, participants with advanced cancer may be asked to respond to a rating scale of chronic pain and then be grouped as those who experience moderate to severe pain and those whose pain is mild or intermittent.

STRUCTURED AND SEMISTRUCTURED ANALYSIS

Coding

Coding is "a deliberate and thoughtful process of categorizing the content of the text," (Gibbs, 2007, p. 39). Two purposes for coding will be discussed: coding of responses to structured and semistructured questions for the purpose of quantifying them is our immediate interest. Later in the chapter, the coding of text for qualitative analysis will be illustrated.

Even more specific, Miles and Huberman describe codes as "tags or labels for assigning units of meaning to the descriptive or inferential information compiled during a study" (1994, p. 57). They identify several types of codes that can be affixed to responses or portions of text:

- *Descriptive codes:* These are the most concrete level of labeling data that simply divide data into various categories or groups of phenomena.

- *Interpretive codes:* These codes are more abstract and are based upon your understanding of the meaning underlying what has been said or done.

- *Pattern codes:* Even more abstract and complex, these codes suggest connections between various patterns or meanings and are indicative of possible themes within the data.

A simple example will be used to illustrate the use of coding to quantify qualitative data at relatively concrete levels of analysis—the descriptive and interpretive.

A semistructured interview guide using investigator-constructed questions was administered to 119 adults who came to senior centers, places of worship, and other community locations for memory screening (Williams, Tappen, Rosselli, Keane, & Newlin, 2009). This sample was composed of African-American, Afro-Caribbean, European American, and Hispanic American adults whose average age was 68 but had a very wide range from the 40s to the 90s. Participants were asked, "If, after screening, you are told that you might have a memory problem, what do you think you will do about it?" Here are a few of their responses:

ID 1	Consult my primary physician for additional tests.
ID 2	I don't know.
ID 3	Whatever I can.
ID 4	Go to the doctor.
ID 5	I'd like to go into it and find out what can be done.

To create the coding scheme, three members of the research team read and reread all of the deidentified responses (names were removed but responses were also deidentified as to ethnic group membership so that this information could not influence the coding decisions). A framework for coding was created in Atlas.ti. Two of the researchers tested the coding scheme, revised it and independently coded all responses. Any differences in codes were reconciled through review with a third coder so final coder agreement was 100%.

The first level of coding of these responses was very concrete. For this question about what participants would do if they screened positive, the following codes were applied:

Code 1	Seek professional help
Code 2	Self-help: mainstream or alternative, complementary
Code 3	General, just "will get help"
Code 4	Not sure, unclear
Code 5	None. Will not seek help

Referring back to the sample responses, each would be coded as follows:

ID 1	Consult my primary physician for additional tests.	Code 1: Seek professional help
ID 2	I don't know.	Code 4: Not sure
ID 3	Whatever I can.	Code 3: General
ID 4	Go to the doctor.	Code 1: Seek professional help
ID 5	I'd like to go into it and find out what can be done.	Code 3: General

Thirty-nine percent of the total sample said they would seek professional help if they screened positive, 5% said they did not know what they would do.

This level of coding was not entirely satisfactory to the researchers because it did not indicate how sure people were about what they would do yet the responses suggested a wide range from people who were unsure to people who were very definite about what they would do. So an additional code was created for degree of certainty and whether or not they would deliberate (think about it) before taking action: (1) take action, (2) deliberate, and (3) unsure, unclear. This is a little higher level of abstraction, requiring some interpretation of the responses:

ID 1	Consult my primary physician for additional tests.	Code 1: Take action
ID 2	I don't know.	Code 3: Unsure, unclear
ID 3	Whatever I can.	Code 2: Deliberate
ID 4	Go to the doctor.	Code 1: Take action
ID 5	I'd like to go into it and find out what can be done.	Code 2: Deliberate

The initial two coders did not agree on the coding of the response for participant with ID 3. After some discussion, the code was changed to 1, "take action."

Once the selections were made for each coding category for each participant, the data were entered into a quantitative analysis program. Chi-square statistics were used to compare responses across the four ethnic group subsamples. More Hispanic Americans planned to seek help right away than did the others, $\chi^2 [9, N = 119] = 30.80$, $p = .0003$. European Americans, on the other hand, were less certain about what they would do than were members of the other three ethnic groups. Very few participants (6%) preferred complementary or alternative treatment over conventional treatment, mentioning herbs, vitamins, special foods or juices they would try (Williams et al., 2009, p. 5).

Content Analysis

Content analysis and its kin, narrative, conversation, and discourse analysis, are a special case in qualitative analysis.

Content analysis is "a family of analytic approaches ranging from impressionistic, intuitive, interpretive analysis to systematic, strict textual analyses" (Hsieh & Shannon, 2007, p. 61). In other words, content analysis may range from highly structured, quantitative analysis to unstructured qualitative analysis. Words in naturally occurring verbal material (text), whether recorded conversation, diaries, reports, electronic text, or books, constitute the data used in content analysis (McTavish & Pirro, 2007, p. 217).

Although both narrative and discourse analyses use text, they differ in their perspective on what the text represents. In *narrative analysis*, the text is conceptualized as a means for sharing experiences with others, exemplified by storytelling. In *discourse analysis*, text is conceptualized as a linguistic tool. Both recognize the social and cultural influences on the way we construct texts (Thorne, 2000). *Conversation analysis* examines the interaction itself: taking turns, opening a conversation, ending a conversation, and so forth (ten Have, 1999).

Krippendorff (2004) lists a number of useful principles to keep in mind when doing content analysis:

- Texts are created for the purpose of communicating with others.
- Texts have multiple meanings, not a single one. The meaning is brought to the text by the reader and may not be agreed upon by all readers.

- Texts can elicit a wide range of responses, but the *response* arises from the reader and cannot be found within the text. This is one of the reasons why computer-based analysis alone does not adequately address many of the research questions directed toward analysis of textual data.

- Consider context when doing content analysis: Why was this text created? By whom was it created? For whom was it created? What was the expected (hoped for) response?

Analyzing the Text

Selecting an approach to the analysis of text begins with a well-constructed research question. As Krippendorff (2004) reminds us, texts convey many different meanings. Several questions need to be answered in constructing the research question.

- What am I looking for in this text?
- Is the focus on content, interpersonal interaction, or both?
- Will I be working at the micro level or macro level of analysis? How micro or macro?
- What type of content analysis best answers my question?
  - ○ Quantitative or qualitative?
  - ○ Analysis of the story or experience or the interactional processes that occur?
  - ○ Strong emphasis on the influence of context or minimal attention to specific context?

Answering these questions thoughtfully will direct you to the appropriate content analysis approach. The following provide examples of three ways a single set of transcribed conversations can be analyzed:

1. As Alzheimer's disease advances, interpersonal communication becomes increasingly difficult or dysfunctional in several ways. For example, vague pronouns are often used to refer to people, places, and things, making it difficult to decipher what is being said. Other problems include word finding (remembering the name or word for specific items) and perseveration (repetition of the same idea). Yet sentence structure remains grammatically correct, and the person is usually able to read a passage of text quite well. These characteristics of the communication dysfunction of Alzheimer's disease provide direction for analyzing conversation of people with Alzheimer's disease. One established approach is to carefully read and then code transcribed conversation for repetitions, word substitutions, and production of content relevant to the subject under discussion. This coding can be done by hand or using a qualitative data analysis program. It is a very specific, quantifiable approach to discourse analysis (Tappen et al., 2001).

2. A very different approach is to read the same transcriptions of conversations for themes and expressions of meaning people with advancing Alzheimer's disease are still able to find in life. Reading such conversations reveals some frequent themes across many one-on-one conversations with an interested listener:

   • Interest in and concern for family
   • Awareness of his or her surroundings and the people in it
   • Everyday activities such as having a meal, taking a walk, and visiting
   • Awareness of his or her cognitive limitations and expressions of concern about them

3. A third way to analyze the same conversation-based data is to examine the effect of the interviewer on the response of the interviewee. If the interviewer asks an open-ended question, can a person with moderate or severe Alzheimer's disease answer it? Is the person more likely to answer a closed-ended question? Are opinion-seeking questions answered more rapidly or more often than fact-seeking questions? (For example, "Do you enjoy your daughter's visits?" versus "How often does your daughter visit?") Are present-oriented questions more likely to elicit a relevant response than questions about the past? Does the interviewee reciprocate with questions for the interviewer (Tappen et al., 1997)?

All of these research questions and more can be addressed by analyzing a single set of transcribed conversations. The analytical approach is determined by the question posed.

Data Transcription

Data transcription should reflect the analytical purpose. For some purposes, especially conversation and linguistic analyses, you need to have every inflection, pause, vocalization, and contraction noted precisely. Timing might even be an issue (you may need specialized software to make the timing accurate). In other cases, some smoothing of the utterances helps the reader focus on the bigger picture (macro) perspective and avoid getting caught up in the accents and mannerisms of a particular individual.

Data Exploration

After transcription is completed and checked for accuracy, read and reread the entire data set, making notes on general impressions, possible coding schemes, and the different perspectives from which you could analyze the data. If you plan to do a conversational analysis, ten Have (1999) suggests looking at turn-taking including pauses and overlaps; sequencing including the beginning and end of a particular sequence or "chunk" of the conversation that follows a specific thread; what each participant is doing on each turn, and the form chosen, for example, what type of greeting is used from the many variations that could have been selected; and how all of this implies a relationship between the interactants (participants) (pp. 105–106). This is done initially for a segment or several segments of the dataset in order to fully develop the coding scheme before analyzing the entire dataset.

Complete the Analysis

Once the coding scheme has been created, it is time to apply it to the entire dataset. If the dataset is large, use of a qualitative data analysis program is very helpful. Following is a list of some of the activities they can support (Krippendorff, 2004, p. 262):

- *Dividing the text into analytical units:* These units could be syllables, words, phrases, sentences, or even paragraphs.

- *Searching the text:* Find, list, sort, count, retrieve, and cross-tabulate the identified analytical units (Krippendorff, 2004, p. 262).

- *Computational content analysis:* The results of the coding can be analyzed quantitatively in some cases.

- *Interactive hermeneutic approaches:* This is the interpretive phase of the analysis. Second- and third-level coding is supported by most qualitative analysis programs.

Some will even generate diagrams of the relationships between the codes.

UNSTRUCTURED ANALYSIS

Coding and Thematizing for Qualitative Analysis

The goal of most qualitative analysis is to move beyond the most concrete, descriptive, level to higher levels of abstraction and interpretation, identifying the themes and sometimes constructing new concepts or theoretical propositions from the results. As mentioned earlier in this chapter, Miles and Huberman (1994) identified three levels of coding: descriptive, interpretive, and pattern. Gibbs (2007) also identifies several levels of increasing abstraction: description, categorization, analytic, and theoretical. *Categorization* creates higher-level groups of similar or related phenomena. *Analytic* codes are more interpretive and may lead to *conceptual* or *theoretical* levels of coding in some studies.

There are two different ways to approach coding. The first is *data driven* or *open* coding. Using open coding, the researcher approaches data without preconceived ideas about how to code the data. Reading and rereading the data is done to begin building the coding scheme. The second approach is *concept-driven, framework,* or *template* analysis. In this second approach, the researcher begins with codes and themes derived from the literature, either theoretical or research. The predetermined coding scheme is modified as new ones emerge from the data. This second approach may limit generation of new insights.

It will quickly become apparent why qualitative coding without quantification is appropriate for most of the data obtained through unstructured observation and interviewing. Following is an excerpt from transcriptions of a set of unstructured interviews. These interviews were done with registered nurse staff of a rehabilitation unit who had been part of a 3-year project to prepare the unit patients for discharge home and follow them home after discharge with the goal of preventing rehospitalization or institutionalization. As hospital stays grow shorter, many people who have had strokes, fractures or amputations are not sufficiently recovered at discharge to be fully independent so an increasing number are being sent for extended inpatient rehabilitation in a long-term care facility. Most of the nurses who staffed this facility had not had any community-based or home healthcare experience prior to this project. The purpose of these interviews was to learn about the experience from their perspective.

The interviews began with an orientation to the study and explanation of confidentiality. Consent for the interview had already been signed. Note that in the tables the symbol R = researcher and P = participant. A little smoothing has been done to make the transcripts readable, but the words used are those of the interviewer (researcher) and interviewee (participant) unless they are bracketed. Remember that this is conversation and that people do not speak as carefully as they write. The first segment (sequence) is the interviewer's introduction, setting the stage for the interview itself.

1	R:	I would like to thank you for agreeing to be interviewed
2		this afternoon and as we go through with this you can
3		feel free to call me C_____. If our names are
4		used, when the tapes are transcribed the transcriptionist
5		deletes my name as well as [yours and] any patient
6		names for confidentiality. So why don't you start by just
7		telling me a little bit of your background as a nurse.

Once the nurse being interviewed relaxes a little, the interviewer proceeds to questions designed to elicit the desired information. An open-ended question (a mini-tour question) begins this part of the interview. The right column illustrates the type of coding that can be done. The first level is the descriptive code. These are the most frequent. Second level codes are in *italics*; third level codes are in CAPITAL LETTERS. A few obvious abbreviations are used—you can use many more in your own work if you can keep track of them. The second- and third-level codes are explained further following the excerpt.

8			
9	R:	Why don't you tell me about your first experience as a nurse providing care within the home environment then.	
10	P:	Well, I was a bit shy when I got to the house. I was	Bit shy. *Initial response RN*
11		careful how I present myself in the home	Careful presenting self. *Initial response*
12		environment. It is very different from the hospital	*RN*
13		environment. I visited, my first visits, was on, I	Different from hospital. *Comparing*
14		visited an elderly couple. The husband was 92 and	Elderly couple. *Pt characteristics*
15		the wife I think was 86 years old and was totally	Wife dependent on husband. *Pt*
16		dependent on her 92-year-old husband who was	*characteristics*
17		not well himself. I was very frightened from seeing	Frightened. *Initial response RN*
18		how the elderly live. It is so different from inside	UNEASE
19		the institution, like the nurses are there in the	Different from inpatient work. *Comparing*
20		institution. We take care of them, but when they go	Pt mobility problem. *Pt characteristics*
21		outside I can see the differences are very hard for	Differences make it hard for pts. *Pts*
22		them. I was very frightened. This old man was	*situation. Comparing*
23		walking almost on his face and his wife was crying	Frightened. *Initial response RN.* UNEASE

24	and she said if anything happens to him God	Crying. *Pt characteristics*
25	knows what would happen to her. They both were	HELP
26	alone, and we have to make referrals to home	Alone. *Pt situation*
27	health agencies to get somebody to go in 5 or 6	Referred home health. *Interventions*
28	days a week to take care of the patient. Husband	
29	needed care too but we get home health to go in	Both needed care. *Pt situation*
30	and provide services for both of them. They cook	Obtain services for both. *Interventions*
31	for them and give personal care to the patient.	Get help cook & personal care.
32	When I got there I noticed her legs were very very	*Interventions*
33	swollen. She looked very sick so we start [project	Legs very swollen. *Pt characteristics*
34	nursing coordinator] and myself, we elevated her	Very sick. *Pt characteristics*
35	legs and we called the doctor. She was on Lasix	Elevated legs, called MD. *Interventions*
36	and apparently she was not taking her medication	Not taking medication well [correctly]. *Pt*
	very well so we elevated her legs and called her	*actions.* HELP
	doctor and we made referrals and go over [the need	Called MD. *Intervention*
	for Lasix].	Made referrals, review need for Lasix.
		Intervention
37	R: What has this experience meant to you as a nurse?	
38	P: Well in my discharge planning now I think	Think differently. *Effect of experience RN*
39	differently, especially when these people are old. I	Especially if old. *Pt characteristics*
40	try to make them more careful about discharge	Make them [other staff] more careful in
41	planning, make sure the social worker is involved,	discharge planning. *Change practice*
42	and they send these people home without help.	Ensure social worker involved. *Change*
43	'Cause if we didn't get there on time I think that	*practice.* CHANGE
44	lady would end up back in the hospital. You have	Not send home without help. *Change*
45	to, you can't just focus on the patient when they	*practice*
46	[are] here. You have to get information from them,	The woman would have been back to
47	who is taking care of them at home and find out if	hospital. *Outcome of RN's care*
48	that person the caretaker at home is qualified.	Not just focus on pt [but on whole family].
49	'Cause sometimes the caregiver is not qualified to	*Change practice*
	take care of the patient.	Ask about home environment. *Change*
		practice. CHANGE
		Sometimes caregiver not qualified. *Pt*
		situation

After this first response from the nurse participant, the interviewer follows-up on the "think differently" comment from the interviewee (participant) that speaks directly to what is sought in this interview: the nurses' experience on this project.

50	R: How are you thinking differently?	
51	P: Well, they come in the hospital, and I interview	
52	them if they are capable of answering the	Ask them if live alone. *Change in practice*
53	questions, and I ask sometimes "Do you live	If yes, assess if capable going home alone.
54	alone?" And the patient will say, "Yes, I live	*Change in practice.* CHANGE
55	alone." So when I am making my discharge	Am very careful. *Effect of experience.*
56	planning I am very careful: is this person capable	Sometimes they are not capable care for
57	of going home by herself? Sometimes they are not	self.
58	capable of going home by themselves, but if you	HELP
	don't have the experience of outside you wouldn't	Without experience would not know what
	know what to do.	to do. *Effect of experience*

The interviewer now guides the dialogue toward exploration of the meaning of the experience.

59 R: Can you tell me about your most memorable patient
60   that you have had?
61 P: Oh well, my most, that S_____ and the one I just
62   told you about that is one of them. I have quite a few of
63   them. I remember a 51-year-old lady she [had] a
64   laminectomy, she was totally disabled, not getting any
65   income from anywhere, and her husband was
66   terminally ill and he had ??? [cannot hear] of the
67   testicles and whenever . . . she was living with three
68   grandchildren, daughter. And the husband and the
69   daughter weren't working. She was on public
70   assistance, the husband was on disability, and she was
71   really in a mess with her finances. She couldn't pay her
72   bills, and her mental status was very very poor because
73   she had all these things on her mind. She couldn't do
74   anything for herself 'cause she used to be very mobile.
75   Because of the laminectomy and the husband was
76   walking around in a daze in the house, and this woman
77   was pretty sharp, and then they wouldn't have enough
78   food to eat, so we had to find a community resource
79   like the church to help. I remember for Thanksgiving
80   a church gave us food, you know turkey, and different
81   types of food and foods to bring to these people. Their
82   light bill, they were cutting off their lights, and [we]
83   had to tell them where to go to get help. I think the
84   government paid that month light bill, and we were
85   there at a time when she was on the edge of committing
86   suicide. And I think we were a great help to her. Well,
87   she did say that. Many nights she would like to go
88   to bed and not [want to] wake up. We were very
89   supportive of her. I even bought her some iron pills
90   out of my own money 'cause she was anemic, and she
91   didn't have enough money to buy the iron tablets that
92   she was supposed to get, and she was very grateful. I
93   was very afraid to buy it for her because I didn't want
94   to hurt her feelings. But then I asked her first is it okay
95   that bringing a bottle of iron and vitamins, and she
      said yes it is okay.

Laminectomy, totally disabled. *Pt characteristics*

No income. Husband terminal. *Pt situation Pt characteristics*. HELP

Living with 3 grandchildren. *Pt situation*

None working. *Pt situation*

Wife—public assistance. Husband—disability. Finances a mess. *Pt situation*

Unable pay bills. Mental status very poor. *Pt situation, characteristics*

All on her mind (pt). Could not care for self. *Pt characteristics*. HELP

Immobile. Spouse dazed. *Pt characteristics*

Woman sharp. *Pt characteristics*

No food. *Pt situation*

Found church to provide food. *Intervention*

Thanksgiving—church provided meal *Interventions*

Lights being cut off. *Pt situation*

Told them how to get help. *Intervention*

Government paid 1 mo light bill. *Outcome of care*

On edge of committing suicide. *Pt characteristics*. HELP

We were great help. Pt said that. *Outcome of RN care*. FULFILLMENT

She not want to wake up. *Pt characteristics*

We were very supportive. *Intervention*

Bought her iron pills out of nurse's pocket. *Intervention*

She said yes. *Pt response.* FULFILLMENT

No money to buy iron tabs. *Pt situation*

She was very grateful. *Pt response*

Nurse was afraid would hurt feelings. *Initial response RN*

Asked woman first regarding iron pills. *Intervention*

Since the experience of the nurse is the focus of these interviews, the interviewer guides the discussion in that direction.

96   R: How did you feel as a nurse when all this was going
97   on? In the family?

98   P: I felt good because I was there to help. I was very   Felt good. *Effect of experience.*
99   happy that I could help. 'Cause I know if we didn't   FULFILLMENT
100   go there all the time when we went there something   Happy. *Effect of experience*
101   would have happened. This woman was distraught.   Woman distraught. *Pt characteristics*
102   So but I felt good that I was able to help her. At the   HELP
103   last visit she was able to walk around. She couldn't do   Felt good ← able to help. *Effect of*
104   much housework, but she was able to walk around   *experience.* FULFILLMENT
105   without using her walker.   At last visit, able to walk. *Pt outcome*
                                                                      Still not able to do housework. *Pt outcome*

106 R: And this was an improvement from the first time
107   you saw her?
108 P: Yes. It was a great improvement, her mental status   Great improvement. Mental status ↑. *Pt*
109   was improved, her skin color was better because at   *outcome*
110   one time she was very very pale, and she started to   Skin color ↑. *Pt outcome*
111   eat and taking her vitamins, and I had seen great   Began to eat. Took vitamins. *Pt outcome*
        improvement.   Great improvement. *Pt outcome*
112 R: What were some of your thoughts and feelings when
113   you were on your last visit as compared [with] how
114   you felt when you went out the first time?
115 P: I was more into visiting patients and giving more   More into visiting. *Effect of experience.*
116   assistance on my last visits. I was pretty new, brand   Brand new. *Initial response.* UNEASE
117   new when I out there the first time. The last visit I   PRACTICE CHANGE
118   felt I was fulfilled because I did a lot during the time   Giving more assistance. *Change practice*
119   I was visiting the patients. I felt fulfilled that I was   Last visit felt fulfilled. *Effect of experience*
120   doing something meaningful in the community.   Did a lot → fulfillment. *Effect of experience.*
                                                                      FULFILLMENT
                                                                      Doing something meaningful in the
                                                                      community → felt-fulfilled. *Effect of*
                                                                      experience

121 R: You have talked a lot about feeling good and fulfilled
122   when you are doing the home visits. How does that
123   compare to your feelings as a nurse when you are
124   delivering care within the hospital setting?
125 P: Oh well, the hospital setting is different because going   Hospital setting different. *Comparing*
126   out there is a one to one. Mostly one to one you have   In community is one to one. *Comparing*
127   more time to sit and allow the patient to ventilate.   Mostly one-to-one. *Comparing*
128   Many times I just sit there, and they just keep talking.   Time to sit, allow patient ventilate. TIME
129   In the hospital you don't have time to sit for a half   *Comparing*
130   an hour with somebody to cry on your shoulders and   I just sit, they keep talking. *Intervention*
131   for you to listen, so it is totally different. It is more   In hospital no time to sit. *Comparing.* TIME
132   relaxing in the home environment. You get to talk   No time let someone cry, no time to listen.
133   more about the patient, find out more their needs.   *Comparing*
134   In the hospital it is different. 'Cause you don't have   Home environment more relaxing.
135   that time, that amount of time.   *Comparing.* TIME
                                                                      Talk more about patient. *Comparing*
                                                                      Find out more regarding their needs.

Comparing
Hospital is different. *Comparing*
Don't have that time. *Comparing.* TIME

The interviewer now guides the dialogue toward summary and conclusion. Asking what the interviewee has to add in this instance generates useful data.

136 R: Is there anything about the project, about your visits
137   that you would like to share with me that I haven't
138   asked you?
139 P: I have different insight now. Because I got to learn
140   what is happening outside when they get out of the
141   institution. It makes me think now when they come in
142   as an admission it gives me a different attitude about
143   them going home. Because I have seen things during
144   my visit that I never knew could happen. I didn't know
145   people could live like that, no family member, nobody,
146   so as a nurse it makes me think I get to . . . now more
147   [often] I think deeper when I am planning the care of
148   these people.

Different insight. *Effect of experience*
Learned what's happening outside. *Effect of experience*
Think now when patient comes in. *Effect of experience.*
Different attitude regarding them going home. *Effect of experience.* CHANGE
Never knew what could happen in the home. *Effect of experience*
Didn't know people lived like that (no family, no help). *Effect of experience*
Think deeper when planning their care now. *Effect of experience. Change practice.* CHANGE

149 R: You also mentioned saying good-bye is difficult.
150 P: It is very difficult, and then you wonder what happened
151   to them after you leave. Who are they going to depend
152   on, who are they going to ask questions? Who is going
153   to sit down and listen to them? It is difficult to leave. I
154   enjoy my home visits. I really do. I really do. We went
155   to a home, and it was so cluttered all kinds of things. I
156   mean from the day they were living maybe for 50 years
157   the whole place was cluttered with garbage and pile up
158   and we advised the husband to even get somebody to
159   come in and help him and the last day we visited them
160   the whole place was different. There was more air, the
161   patient was looking better, and he himself was looking
162   better. So I think going out there is very very
163   important. Very important for these people. Especially
164   when they have no one. No family member, and they
165   have to depend on themselves. It is hard. So they are
166   glad to have us.

Very difficult (saying good bye). *Leaving*
Wonder what happened to them. *Leaving*
Who can they depend on? *Leaving*
Who can they ask questions of? *Leaving*
Who will sit down? Who will listen? *Leaving*
Enjoy home visits, really do. *Effect of experience*
One home so cluttered-50 yrs worth. *Pt situation.* HELP
Garbage piled up. *Pt situation*
Advised husband get somebody to help. *Intervention*
Whole place different. *Outcome*
More air. *Outcome*
Patient looked better. Husband looked better. *Outcome*
Going out there is very important. FULFILLMENT *Effect of experience*
Very important for these people. *Outcome*
Especially if they have no one.
No family. Have to depend on themselves. It is hard [for them]. *Pt situation* HELP
They are glad to have us. *Outcome care*

The following is just an ending for the interview. It is important in terms of conducting a complete interview, but it is not usually necessary to code it unless new information appears here.

167 R: I am glad that you were able to participate in this
168 interview. If I think of any other questions that I would
169 like to ask you as I am analyzing the data, can I get in
170 touch with you again?
171 P: Sure.
172 R: Thank you.
173 P: You're welcome.

Altogether, 10 categories were created to code at the second, categorical level:

1. Initial response from RN
2. Comparing home and inpatient work environment (shortened to comparing)
3. Pt characteristics
4. Pt situation
5. Interventions
6. Pt actions
7. Change in practice
8. Outcome of RN's care
9. Effect of experience
10. Leaving pt and family

The two main threads in the nurse's responses are (1) patient and family descriptions, their problems, concerns, actions, and eventual outcome; and (2) personal response, feelings, and thoughts of the nurse in relation to this new practice environment. In between or connecting these two are the interventions (care) provided to the patient and family by the nurse (see Figure 21-1).

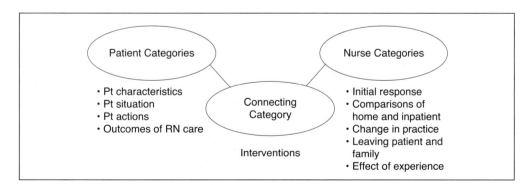

Figure 21-1 Categorical coding from interview excerpt.

A third, higher level of analytic codes can be identified as well for this interview. These are more interpretive:

- Initial unease of the nurse created by moving practice from inpatient to home environment: UNEASE.

- Patients and family needed help, desperately, in some instances, not provided until nurse visited: HELP.

- Home visit characteristics including more time for each patient led to greater nurse satisfaction with practice: TIME.

- Expressed fulfillment: FULFILLMENT.

- Having had the experience led to changes in inpatient practice: PRACTICE CHANGES.

These codes address primary themes of the interview that are of interest to the researcher. They are not exhaustive of the many possible themes that could be identified.

Assuming that the interviews of the other nurses who also followed their patients' home are similar, it would be possible to move to the conceptual/theoretical level as well as to generate some hypotheses for further research. A few examples:

Concepts	*Time constraints* exist on nursing care.
	Nurse experienced *professional fulfillment.*
	Transitions between care settings require preparation and support.
	Experiential learning can produce *changes in practice.*
Hypothesis	Opportunity to care for patients one at a time as some other health professionals do (physicians, therapists, social workers) would increase nurse satisfaction and professional fulfillment.
Hypothesis	Experience with postdischarge follow-up care raises nurses' awareness of the needs for comprehensive discharge planning.

This is an example of a general or generic qualitative coding approach that could be done by hand or using a qualitative data analysis program. Reference will be made to this interview again as we proceed to consider ethnographic, grounded theory, and phenomenological analyses.

ETHNOGRAPHIC ANALYSIS

The ethnographic approach to data collection and analysis is designed to achieve understanding of other cultures. Originally employed by anthropologists who often devoted years to the study of remote places and people, it has also been used to study subcultures closer to home: street people, gay and lesbian groups, hospital environments, health beliefs of minority and disadvantaged populations, and so forth.

For example, there are different subcultures within the world of health care including the traditional biomedical subculture and the nontraditional, complementary and alternative treatment subculture. Kokanovic and colleagues (2009) found these two subcultures clashing within a health center: a research assistant they had hired promoted a type of treatment for depression that other providers in the center saw as "anti-pharmacotherapy" and "anti-psychiatry," while a center welfare worker held a strong "biomedical/ biopsychiatry," perspective (p. 712). Even more interesting, in one ethnic community they found that people believed depression had demonic causes, affected those who offended their ancestors, or was the result of a tragic event. In another ethnic community they studied, they found there was no equivalent term for *depression* in their language, only the equivalent of the English word "crazy" (p. 712).

Ethnography is concerned with culture. It is defined by this focus rather than by a particular method (Chambers, 2003, p. 380). Although the ethnographic interview is the core source of information, ethnography employs many other sources as well. Observation is another major source of ethnographic data. Artifacts, documents, arts, and language are additional sources.

The task of the ethnographer is to make sense of cultural beliefs, values, norms, structures, and functions (Wolf, 2007, p. 312). In more technical terms, the task is to "decode cultural symbols and identify the underlying coding rules," which is done by uncovering the relationships among them (Spradley, 1979, p. 99). Spradley uses the term *symbol* very broadly to refer to any object or event we can see or experience (p. 95).

The researcher usually finds it necessary to identify and follow a particular thread through the data rather than attempting to use all of the information available. For example, in the nurse interview, the analysis focused on the thread of the nurse's experience rather than the experience of the patient who is inadequately prepared for discharge home.

Coding

Analysis begins with the first interview or observation undertaken in an ethnographic study (Gobo, 2008). In fact, it should begin even earlier as you are negotiating entry into the field. Your notes taken at that time and thoughts about what you are seeing and experiencing are the beginning of your data collection and analysis. The data that you have collected should provide the "thick description," that Geertz (1973) recommended (deriving the concept from Ryle, 1971) and you need to try to remain as faithful to informants' perspectives as possible throughout data collection and data analysis (Wolf, 2007, p. 32).

All of the data amassed should be read in its entirety, then reread and contemplated before beginning the coding. The ethnographic analysis begins with the type of coding and thematizing already described in the previous section. Data are separated into units for coding, sorted by code and larger categories, searched, and then reconstituted into a narrative that reflects and explains the informants' world (Wolf, 2007).

There are varying degrees of formality and detail in different ethnographic analyses. In some instances, chunks from the transcripts are grouped or indexed by topic and chains of relationships (for example, staff relationships in an agency) are mapped out (DeVault & McCoy, 2001).

All of this needs to be done within the *context* of the people and events that you are studying (Morse, 1992). In fact, in some instances, the analysis will move back and forth between context and content. For example, if you are studying processes of care in a free-standing clinic, the context may include the neighborhood where the clinic is located, sources of funding for the clinic (a governmental agency, benefactors, free care or fee-for-service), the clientele served (homeless, pregnant women, people with HIV), and so forth. Describing the processes without this context would generate a very thin description and shallow analysis.

Interpretation

As you code, create categories and search for themes. Bernard (1988) reminds us to be constantly checking and rechecking the ideas that are forming. In particular, look for the following:

- Inconsistencies in statements of different informants may reflect real differences, differences in perspective, or misunderstanding on your part. The inconsistencies need to be checked out and corroborating evidence sought.

- Similarly, negative evidence should not be ignored. Instead, it should be evaluated and explained.

- Alternative explanations should be considered. For example, it is generally assumed in Western societies that more women are working now because of the emphasis on equality and women's rights. An alternative explanation would be that they were forced to work because the purchasing power of their spouses' income was declining or their families' expectations were rising faster than one income could accommodate (Bernard, 1988).

- Also, consider the extreme cases and why they are extreme: do they represent outliers, or are they markers for the far ends of a continuum?

The importance of moving beyond the most concrete level of description is frequently emphasized. Gubrium (1988) for example, cautions that what people say is not necessarily what they mean. Consider an example from everyday life: If a friend of yours made dinner for you but the meal was burned, would you tell your friend that it tasted bad or would you say the food was terrific? It takes understanding of what we call being polite or sparing someone's feelings to understand why someone would say burned food tasted terrific.

Triangulation is an important way to address these questions of validity. Multiple sources of information are sought to provide confirmation of what is said by an initial informant. This provides different points of view on the same information. In particular, it provides more perspectives from which to view and interpret the original information (Fetterman, 1989). In the burned food scenario, for example, the astute ethnographer would ask another person after dinner, "Did J____ really think that burned food tasted good?" This second informant is likely to say "Of course not. She was just sparing the cook's feelings."

Additional Strategies

There are several more complex analytic strategies that go beyond simple coding schemes: domain analysis, taxonomic analysis, structural and contrast questions, and componential analysis (Bernard, 1988; Spradley, 1979). We will consider each of these briefly to give you an idea of what can be done in an in-depth ethnographic analysis. All of these analyses are based upon the assumption that there is a *system* of symbols within a culture or subculture and that the relationships between symbols can be discovered (Spradley, 1979).

- *Domain analysis:* We have already talked about creating categories. Domains can be thought of as sets of categories within categories. The *cover term* is the name of the larger category or domain; *included terms* are those included within that domain (Spradley, p. 100). For example, the term *patient* is an important domain within health care. Included terms may be *inpatient, outpatient, ambulatory patient, pediatric patient,* and so forth. The categories within categories are age of the patient, type of care needed, condition, or location of the patient.

- *Structural and contrast questions:* These questions lead to further exploration of a particular domain. The structural questions explore what is included within a category or domain. For example, you could ask, "If I went to the clinic for a flu shot, would that qualify me as a patient?", "What if I just called a physician's office with a question?", or the more complex question, "Do I have to be sick to be a patient?" This last question leads to the idea of contrast questions:

  ◦ "Who is a patient and who is not?"

  ◦ "If I cut my finger chopping parsley, does that make me a patient?"

  ◦ "If I cut my finger and it will not stop bleeding, does that make me a patient?"

  ◦ "Or do I become a patient only if I need stitches? Do I have to need care to be a patient? Not only need but also ask for care? Or do I have to receive care to be a patient?"

- *Taxonomies:* When you begin putting together the information from all of these questions, the relationships can become very complex. Bernard (1988, p. 337) points out that we use "folk" taxonomies all the time. For example, supermarkets group dairy items in one place, fresh produce in another, and ready-to-eat cereal in another. We do the same in health care, putting surgical units together, laboratories in another place, and x-ray in another place. The diagram in Figure 21-1 is an example of a very small taxonomy of patient and nurse-related topics touched upon by the nurse in the interview excerpt presented earlier. These taxonomies are very helpful not only in organizing information but also in showing how the items relate to each other.

- *Componential analysis:* Componential analysis addresses the various attributes of a cultural symbol (Spradley, 1979, p. 174). For example, what are the attributes of a pediatric patient? Attributes may include youth (child, not an adult); sick, injured, or in need of preventive care; unable to provide his or her own consent for treatment; usually accompanied by an adult; and so forth.

It is not necessary to include all of these analyses in one study, but they suggest what may be helpful in analyzing ethnographic data.

Writing the Narrative

Writing the final narrative is an important part of completing the analysis. New insights may occur to you even as you are writing what you think are the final results. This is not unusual and should not be considered a fault in your analysis.

Bernard (1988) reminds us that, contrary to the popular saying, "Data do not speak for themselves" (p. 323). Your job is to present the analysis in such a way as to clearly convey the aspect of the culture under study to the reader so that the reader may understand the meanings underlying cultural beliefs, norms, values, and related behaviors of the people of that culture. Some choose to report using the voice of the researcher; others elect to emphasize the voice of the informants supported by judicious use of examples, excerpts from the transcripts, and quotes from informants (DeVault & McCoy, 2001). Flow charts, concept or meaning maps, and other diagrams summarize structures and illustrate relationships and are helpful supplements to the written narrative. The ideal ethnography not only describes an aspect of the culture of interest with great clarity but also sheds light on the meanings of the symbols described.

GROUNDED THEORY

Grounded theory is distinguished from other types of qualitative research by its method and intent, which is to develop theory grounded in data (Corbin, 2009, p. 52), particularly middle-range theory (Charmaz, 2001). This is in contrast with ethnography, which is distinguished by its focus on culture. Much grounded theory research is concerned with social and psychological processes related to health. For example:

> Evans and Robertson (2009) conducted a grounded theory study of older women's search for the right physician. This focus on the search for the right physician emerged from the first round of interviews. They actually had begun by asking participants to talk about their chronic health problems. The progression of the questions toward increasing understanding of the search for the right physician is illustrated by an example of a question from each session (p. 413):
>
> First interview: Describe your health over the last year.
>
> Second interview: Give some examples of your interactions with your doctor.
>
> Third interview: What things are keeping you from getting the kind of care you desire?

After the interviews were transcribed line by line, open coding was done, then selective and axial coding. The researchers felt that they had not reached saturation after

the first eight women were interviewed, so they enrolled an additional three participants. One woman told of being haunted by an incident of overmedication during a
hospitalization that nearly killed her. Because of this, she felt she could no longer
trust her physician or that hospital. The researchers note that this story crystallized
their hypothesis of a need for two-way physician–patient communication and having
a voice in healthcare decisions (p. 426). Based upon their analysis of all of the interviews, the researchers concluded that the women sought participation in planning
their health care.

Sociologists Glaser and Strauss (1967) are credited with the development of grounded
theory, which emerged from their study of dying patients and the ways in which professional staff, the patient, and the family handled their knowing that the patient was dying,
particularly whether they discussed it openly or kept their awareness to themselves. Glaser
and Strauss (1967) emphasize the usefulness of grounded theory in generating theory systematically. The resulting theory, they say, should be well integrated, clear in its purpose
and based upon thick description. It can generate interpretation, explanation, application, and prediction (p. 1).

Distinguishing features of the grounded theory approach are constant comparison,
theoretical sampling, and a guiding principle called theoretical saturation (Boeije, 2007).
These ideas have been widely adapted in generic studies as well. However, many of the
generic studies remain at a relatively concrete level, and do not progress to the generation
of concepts and theories.

We will consider constant comparison, theoretical sampling, and saturation here as
part of the process of concurrent data collection and analysis that is grounded theory.

Constant Comparison Method

In grounded theory, data collection and analysis are not done separately or sequentially,
one after the other. Instead, they are part of a cyclical process that moves from data collection to analysis and back to data collection (Boeije, 2007). What is learned in the first
interview, for example, guides the type of questions asked at the next interview. You may
recall from the interview excerpt presented earlier, that the nurse said she was frightened
when she first visited her patients at home. Think about this for a moment: Why would
an experienced, highly competent nurse be frightened at the prospect of seeing one of her
discharged patients at home? We can speculate, of course, but wouldn't it be preferable to
explore this further in a second or third interview and to find out if other nurses felt the
same way? By conducting several interviews with the same person, you can explore a topic
like this in depth. Interviews with additional participants allow you to compare their
responses to the description given by the first nurse: Is this a common reaction among
experienced inpatient nurses when first confronted with making a home visit? If it is a
common reaction, what contributes to this reaction? As you continue to explore this
topic, moving from data collection to analysis and back to data collection, creating
memos recording your best guesses (hypotheses) for example, as to why this new

experience is frightening, you will begin to develop a theoretical explanation for this phenomenon.

Suppose, for example, that the interviewer asked the nurse why she felt frightened. On the first interview, the nurse responded, "Oh, I don't know. Just feeling a little shy seeing my patients in their own home. This was new to me." On the second interview she elaborated on the explanation. "It's not the same as on the unit. Here, I am walking into their private home. Maybe they resent my intrusion but don't want to say so." On the third interview, the nurse elaborated much more. "Home is their space, not mine, and what if an emergency occurred? Here there's no crash cart. What if they need a new dressing, a lab test, or new medication? It's just so different out there in the community. I don't have control over what medications they take, being sure they change the dressing daily, making sure they see their doctor. I can tell them what to eat, but I can't order a new tray for them or check to see if they've eaten enough. At first, I didn't know how I was going to get anything done out there."

Now we have some indication of the factors that contributed to this nurse's response:

- While she was experienced at inpatient care, she was not experienced at home visiting.

- At first, she did not know how she could be of help to her patients in this setting, leaving her feeling like a potentially unwanted guest, even worse, an intruder.

- She was accustomed to having equipment and services within reach or available with a telephone call and did not know how to obtain them in the home, leaving her feeling ill equipped.

- She was "the boss" on the inpatient unit, in control of what was happening. But in the home, she shared control with her patients.

We can hypothesize, then, that her prior experience had only partially prepared her for this new setting and that she was, on some level, aware of this, leading to feeling that the situation was not well under control. Her high confidence level on the inpatient unit was severely diminished because of this. However, this was a temporary diminishment as she rapidly regained confidence with guidance and experience. These ideas, by the way, would be what you record in the memos.

Of course, this emerging theoretical statement has to be tested and retested with other interviewees. It has to be further developed and further refined into a much more cogent statement or concept. It may be qualified if it is found that some nurses do not experience this same response. The degree of uneasiness may also be quite varied from nurse to nurse, further qualifying the concept.

Coding

Coding emerges from the data. Charmaz (2006) recommends staying close to the data when doing the initial coding and using action language whenever possible, not topics as was done in the generic coding of the interview illustrated earlier. Action coding uses *changing* instead of *change*, *responding* instead of *response*, *experiencing* instead of *experience*, and *fulfilling* instead of *fulfillment*. This is done to stay as close to the data as possible and to avoid applying existing ideas and concepts instead of allowing them to emerge from the data. Stern (2009) also warns against using "pet codes," favorites that are not necessarily the best fit for your data.

As the coding is done, the researcher is also comparing one incident with another, one comment with another. This is the constant comparison method that begins to develop theory. For example, Glaser and Strauss (1967, p. 106) noticed through comparisons across observations that nurses perceived some dying patients as a high social loss but others as a low social loss. When an important difference like this is noticed, the researcher should write a *memo* about it to record the idea for future reference.

Focused coding is the next level of coding. These codes are more general, more conceptual, and more abstract. They are generated by comparing codes across incidents or people (Charmaz, 2006).

Axial coding brings the data together again, although in a different form. Large amounts of data are synthesized, connections and links identified, and dimensions described. One framework for doing this considers the following (Charmaz, 2006, p. 61; Corbin & Strauss, 2007, p. 101):

- Conditions that lead to the phenomenon
- The context in which it occurs
- Responses of the participants to this phenomenon
- Outcomes of the responses

This framework of conditions, context, strategies, and consequences is just a suggested one. You may find that the phenomenon that you are studying could be better framed with a different set of dimensions.

Theoretical Sampling

Although the researcher begins a grounded theory study with a general idea of what the sample should be like, the specifics of exactly who should be interviewed and how many should be interviewed evolve as the study progresses. For example, the researcher who interviewed the nurse might decide that the coordinator of the project could have a different but helpful perspective on the nurses' initial responses. Obtaining different perspectives (the patient, nurses, and family, for example) is a type of *triangulation* (Boeije, 2007). The following is another example:

Corbin (2009) described what occurred near the beginning of a study of [American] participants in the Vietnam War. She began with an interview of an army nurse and was struck by the fact that he said his experience in Vietnam was "not so bad" (p. 44). How could this be? She thought it might be because he had not been a combatant, so he had not had to fight or to kill others. The experience could have been much different for those who were combatants. This directed the choice of the next interviewee, an American combatant in the Vietnam War.

Saturation

Unlike most quantitative research studies in which the desired number of participants is specified at the outset, the sample size in unstructured qualitative research is somewhat indeterminate at the outset. When employing the grounded theory approach, the goal related to sample size is to include as many participants as necessary to achieve saturation. How do you know this has been achieved? Saturation is achieved when new cases do not bring any new information or insights to light (Boeije, 2007, p. 267).

In fact, Glaser and Strauss (1967) suggest you do not even have to continue coding the same idea or experience again and again if you have already coded it several times and no new aspects of it appear any more. Of course, if you plan to talk about the frequency of an idea or experience or even quantify it, then you do have to continue coding it. If not, then you may stop coding when you have reached *theoretical saturation* (p. 111).

Writing Theory

When you have completed coding at all three levels, have an ample set of memos, have achieved that higher level of abstraction we call theorizing, and you have then completed a process of *induction* proceeding from many disparate bits and chunks of data to a reconstituted, explanatory whole, you are ready to begin writing theory (Glaser & Strauss, 1967). To simplify this somewhat, the codes and categories provide the structure, and the memos provide the explanation and discussion. Too often, researchers provide the results without walking the reader through the thought processes that led to the result. This lack of transparency reduces the reader's ability to evaluate the trustworthiness of the findings.

Corbin and Strauss (2007) offer a set of criteria for evaluating the outcome of a grounded theory study. They provide a helpful guide for both the researcher and the reader of the final product, whether a report, journal article, or book (pp. 106–107):

- Were concepts generated?
- Are the concepts systematically related?
- Are the categories dense and well developed?
- Is variation (i.e., the degree to which a phenomenon varies between groups) addressed?
- Are macrosocial conditions and context linked to the phenomenon?
- Do the findings have significance in terms of explaining a phenomenon or suggesting direction for further research?

These questions are designed to address how well the reported results are grounded in the data.

PHENOMENOLOGICAL ANALYSIS

This approach to qualitative research is closely tied to the underlying philosophies that have informed their development. Those who use the method without the philosophical underpinnings are frequently criticized for doing so (for example, Giorgi, 2006a).

Many nurse researchers find phenomenological analysis intuitively appealing because it focuses upon the individual's experience and the context of that experience. This is a central concern for nursing, thus the frequent use in qualitative nursing research.

The basic principles of unstructured qualitative analysis have already been addressed. In this last section of Chapter 21, we will focus upon the unique features of descriptive and interpretive phenomenological analysis. The two primary traditions are described here.

Two Schools of Thought

It may come as no surprise to you to find that there is more than one school of thought within phenomenology. In fact, as many as 18 different forms of phenomenology have been identified (Norlyk & Harder, 2010, p. 1).

The first is the *eidetic* or *descriptive* tradition derived from Husserl's philosophy. No specific research question or hypothesis is formulated when launching this type of inquiry but identification of the phenomenon of interest is appropriate (Lopez & Willis, 2004). *Bracketing* is an essential part of this approach. To do this, the researcher refrains from searching the literature before embarking upon the study. Further, the researcher is expected to bracket or set aside any existing knowledge or personal experiences related to the subject of the inquiry. Writing down your expectations and preconceived notions on the outcome of the study may help remind you of what they are and help to prevent you from finding only what you expected to find and hearing only what you expected to hear from interviewees. Keeping an open mind is essential, but in reality it is very difficult to do. In fact, Giorgi (2006b) warns it may create a false sense of security that one's preconceived notions, biases and prejudices are not influencing the interpretation just because they were recognized. Hidden biases may not be brought to consciousness at all and may not be listed. Dahlberg and Dahlberg (2004) call these preconceived notions *pre-understandings* and warn the researcher of the danger of these ideas influencing the analyses in an uncontrolled manner.

The search for *universal essences* (eidetic structures) that are a part of everyone's experience is a second element. These essences are commonalities thought to be shared by each person who has this experience. The context that the experience occurs in is not a primary part of a descriptive phenomenological analysis. It is thought that the essences can be extracted from participants' experiences and that those essences "represent the true nature of the phenomenon being studied" (Lopez & Willis, 2004, p. 728).

The *interpretive tradition,* derived from the works of Heidegger, goes beyond description to search for "meanings embedded in common life practices" (Lopez & Willis 2004, p. 728). This is the interpretive aspect of the approach, moving beyond the words of the participant to seek the meaning in them. Context is part of this analysis because the way we experience a phenomenon, whether it is chronic pain, being overweight, or adopting a child is influenced by the people and circumstances surrounding us, our *life world* (Lopez & Willis, 2004, p. 729).

Instead of bracketing or setting aside experience and personal opinion, the interpretive phenomenological researcher can use them as guides to shaping the inquiry. Further, a theoretical perspective or framework may be used so long as it is made clear that it is the lens through which this experience was viewed. In fact, Dahlberg and colleagues (2001) suggest you keep several possible theories in mind and "let them compete" (p. 208) during the analysis phase. The interpretation, then, becomes a "blend" of the meanings of the researcher and the participants, which is called *intersubjectivity* (Lopez & Willis, 2004, p. 730).

Intersubjectivity is explained by Munhall (2007) as the intersection of the subjective worlds of, in this case, the researcher and participants. This subjective world includes feelings, thoughts, opinions, ideas, and so forth. The portion of this subjective world that is revealed in the interview is the *shared perceptual space of intersubjectivity* (Munhall, 2007, p. 173).

Planning and Conducting the Inquiry

Munhall (2007) and van Manen (1990) have described the conduct of a phenomenological inquiry in very clear terms, which are sometimes difficult to find in writing about phenomenology. The following sections outline the process of phenomenological inquiry.

Immersion

First, you must become well acquainted with the underlying philosophy, and be certain there is a good fit between that philosophy and your approach. There are multiple ways to look at the world and to interpret the meaning of people's experiences in the world. You may need to begin with secondary sources to help you understand the many forms of phenomenology. Consider beginning with the work of Munhall (2007) and van Manen (1990), whose writing is accessible.

Aim of the Inquiry

An aim is a more general statement than a research question or hypothesis. It defines the focus of your study as well as the context. For example, you might be interested in the experience of adopting a child. This is an appropriate topic but so broad that it needs some delimiters. So, with further thought about the subject and reflection on why you chose it for your inquiry, you might add these delimiters: *international* adoption of a child with *chronic health problems* by a *single parent*. Before proceeding, it is also important to reflect on why you selected this topic (you know someone who has adopted a child with cardiac disease who was born outside the United States) your thoughts, feelings, opinions, theories, and so forth on this subject. This is important because it is essential to remain open to new ways of thinking about the phenomenon you are studying. It requires a great deal of introspection and self-honesty to do this. Munhall (2007) emphasizes this as:

knowing that you do not know something, that you do not understand someone who stands before you and who perhaps does not fit into some preexisting paradigm or theory, is critical to the evolution of understanding meaning for others. (p. 172)

The researcher who cannot achieve this state of openness risks predetermining the outcomes of the study, a severe threat to its credibility and trustworthiness.

Inquiry and Processing

As is done in grounded theory, these are done concurrently. Interviews are fundamental to the inquiry, but observations, reading of texts, and other sources of information may be used. The interviews or dialogues are transcribed and the text is analyzed. However, this is not an analysis of the language used as it might be in a discourse analysis but an analysis of the phenomenon under study (Spiegelberg, 1975; Starks & Trinidad, 2007). More than one person should generally be interviewed to avoid reaching conclusions due to the choice of individual rather than to the choice of phenomenon (Giorgi, 2006a; 2006b). The following are the types of questions that may be helpful in conducting the interview:

- Can you give me an example?
- How did you feel when that happened?
- Tell me more about. . . .

These are very open ended and designed to avoid suggesting an interpretation or "appropriate" response. Concurrently, you will be reviewing and "dwelling" with the data, beginning to write the narrative of the participants' experience, searching for and thinking about the meaning of the experience that goes beyond what the interviewees actually said.

Van Manen (1990, p. 101) suggests that four existentials (fundamental themes of our life world, not specific to a particular experience but generally applicable) may be used as a guide for reflection.

- *Lived space:* Felt space, whether open or confined, homelike or strange
- *Lived body:* The corporeal presence in the world
- *Lived time:* Subjective, not clock time
- *Lived other:* Human relations

Analysis

Remember that the purpose of the interpretive type of phenomenological study is not to just relate the facts of an experience (describe the phenomenon) but to discern the meaning of the experience as well. This is eventually communicated to others through writing, one reason why writing pieces of the narrative begins so early in this process. The analysis phase is one of reading, reflecting, discussing, and writing. Van Manen (1990) speaks of *reflecting phenomenologically*, attempting to grasp the essence of the experience

(p. 78). Discussion may take place with colleagues, members of the research team, or with participants. Reading may be limited to related theoretical and research publications or may be extended to experiential literature.

An example from the now familiar nurse-managed family follow-up study may help to illuminate this process:

> Turkel, Tappen, and Hall (1999) conducted a phenomenological study of the experience of five long-term care nurses whose roles were reconfigured to include home-based follow-up care. An excerpt from transcriptions of the interviews conducted for this study was included earlier in this chapter. Interviewees were asked to describe their experiences visiting patients at home and what this experience meant to them. Following guidelines suggested by van Manen, the researchers read and reread the full transcripts of the interviews, marking text and adding thoughts in the margins. They discussed the transcripts, reflected upon them, and began writing. Themes that are described by van Manen as "threads that weave the experiences together" (p. 63) began to emerge from this process, which is not a "rule-bound process but a free act of 'seeing' meaning" (p. 79).
>
> Several themes emerged from this time of reading, reflection, and writing:
>
> • Transformation from insecurity to increased competence
>
> • Making a difference for their patients
>
> • Feeling rewarded
>
> • Changes in patterns of practice within the facility
>
> • Developing mutual relationships with patients and families

The overarching theme or meaning for the nurses' experience was expressed as *moments of excellence* that "gave nurses a renewed passion for professional practice as they realize the impact they had on their patients' lives" (Turkel et al., 1999, p. 11).

The process of analysis may become more complex than this description of a very simple study suggests. Colaizzi (1978) breaks the process down into stages:

1. Read the text in its entirety. The purpose of this is to see the whole of the text at one time, to get a global sense of it (Giorgi, 1997).

2. Go back to the text and extract the significant statements (phrases usually or sentences) relating to the phenomenon you are studying. This second reading will take more time. These statements are still in the words of the participants at this point. Caution must be taken to do this without decontextualizing the statements (Giorgi, 2006b).

3. Begin the process of the transformation of these statements from the participants' words to your "creative insights" (Colaizzi, 1978, p. 59) on the meaning of these statements but keep them connected to the data as well.

4. The "meaning units" (Giorgi, 1977, p. 247) created are now aggregated into clusters and themes that need to be validated against the text (Colaizzi, 1978).

5. Discrepancies, contradictions, disagreements and different perspectives should be studied, not ignored. Try to find the underlying reason or the interpretation that connects them. Leaving them unexplained weakens the final conclusions (Dahlberg et al., 2001, p. 209).

6. Integrate all of this into a comprehensive narrative that describes the structure of the phenomenon. Support with pieces from the text—participant comments, your observations.

7. Colaizzi (1978) recommends asking the participants to review and comment on these conclusions. Giorgi (2006a) on the other hand calls the use of outside experts or feedback from the participants "misguided" (p. 357). Why so negative about obtaining this feedback which is generally considered a strategy for establishing trustworthiness? Giorgi (2006a) explains that, while people certainly know what they are experiencing, they have not necessarily reflected on the meaning of their experience.

Hermeneutic Writing

Writing begins early in the process of a phenomenological inquiry. The goal of the final product is to permit us to see the "deeper significance, or meaning structures of the lived experience it describes" (van Manen, 1990, p. 822).

Munhall (2007) suggests an approach to accomplishing this:

- Condense the phenomenological writing that you've been doing into a summary of the major interpretations.

- Show how you arrived at these interpretations. Include the stories or a quote from the participants, your reflections, and your interpretations.

- Relate the findings to social and political issues and to the provision of health care (i.e., the implications of your findings).

- Discuss the potential consequences of your findings. Munhall (2007) suggests that a call to action can be an appropriate conclusion.

Misunderstandings and Misconceptions (About Phenomenological Inquiry)

Norlyk and Harder (2010) reviewed 38 articles identified by the authors as having been done using the phenomenological method of research. They found a number of misunderstandings and misconceptions about the phenomenological approach that may provide some useful reminders for other researchers:

- Make clear how the study is phenomenological in its approach.

- Distinguish between descriptive and interpretive inquiry.

- Identify the philosophical assumptions on which the study is based.

- Quotes from participants support but do not replace narrative.

- Make sure the aims are appropriate to phenomenological inquiry. Purposes that are generally not appropriate include finding or testing solutions to identified problems.

- Do not use terminology specific to other traditions such as *theoretical saturation* from grounded theory or *selection bias* from quantitative sampling.

In general researchers are cautioned to use the appropriate methods and terminology specific to phenomenology if they choose to conduct a phenomenological inquiry.

CONCLUSION

While there are commonalities among the many types of qualitative analysis described in this chapter, each approach has its distinctive features, methods, goals, and terminology. Many are based on long-established traditions that should be respected when using them. Others are more contemporary, borrowing the most useful strategies from the more traditional approaches.

To some beginning researchers, qualitative analysis appears easier to accomplish than does quantitative analysis. This is deceptive. An elegant, insightful qualitative analysis is like a work of art: inspiring the beholder (the reader) but representing a mighty effort on the part of the artist (the researcher).

REFERENCES

Bernard, H. R. (1988). *Research methods in cultural anthropology*. Newbury Park, NJ: Sage.
 ◇ The flow charts and other organizers of ethnographic data in chapter 14 are worth a look.
Boeije, H. (2007). A purposeful approach to the constant comparative method in the analysis of qualitative interviews. In S. Sarantakos (Ed.), *Data analysis* (pp. 265–285). Los Angeles, CA: Sage.
 ◇ Detailed description of theoretical sampling and the constant comparison method using interviews of couples dealing with multiple sclerosis as an example. The focus is practical.
Chambers, E. (2003). Applied ethnography. In N. K. Denzin and Y. S. Lincoln (Eds.), *Collecting and interpreting qualitative materials* (pp. 389–418). Thousand Oaks, CA: Sage.
Charmaz, K. (2006). *Constructing grounded theory: A practical guide through qualitative analysis*. Los Angeles: Sage.
Charmaz, K. (2001). Qualitative interviewing and grounded theory analysis. In J. F. Gubrium & J. A. Holstein (Eds.), *The Sage handbook of interview research* (pp. 675–694). Thousand Oaks, CA: Sage.
Colaizzi, P. F. (1978). Psychological research as the phenomenologist views it. In R. S. Valle & M. King (Eds.), *Existential-phenomenological alternatives for psychology* (pp. 48–71). New York, NY: Oxford University Press.
 ◇ Uses an example unrelated to nursing (reading van Gogh's letters) but the process (especially the thinking behind the interpretation) is clearly explicated.
Corbin, J. (2009). Taking an analytic journey. In J. M. Morse, P. N. Stern, J. Corbin, B. Bowers, K. Charmaz, & A. E. Clarke, *Developing grounded theory: The second generation* (pp. 35–53). Walnut Creek, CA: Left Coast Press.
 ◇ Corbin tells how she began a grounded theory study—a nice introduction to constant comparison and theoretical sampling.

Corbin, J., & Strauss, A. (2007). Grounded theory research: Procedures, canons and evaluative criteria. In S. Sarantakos (Ed.), *Data analysis* (pp. 91-109). Los Angeles, CA: Sage.

Dahlberg, K., Drew, N., & Nystrom, M. (2001). *Reflective lifeworld research*. Lund, Sweden: Studentlietteratur AB.
   ✧ Speaks to the beginning researcher who wants to conduct a phenomenological study. Blends the philosophy and research method well.

DeVault, M. L., & McCoy, L. (2001). Institutional ethnography. In J. F. Gubrium & J. A. Holstein (Eds.), *The Sage handbook of interview research* (pp. 751-775). Thousand Oaks, CA: Sage.

Evans, K., & Robertson, S. (2009). "Dr. Right": Elderly women in pursuit of negotiated health care and mutual decision making. *Qualitative Report, 14*(3), 409-432.

Fetterman, D. M. (1989). *Ethnography: Step by step*. Thousand Oaks, CA: Sage.

Fisher, M. J. (2009). 'Being a chameleon': Labour processes of male nurses doing bodywork. *Journal of Advanced Nursing, 65*(12), 2668-2677.

Geertz, C. (1973). *The interpretation of cultures*. New York: Basic Books.

Gibbs, G. R. (2007). *Analyzing qualitative data*. London: Sage.
   ✧ Very practical, detailed guide to qualitative analysis.

Giorgi, A. (1997). The theory, practice and evaluation of the phenomenological method as a qualitative research procedure. *Journal of Phenomenological Psychology, 28*(2), 235-260.

Giorgi, A. (2006a). Difficulties encountered in the application of the phenomenological method in the social sciences. *Analise psicologica, 3*(24), 353-361.
   ✧ A critique of six dissertations, three from psychology and three from nursing, whose authors claimed they had used the phenomenological method.

Giorgi, A. (2006b). Concerning variations in the application of the phenomenological method. *The Humanistic Psychologist, 34*(4), 305-319.
   ✧ Discusses differences among several phenomenological research methods.

Glaser, B. G., & Strauss, A. L. (1967). *The discovery of grounded theory: Strategies for qualitative research*. New York: Aldine de Gruyter.
   ✧ Written by the developers of grounded theory.

Gobo, G. (2008). *Doing ethnography*. Los Angeles: Sage.

Gubrium, J. (1988). *Analyzing field reality*. Newbury Park: Sage.

Hsieh, H. F., & Shannon, S. E. (2007). Three approaches to qualitative content analysis. In S. Sarantakos (Ed.), *Data analysis* (pp. 61-75). Los Angeles, CA: Sage.

Kokanovic, R., Furler, J., May, C., Dowrick, C., Herrman, H., Evert, H., & Gunn, J. (2009). The politics of conducting research on depression in a cross-cultural context. *Qualitative Health Research, 19*(5), 708-717.

Krippendorff, K. (2004). *Content analysis: An introduction to its methodology*. Thousand Oaks: Sage.

Lopez, K. A., & Willis, D. G. (2004). Descriptive versus interpretive phenomenology: Their contributions to nursing knowledge. *Qualitative Health Research, 14*(5), 726-735.

McTavish, D. G., & Pirro, E. B. (2007). Contextual content analysis. In S. Sarantakos (Ed.), *Data analysis* (pp. 217-237). Los Angeles: Sage.

Miles, M. B., & Huberman, A. M. (1994). *Qualitative data analysis*. Thousand Oaks, CA: Sage.

Moncrieff, D. W. (1978). Aesthetic consciousness. In R. S. Valle & M. King (Eds.), *Existential-phenomenological alternatives for psychology* (pp. 358-376). NY: Oxford University Press.
   ✧ A wonderful essay on consciousness. Especially worth reading if you plan to conduct a phenomenological research study.

Morse, J. M., Stern, P. N., Corbin, J., Bowers, B., Charmaz, K., & Clarke, A. E. (2009). *Developing grounded theory: The second generation*. Walnut Creek, CA: Left Coast Press.
   ✧ In this book are some excellent examples of qualitative studies done within each of the great traditions and more. The classic "On being sane in insane place" by Rosenhan is just one example.

Morse, J. M. (1992). *Qualitative health research*. Newbury Park, NJ: Sage.

Munhall, P. L. (2007). A phenomenological method. In P. L. Munhall (Ed.), *Nursing research: A qualitative perspective* (pp. 145–210). Sudbury, MA: Jones and Bartlett.
 ✧ The review of the process of conducting a phenomenological study from beginning to end is very helpful, easy to follow.

Norlyk, A., & Harder, I. (2010). What makes a phenomenological study phenomenological? An analysis of peer-reviewed empirical nursing studies. *Qualitative Health Research*. Advance online publication. doi: 10.1177/1049732309357435.

Ryle, G. (1971). *Collected papers: Collected essays 1929–1968*. UK: Hutchinson.

Spiegelberg, H. (1975). *Doing phenomenology: Essays on and in phenomenology*. The Hague: Martinus, Nijhoff.

Spradley, J. P. (1979). The ethnographic interview. New York: Holt, Rinehart and Winston.
 ✧ If you can get past a few dated examples, Spradley's work is one of the most readable, helpful guides for conducting an ethnographic interview.

Starks, H., & Trinidad, S. B. (2007). Choose your method: A comparison of phenomenology, discourse analysis and grounded theory. *Qualitative Health Research, 17*(10), 1372–1380.
 ✧ Finding the different types of qualitative methods confusing? The figure on the second page of this article might help you sort them out.

Stern, P. N. (2009). Glaserian grounded theory. In J. M. Morse, P. N. Stern, J. Corbin, B. Bowers, K. Charmaz, & A. E. Clarke, *Developing grounded theory: The second generation* (pp. 55–65). Walnut Creek, CA: Left Coast Press.

Tappen, R. M., Williams, C. L., Barry, C., & DiSesa, D. (2001). Conversation intervention with Alzheimer's patients increasing the relevance of communication. *Clinical Gerontologist, 24*(3/4), 63–75.

Tappen, R. M., Williams-Burgess, C., Edelstein, J., Touhy, T., & Fishman, S. (1997). Communicating with individuals with Alzheimer's disease: Examination of recommended strategies. *Archives of Psychiatric Nursing, 11*(5), 249–256.

Tashakkori, A., & Teddlie, C. (1998). Mixed methodology. Thousand Oaks, CA: Sage.

ten Have, P. (1999). *Doing conversation analysis*. London: Sage.

Thorne, S. (2000). Data analysis in qualitative research. *Evidence Based Nursing, 3*, 68–70.

Turkel, M., Tappen, R. M., & Hall, R. (1999). Moments of excellence. Nurses' response to role redesign in long-term care. *Journal of Gerontological Nursing, 25*(1), 7–12.

van Manen, M. (1990). *Researching lived experience: Human science for an action sensitive pedagogy*. London, Ontario: State University of New York Press.
 ✧ A classic on phenomenological research. The focus is on pedagogy (teaching), but is transferable to nursing.

Williams, C. L., Tappen, R. M., Rosselli, M., Keane, F., & Newlin, K. (2009). Willingness to be screened and tested for cognitive impairment: Cross-cultural comparison. *American Journal of Alzheimer's Disease and Other Dementias, 25*(2), 160–166. Advance online publication. doi: 10.1177/1533317509352333.

Wolf, Z. R. (2007). Ethnography: The method. In P. L. Munhall (Ed.). *Nursing research: A qualitative perspective* (pp. 293–330). Sudbury, MA: Jones and Bartlett.
 ✧ A nice introduction to ethnography. Includes a table of ethnographic studies done by nurses.

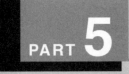

PART 5

Reporting

CHAPTER 22

Presenting Your Research Findings

A presentation of research findings can be dry, dull, and sleep inducing, or it can be compelling, riveting, and eye-opening. We will try to achieve the latter by suggesting some guidelines for producing posters and podium presentations that are both interesting and of professional quality.

Even at national conferences, you can encounter disorganized, handwritten transparencies projected on a screen or handwritten pages tacked to the display stand provided for poster presentations. With the digital technology and user-friendly software available, there is no excuse for these poor presentations. On the other hand, we are flooded every day by incredibly creative media designed to teach, entertain, or persuade. Your presentation is unlikely to be able to compete with these masterpieces of imagination, but your audience does not expect it to. They have come to learn about your study; your job is to effectively share the information with them.

We will address poster presentations first and then direct our attention to making a podium presentation.

POSTER PRESENTATIONS

Some people are disappointed when their submitted abstract is designated a poster presentation; others are relieved that they will not have to stand in front of a group and speak. The advantage of a poster presentation is that once the poster has been created, most of your work is done. At the conference, you can relax and engage in conversations with the people who come by to see it. This assumes, of course, that you have created an attractive and informative poster.

Organizing the Information

You could conceivably have hundreds of pages of literature review, proposal descriptions, and data from your study. This has to be condensed to fit into a 3 ft × 6 ft space. It may help to set aside those hundreds of pages of notes, proposals, and printouts and begin by using the acronym TIMRAD to organize your presentation (American College of Physicians, 2009; Purrington, 2007; Milutinovic, 1996):

Titles
Introduction
Method
Results
Analysis
Discussion

Once you have organized your main ideas, you can fill in more (but not too much) detail. The following list is one way to do this.

1. *Titles:* Include the title of your study and the investigators with their credentials and affiliations. If the study was funded, recognize the source of the funding. There may be other acknowledgments you want to add here, but keep them brief.

2. *Introduce the study:* Include purpose, objectives, or goals of the study but not all three (all three would be too many words for a poster). Then connect the study with previous work, very briefly sketching the theoretical background, particularly if there was a choice of theoretical perspectives or if you are testing or challenging current theory.

3. *Method:* Briefly describe the study design. Describe the characteristics of the sample. List the measures you used, explaining them only if needed (many are well known to professional audiences). Mention any unusual or important procedures. Mention where the study was done such as listing research sites.

4. *Results:* Present the main findings in a logical order. Use tables or graphs for quantitative data where possible. Provide well-chosen quotes, explanations, or examples (just a few) to support your findings.

5. *Conclusions:* Summarize your main findings. Connect the findings to existing knowledge and theory. Discuss implications of the findings for practice and for further study.

Adding Graphics

The outline above is just the bare bones of a presentation. Where appropriate, add a cogent quotation, an important reference or website, or diagrams to illustrate the theoretical framework, an anatomical detail, or a complicated procedure. Photographs may be added as well with permission of those photographed (video clips may be used effectively during a podium presentation). Use your imagination, but do not overembellish the presentation.

The following are some additional suggestions for preparing a poster:

- Check the size and type of display (especially whether it is on a table or display stand) before designing the poster.
- Choose either a bold, bright palette of colors or a soft muted combination, but not both.
- Use large letters that can be read several feet away for the title and for the most important points of information on the poster.
- Arrange graphics that enhance but do not distract from the information.
- Be sure the poster you are creating can be easily transported to where you will be displaying it.

If you still feel uncertain about how to design your poster, ask your classmates, colleagues, or mentors if they will show you posters they have designed. You may also want to consult with graphics design people if they are available in your organization (see Figure 22-1).

PODIUM PRESENTATIONS

If you will be presenting your study in front of a live audience, there are some additional considerations in preparing your presentation.

Organizing the Information

Instead of arranging the information within a specified space, for a podium presentation the information will be presented sequentially, one frame or "slide" at a time. (We still call them slides but people rarely use actual slides—the term has migrated to the electronic environment.) Before you begin, you need to know how much time you are allowed and the type of projection equipment that will be available.

You can use the same outline as you would for a poster, but you will probably be able to add a little more detail in each section.

Each slide should have only two or three points of information on it. Remember that the visuals are meant to be an outline of what you are planning to say, not everything you plan to say.

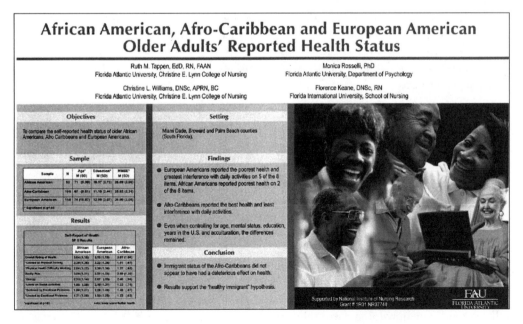

Figure 22-1 Example of poster prepared for a professional conference.

Adding Graphics

Selecting the right graphics for a podium presentation is difficult because most people look at their slides on paper or a computer screen, which is really quite different from the way they will appear on a large screen. For example, red lettering on a black background is very bright on a small screen that is close to your eyes, but it is not the best choice for a large screen in a large room. Yellow letters on a bright blue background are easier to see. For most presentations, dark lettering on a light background is usually a safe choice.

If someone else is designing your graphics, be sure they understand the purpose of the presentation and the expected audience. Here's an example of what could go wrong if you don't:

> Doctoral student Darlene Grabowski was very excited about the opportunity to do her first podium presentation at a regional nursing research conference. Her qualitative study using grounded theory to develop a theory of grieving related to sudden loss of vision in both eyes was recently completed. Darlene's mentor helped her prepare the outline for the presentation and her employer offered to have the graphics department prepare the PowerPoint presentation. Unfortunately, the PowerPoint presentation was not completed until the afternoon before the conference. Darlene just picked up the CD and took it home without looking at it. That evening, she reviewed it on her laptop. She was horrified to see that a well meaning but misinformed graphics designer had given her slides a rosy pink background. At the top and bottom of each slide was a telephone wire graphic on which a half dozen cute little chirping bluebirds sat. Darlene did not have the software on her laptop to change the graphics. All she could do was tell the audience that the designer had not been aware of the topic and apologize for its inappropriateness. A few sympathetic chuckles from the audience helped her to relax and present her study well despite the graphics mishap.

Overly busy slides, small lettering (often because a document was scanned to make a slide) and poor contrast between lettering and the background are the most common mistakes made in creating the graphics design for a podium presentation. Remember, the graphics are there to support and highlight the information.

Speaking

A frequently quoted survey of people's worst fears found that most thought only death was scarier than public speaking. This is not true of everyone, of course, but many people become very nervous when they have to speak to a large audience. The result can be a dry mouth (use a throat lozenge or sips of water to counteract this) and speaking too fast. One nervous speaker finished an hour lecture in 17 minutes! If you are new to public speaking, practice your talk in front of the mirror and then in front of family or friends. Time your talk so you know how long it will take at normal speed. Another helpful preparation tip is to mark the information in your notes as (1) essential, (2) an elaboration of the essential, or (3) would be nice to say if there's time (American College of Physicians, 2009). Still need more help to relax? While you are speaking, look for two or three interested appearing faces in the audience and talk to them. Their nonverbal encouragement will help you feel more comfortable.

The following are some additional do's and don'ts for effective presentations:

Do	**Do Not**
Know what you want to say and practice it	Memorize your talk, or read your notes unless you are not speaking in your native language and have to do this
Look at people in the audience and talk to them	Turn your back to the audience to see the slides (Emerald, n.d.)
Speak at your usual rate	Speak too fast or too slowly
Tell stories related to your study	Tell jokes that have no relation to your study
Be yourself	Try to be very formal
Stay focused	Wander away from your topic
Watch the time or ask someone else to be your timekeeper	Speak past your allotted time
Try to enjoy your time in the limelight	Worry about making a good impression

Most audiences love handouts. Selecting a key image, diagram, or an outline of your key points to copy and distribute to your audience will please most listeners (Herman, n.d.). Often people in the audience will be interested in speaking with you about your research, so plan to stay after the presentation for a few minutes to talk with them. You may also want to provide an e-mail address so people can contact you later. These informal exchanges are not only enjoyable but sometimes lead to new ideas for your research and new opportunities for collaboration.

CONCLUSION

The conversations that occur with poster and podium presentations are a very valuable and energizing exchange of information among scientists with similar interests. They are not, however, a substitute for publishing your findings. Publication reaches a wider audience and provides a more permanent record of your work.

REFERENCES

American College of Physicians. (2009). *Preparing the research presentation*. Retrieved January 23, 2009, from http://www.acponline.org/residents_fellows/competitions/abstract/prepare/res_pres.htm
  ◇ A detailed "generic" outline using tanning salons and AIDS as examples for presentations is very well done. If you are having trouble outlining your presentation, you might want to look at this.

Emerald Group Publishing. (n.d.). *How to . . . Give a research presentation*. Retrieved January 21, 2009, from http://info.emeraldinsight.com/research/guides/research_presentation.htm?PHPSESSID= c16u9kplbbdj7jmd7ullla2p60&
  ✧ The section "Giving the Presentation" addresses being nervous about presenting. There is also some good information about being sure everything is ready and working well before your presentation.
Herman, E. (n.d.). *Guidelines for research presentations*. Retrieved January 23, 2009, from http://www. uoregon.edu/~eherman/writing/Research%20Presentation%20Guidelines.htm
Milutinovic, V. (1996, September). The best method for presentation of research results. *IEEE TCCA Newsletter,* 1–6. Retrieved January 23, 2009, from http://tab.computer.org/tcca/NEWS/sept96/ bestmeth.pdf
Purrington, C. (2007). *Gratuitous advice on giving a talk*. Retrieved January 23, 2009, from http:// www.swarthmore.edu/NatSci/cpurrin1/powerpointadvice.htm
  ✧ Humorous with lots of practical suggestions (although it does focus more on mice, lizards, and insects than most nursing presentations do).

CHAPTER 23

Publishing Your Research Results

Have you completed your study? You are not finished until you have shared the outcomes with the people who supported your study, colleagues who would be interested in your results, and, in some instances, the public.

REPORTING TO FUNDERS

Reporting to your funder is an obligation if you have received financial support for your study. Funders usually want two types of information: how their money was spent, and what was accomplished. Each funder will have a different reporting format that you should follow as closely as you can in preparing your reports. Sometimes funders also want to be involved in releasing the results to the public, a request that should be respected.

REPORTING TO THE PUBLIC

There is a great interest in health matters among members of the public, but there are also several precautions to keep in mind if you decide to go directly to the public with your findings:

- You will have to "translate" your findings from technical language into language a layperson can understand.

- Remember that knowledge is cumulative. Your study's results need to be connected to what is already known.

- Remember also that it is rare for a single study to be definitive. Results need to be replicated, that is, to be confirmed in other studies before they are used to change practice.

- When you speak with reporters, you may not have the final say on how the results are written up and made known to the public. Misquotes can distort your results, so be sure you are very clear in describing your results and in explaining what the results mean. Some publishers will let you review a draft of what will be in print, others will not.

- Going directly to the public bypasses peer review, that important source of critique that provides an objective evaluation of the credibility of your study results and its importance to health care.

PUBLISHING IN PROFESSIONAL JOURNALS

Reports to funders and press releases to the public are not substitutes for publishing in a professional journal. For most people, writing a research-based article is hard work. The following is a guide to help you prepare a manuscript for submission once the study is done:

1. Select a target journal. Some points to consider in making this important decision:
   - Does the subject of your study match the subject matter of the journal?
   - Does the journal primarily publish research?
   - Is it an interdisciplinary journal? A nursing journal? A journal targeted to another profession?
   - What is the rejection rate of the journal? You can find this out by checking the journal's home page or one of the published articles on manuscript acceptance and rejection rates.
   - Have similar articles been published in the journal recently?

2. Download the information for authors from the journal you selected:
   - Review this information to be sure the article you plan to write is of interest to this journal.
   - Carefully review page limits and other requirements of the journal.
   - Follow the required format as you write the article.

3. Assemble your related articles, references, data output, original proposal, and other materials related to the subject of the article. Reread them if you need to refresh your memory before creating the outline.

4. Outline the article. Be sure to include the following:
   - Introduction (one that captures the reader's attention)
   - Importance of the study
   - Review of related theory and research to connect the study to existing knowledge. Select the key studies to describe, do not select them on the basis of publication date as you might for a clinical paper. Synthesize and evaluate the information, don't just repeat it. Emphasize primary sources; avoid secondary sources as much as you can (Galvan, 2006).
   - Purpose of the study
   - Method: Include the design, sampling procedures and sample description, research sites, measures, and procedures, including consent procedures and any other relevant information. Often a summary of the statistical analyses that were done is included in the methods section.
   - Results: Include sample characteristics if not described in the methods section. Focus here on the results of the study and the data analysis that was done, not your interpretation of the results
   - Discussion: This section should begin with a summary of the results and relation to the purpose stated earlier. Then discuss your conclusions based on

the results, limitations of the study, and suggestions for further research. Finally, discuss the implications for practice (that is, how the results might inform practice), and reiterate the importance of the study.

5. Next, make notes about the key points under each item of the outline.

6. Then write the narrative for each section of the outline using your notes regarding the key points but now filling in the details.

7. Read the manuscript from beginning to end. Revise and rewrite where needed.

8. Ask a colleague to review and critique the manuscript, or set it aside for several days to get some distance from it, and then review it as if it were someone else's manuscript.

9. Recheck the formatting, limits on length, and other requirements in the instructions to authors to be sure you have followed their directions.

10. Submit the manuscript with a brief cover letter to the editor, signatures, and any statements regarding authorship required by the journal.

11. Keep track of the article online as it moves through the review process.

12. If you receive a request for revisions, make each one of them carefully, and list them in a letter to the editor (remember, this letter may be sent to the previous reviewers or a new set of reviewers). If there is a change requested that you are not able to make, respectfully explain why you cannot.

13. If the article is rejected, analyze why this happened, taking careful note of whatever reasons were given by the editor. Discuss your next steps (revising and resubmitting to another journal) with colleagues and mentors before proceeding. *Do not* abandon the manuscript.

14. When you receive the acceptance of your article, celebrate. This is an achievement to be proud of.

SPECIAL CONSIDERATION FOR QUALITATIVE RESEARCH MANUSCRIPTS

Clear, concise writing is just as important when preparing a manuscript on the results of a qualitative study, but there are also some special considerations. Restrictions on the length of the article are especially challenging when you want to include many quotes or some of the thick description that characterizes qualitative research. Careful selection of the quotations and descriptions are needed to stay within the space limitations. Devers and Frankel (2001) suggest that additional description can be made available in an appendix or online. They also caution against careless use of qualitative research terms. For example, the term *rigor* is more appropriate than *reliability* and *validity* for most qualitative research. Bracketing is consonant with Husserl's philosophy, but being able to put aside one's own beliefs has been questioned by van Mannen, so it is not appropriate to say your study used van Mannen's approach but also that you used bracketing (Watson,

2003). Despite its respected tradition in many disciplines, there are still journals and reviewers who do not understand or value the contribution of qualitative research to our understanding of health-related phenomena. You may want to check recent articles published in the journal selected to see if they publish qualitative research.

REASONS FOR ACCEPTANCE

Surveys of journal editors and reviewers consistently identify a few important characteristics of manuscripts that are accepted. These are excellent writing, importance or timeliness of the topic, and soundness of the study design (Bordage, 2001).

Reviewers also look for a focused, current review of the literature, implications for practice, and recognition of the limitations of the study.

REASONS FOR REJECTION

Poorly written manuscripts describing poorly designed studies are the major reasons why manuscripts are not accepted. "Wordiness," especially in the introduction and discussion sections, is a common problem (Byrne, 2000), and many manuscripts have too little detail in the method section. These problems can be fixed, but a study that was poorly designed is hard to fix after it is done.

RESUBMISSION AFTER REJECTION

It is never easy to have your work rejected. You may need a few days to recover from your disappointment before revising and resubmitting the manuscript to another journal. Some journals accept only one out of five manuscripts submitted, so occasional rejections should be expected.

It is important to review the reasons for the rejection so that you can make a thoughtful decision about where to resubmit the article and what revisions you should make before resubmission. Consider the following:

1. Is the journal appropriate? Is this a topic of interest to their readers? Do they publish research studies?

2. Is the manuscript of sufficient quality and importance for a top-tier journal, or should you look for a journal that is a little less selective?

3. Is the manuscript well written? Is it clear, organized, succinct, and logical but also compelling? If not, you may need some editorial assistance to make it so.

4. Was the study designed and executed well? If yes, does the manuscript reflect this quality? If no, is there still something worth sharing with others?

5. Is the topic timely? Is it important? Print journals have limited space. Their editors want to print articles on the most important topics, ones that are of interest to their readers.

6. Has the journal you selected recently published an article on the same subject? If yes, the editor might reject an otherwise acceptable manuscript without reviewing it.

Colleagues, teachers, and mentors are usually willing to help you answer these questions. There are also many books and articles about writing for publication that you may find helpful.

CONCLUSION

Sharing the results of your research with others is part of your responsibility as a nurse researcher. Practitioners need to know the results of your research if they are going to make their practice as evidence based as possible.

Consider a different perspective on the importance of publishing the findings of your research that may motivate you to get your findings published: It would be selfish not to share what you learned, wouldn't it?

REFERENCES

Bordage, G. (2001). Reasons reviewers reject and accept manuscripts: The strengths and weaknesses in medical education reports. *Academic Medicine, 76*(9), 889–896.

Byrne, D. W. (2000). Common reasons for rejecting manuscripts at medical journals: A survey of editors and peer reviewers. *Science Editor, 23*(2), 39–44.

Devers, K. J., & Frankel, R. M. (2001). Getting qualitative research published. *Education for Health, 14*(1), 109–117.

Galvan, J. L. (2006). Writing literature reviews. A guide for students of the social and behavioral sciences. Glendale, CA: Pyrczak Publishing.
   ◇ If you need a lot of help writing a review of the literature, this book will guide you through the entire process. Model literature reviews at the end of the book are also worth looking at.

Watson, L. A. (2003). Commentary. *Western Journal of Nursing Research, 25*, 318.

FOR FURTHER READING

Blancett, S. S. (1991). The ethics of writing and publishing. *Journal of Nursing Administration, 21*(5), 31–36.
   ◇ A classic, easy-to-read article on various types of misconduct: fraud, falsification, plagiarism, "honorary" authorship, massaging data, etc.

Bradigan, P. S. (1996). *Writer's guide to nursing and allied health journals.* Washington, D.C.: American Nurses Publications.

Daly, J. M. (2000). *Writer's guide to nursing periodicals.* Thousand Oaks, CA: Sage Publications.

Fahy, K. (2008). Writing for publication: The basics. *Women and Birth, 21*, 86–91. (Also available at http://www.ScienceDirect.com.)
   ◇ A good review of how to write well. The examples use nursing situations and are very helpful.

Happell, B. (2008). Writing for publication: A practical guide. *Nursing Standard, 22*(28), 35–40.
   ◇ Especially helpful. Here are the descriptions of various types of articles, from research and quality improvement to clinical articles and debates.

Publication Manual of the American Psychological Association (6th Ed.). (2009). Washington, D.C.: American Psychological Association.
   ◇ The American Psychological Association's format and guidelines are frequently used in nursing journals. Examples of common abbreviations and how to set up tables are especially helpful.

Nursing Research journal website. Available at: http://journals.lww.com/nursingresearchonline/pages/default.aspx

    ◇ On selected articles, this journal publishes (with the author's permission, of course) the original reviews of a manuscript and the author's response. If you have never submitted a research manuscript before, you might learn a lot from reading a few of these.

San Francisco Edit. (n.d.). *Eleven reasons why manuscripts are rejected.* Retrieved March 16, 2009, from http://www.sfedit.net/newsletters.htm

    ◇ Although written for a more general audience, this website focuses on data based writing and has some very practical advice.

Webb, C. (2003). Editor's note: Introduction to guidelines on reporting qualitative research. *Journal of Advanced Nursing, 42*(6), 544–545.

    ◇ If you are reporting qualitative research, this brief article, especially the basic criteria for acceptability of qualitative research reports, is a must-read. See also http://www.journalofadvanced nursing.com

CHAPTER 24

Preparing Research Proposals

A proposal is *an idea that is put forward for consideration* (Free Dictionary, 2009). There are two types of proposals that are of special interest in nursing research: one is the thesis or dissertation proposal, and the other is an application for funding. In either case, you as the proposer are seeking approval for your research idea and for your plan for conducting the research study.

The hallmark of a good thesis or dissertation proposal is good science. A good research proposal for funding is a combination of good science plus some artful persuasion that your idea is worthy of monetary support.

THESIS AND DISSERTATION PROPOSALS

Written thesis and dissertation proposals focus primarily on the topic selected and how you plan to study it. By the time you write your proposal, the topic should be clearly specified and the work should be of a size and scope that you will be able to complete it in a reasonable amount of time.

Most dissertation proposals are composed of preliminary drafts of what will become the first three chapters of the completed dissertation: the introduction, a review of the literature, and the methods chapter.

The Topic

The topic or subject of the dissertation should be reflected in the title of the dissertation and every section of the dissertation that follows. In addition to the title, several other aspects of the topic should be addressed in the proposal:

1. A statement of the problem, area of interest, research question, or hypothesis, depending upon the type of study proposed

2. The theoretical framework within which the topic will be explored. In some instances, especially in qualitative studies, it is also appropriate to include the philosophical stance.

3. Significance of the study, why it is important, what will be learned and how the study will contribute to the body of nursing knowledge and ultimately to the quality of patient care

4. Existing literature on the topic, that is, what is already known, understood, and has been discovered about the topic

5. Limitations of existing theory and research on the topic including gaps in knowledge, weaknesses or limitations of the studies already done, and how your study will address one of these gaps or limitations

The Methodology

The proposed methods to be used in conducting the study also need to be described in sufficient detail that the reader can judge their appropriateness. Aspects of the methodology to be addressed in the proposal include the following:

1. Whether the study will be a qualitative, quantitative, or mixed methods study

2. The specific design selected, such as case study, ethnography, or clinical trial

3. Sample, including the size of the sample and how the size was determined and the characteristics of the sample, both inclusion and exclusion criteria

4. Participant recruitment, including consenting procedures, how potential participants will be accessed, and your estimate of the number who will be willing to participate

5. Plan for data collection, including the measures used (discussed in some detail including reasons for their selection, the time it takes to administer, reliability, and validity) if a quantitative study, an outline of participant approach and interview questions or observations if a qualitative study, and the time frame for accomplishing this work

6. Data analysis should connect directly to the proposed problem statement, question, or hypothesis. In many qualitative studies, analysis will be done in tandem with data collection, and this should be reflected in the proposal.

If you need a template for writing your thesis or dissertation proposal, you may ask classmates who have already completed an approved proposal if you may read it. Some colleges will maintain a file of proposals or abstracts of thesis and dissertation proposals.

It is not "cheating" to read someone else's proposal. Your proposal will address a different topic and probably use a different method. What you learn from reading an approved proposal is the formatting, typical length, and amount of detail included; the scientific style of writing that is used; and what a successfully completed proposal looks like.

GUIDANCE FOR WRITING A THESIS OR DISSERTATION PROPOSAL

Guidance during the thesis or dissertation work comes in several forms. To the extent possible, you should take advantage of these as much as possible. There is usually a set of written guidelines produced by your college, graduate school or office of doctoral studies. To avoid having to rewrite the dissertation or even having to begin all over again, you should become thoroughly familiar with these guidelines. Members of your thesis or dissertation committee are a second vital source of information and guidance. Individual consultations with each one can be very helpful. The chair of your committee should be your main source of guidance throughout the entire experience.

There are several other sources of guidance that will be of varying degrees of help to you depending upon your circumstances and your topic. The first are your classmates, especially those who have gone before you. They not only can share their experiences with you and explain the seemingly inexplicable rules and norms for master's theses and doctoral dissertations in your college, but they can also inspire you with stories of their successes. It is also helpful to obtain several completed dissertations that were done within your college and read them. Knowing what an acceptable final product looks like can take some of the mystery out of this process.

For students who have a great deal of difficulty writing well, many colleges have writing centers available. The consultants at most centers are very helpful. They can provide helpful written resources and review your work, indicating common mistakes and ways to correct them but expectations regarding their help have to be kept within reason. For individuals who have a great deal of difficulty expressing themselves well in writing, especially in scientific writing, some colleges will permit the use of editors to improve the final product. This may be especially helpful for those for whom English is not their first language.

PROPOSALS FOR FUNDING

The fundamentals of writing a good research proposal remain the same for those that will be submitted for funding, but there are some additional considerations as well. Two major differences between these two types of proposals underlie most of the additional information provided in this section. The first is that when seeking monetary support for your proposed study, you are probably *competing* with others who are also trying to win support for their proposals. The second difference is the *distance* between you and the reviewers of your proposal. Most of the people reviewing your thesis or dissertation proposal not only know you but also your advisor and the environment within which you will be conducting the study. This is not the case with a proposal submitted for funding. Instead, most of this information is likely to be unknown to the reviewers unless you provide it. As a result, a proposal for funding needs to address additional matters that are known or assumed when proposal review occurs within your college or university.

New researchers find it difficult to decide where to begin the long-term process of conducting funded research. Devine (2009) suggests two possibilities: begin with applications for small grants as the principal investigator or join a research team as a co-investigator to give yourself an opportunity to "learn the ropes" before striking out on your own. There is, of course, no reason why you could not do both of these.

Finding the Right Funder

There are a variety of funding sources available to nurse researchers, but it is important to find the right match between (1) your experience level and choice of subject, and (2) the interests and expectations of the funder (Holtzclaw, Kenner, & Walden, 2008).

Funding sources can be divided into several categories:

- *Internal sources:* Usually these are small grants designed to help the researcher get started by supporting pilot work that is often needed before larger grants are sought. These may be called *seed money* grants.

- *Professional association grants:* There are general nursing research grants such as those provided by the American Nurses Foundation (ANF) and those provided by specialty nursing organizations such as the American Association of Critical-Care Nurses (AACN), the National Association of Pediatric Nurse Associates and Practitioners (NAPNAP), or the American Spinal Injury Association (ASIA). Check your own specialty organization website to see if they offer small research grants.

- *Disease-specific associations:* You will know the groups that are associated with the health concern of special interest to you. The American Cancer Society, American Heart Association, the National Parkinson Foundation, and the American Diabetes Association are just a few examples.

- *Private foundations:* There are many private foundations, some quite large, that are interested in health-related projects and research studies. The Robert Wood Johnson Foundation, W. K. Kellogg Foundation, Commonwealth Foundation, and March of Dimes Birth Defects Foundation are examples of large foundations interested in funding certain types of health-related studies. You may also have local foundations in the area where you live and work that support health-related studies.

- *Corporate funders:* Best known of the corporate funders are the pharmaceutical companies. The amounts available are less than they were in the past, but these are still potentially good sources of research studies if there is a match in interests.

- *Federal agencies:* The best known of the federal agencies are the National Institutes of Health (NIH), especially the National Institute of Nursing Research (NINR) but also the National Institute of Mental Health (NIMH), and centers for the study of minority health issues, complementary therapies, and many more. Additional federal sources include the Agency for Healthcare Research & Quality (AHRQ) and the Centers for Disease Control and Prevention (CDC). As you can tell from their names, each has a specific area of interest within the healthcare arena. Opportunities for funding range from support of predoctoral and postdoctoral study to large center grants.

For help in finding a good match, you want to do several things. First, talk with your mentors or advisors, colleagues, and staff of the nursing research office or the office of sponsored research. Those with research interests most closely related to yours and with grant writing experience are likely to be the most helpful. Second, search each of the possible funders' websites for information about the type of grants they offer. These change frequently in some cases, so you should not rely on printed materials that may be out of date. Some have lists of active grants in print or online that can be very informative. Others send representatives to national conferences and even provide opportunities for you to confer with them onsite. You will find that funders vary a great deal in the amount of guidance they are able to offer to new researchers, but virtually all are willing to talk with you about the appropriateness of your proposed topic and your eligibility for their grants. If you are fortunate enough to know someone who has received a grant from one of these funders, this person may also be a rich source of information. Doing this type of homework before writing a grant proposal is essential and will be time saving in the long run.

Information Commonly Requested

Various funders (grant makers or grantors) will ask for different types of information about you and your organization. The following sections cover the most common.

Preparation and Experience

Funders want to know that you have the ability to carry out the proposed research. They also want to know whether, if you encounter a problem, you will know how to resolve it. An experienced mentor is an asset when applying for pre- or postdoctoral grants, which are generally given to new researchers. In a larger study, the other members of the research team are expected to contribute knowledge and experience that is complementary to yours. For example, you may have a strong background in intensive care (ICU) nursing but little mental health experience. A colleague with mental health experience, especially in research related to mental health issues, would be an excellent complement on a study of psychosis or depression in the ICU.

Often, the number of pages in which you can describe your preparation and experience is limited. In this case, include the essential information such as education and employment, and then select the most relevant additional information, particularly any of your publications or previous research that is related to the proposed topic.

Budget

Having to create a budget for a project scares some people, particularly those who are not accustomed to applying time and money valuations to their research activities. The following sequence of steps may help. The steps begin with words and ideas, not numbers, to develop a *conceptual budget* that is gradually converted into numbers, resulting finally in a *detailed budget* that can be submitted with the proposal. The work on the conceptual budget is not discarded, however, because that information is the basis for the detailed budget and can also be used to compose the *budget justification*, a narrative that explains the detailed budget. Note that while you can begin work on the budget early in the development of the proposal, you cannot finalize it until the composition of the research team and the work that they will do has been finalized. The following are steps to constructing the final detailed budget:

- List all the people who will be involved in conducting the study. Begin with yourself, and add anyone who will work on the study including consultants, but

not the participants themselves unless you plan to provide small gifts or monetary incentives.

- Add to this personnel list a list of equipment, supplies, software, lab test fees,
and other expenses that you can expect to incur in conducting the study. Then,
if allowed, add travel costs for presenting results from the study and for
bringing in consultants if that is what you plan to do. These first two lists, with
descriptions of what each person is expected to do and how each piece of equipment or supplies will be used, constitute the conceptual budget.

- There is a category called *overhead* or *indirect costs* that covers such expenses as
office space, building maintenance, grant administration, secretarial support,
and other administrative support. Your finance person will be able to calculate
this for your budget. Most universities have an agreed upon rate for federally
funded research grants. Some private foundations allow a much smaller
amount than does the federal government, others allow none at all.

- As indicated above, it is now time to describe the work that each person will do
in relation to the proposed study: recruit participants, conduct interviews, perform tests, enter data, provide consultation on data analysis, and so forth. Do
the same for all equipment, supplies, travel, or other expenses that you are
asking be covered; explain their purpose and how they will be used to support
grant activities.

- Now, estimate the amount of time each person will require to accomplish their
tasks. It is probably easiest to do this by first thinking in terms of hours per
week. For example, one morning a week of work (a half day) would equal 4
hours, which is a 10% effort within a 40-hour week. This can then be converted
using the formula preferred by the funder. For example, if the funder wants
effort reported as months of the year, 10% of 12 months would equal 1.2
months per year. A second task is to obtain exact costs for travel, equipment,
software, lab tests, copyrighted tests that might be used, and supplies that will
be requested.

- At this point it is best to have a finance person help you because it is time to
apply exact cost figures to your conceptual budget, converting it into the
detailed budget. Once this is done, the finance person will also apply the
allowed indirect cost for the proposed study. These can be found in the research
study budget in Figure 24-1.

- Budget adjustments frequently have to be made at this point. The bottom line
(total) of the first draft of the detailed budget may come as a shock if you have
not done this before and have not yet learned how to estimate costs. Mileage, for
example, is often a very costly item, and you may have to find ways to cover
travel expenses without exceeding the budget limits set by the grantor. Some
transcriptionists, for another example, charge very high rates. If this is the case,
you may have to find an alternative individual. You may also have to trim time

A. Senior/Key Person

Prefix	First Name	Middle Name	Last Name	Suffix	Project Role	Base Salary ($)	Cal. Months	Acad. Months	Sum. Months	Requested Salary ($)	Fringe Benefits ($)	Funds Requested
Dr.					PD/PI	176,020.00	3.00			44,005.00	13,202.00	57,207.00
Dr.					Investigator	107,875.00	3.00			26,969.00	8,091.00	35,060.00
Dr.					Investigator	118,033.00	2.40			23,607.00	7,082.00	30,689.00
Dr.					Investigator	329,600.00	0.90			14,753.00	4,426.00	19,179.00
Dr.					Investigator	131,189.00	0.90			9,839.00	2,952.00	12,791.00
Total Funds Requested for all Senior/Key Person												
Total Senior/Key Person												154,926.00

B. Other Personnel

Number of Personnel	Project Role	Cal. Months	Acad. Months	Sum. Months	Requested Salary ($)	Fringe Benefits ($)	Funds Requested
	Graduate Students						
1	Nurse Practitioner	6.50			36,326.00	11,806.00	48,132.00
1	Psychometrician	6.50			23,839.00	7,748.00	31,587.00
Total Number Other Personnel							79,719.00
Total Salary, Wages and Fringe Benefits (A+B)							234,645.00

C. Other Direct Cost

	Funds Requested
Material and Supplies (Psychological Tests)	350.00
Consultant Services	31,250.00
Subawards/Consortium/Contractual Costs	36,587.00
Office Supplies and Postage	2,000.00
Participant Incentives and Translation Costs	7,750.00
CT Scans and Blood Chemistry	36,900.00
Total Other Direct Costs	114,837.00

D. Direct Costs

	Funds Requested
Total Direct Costs (B+C)	349,482.00

E. Indirect Costs

Indirect Cost Type	Indirect Cost Rate (%)	Indirect Cost Base ($)	Funds Requested
Modified Total Direct Cost (on-site)	44.50	337,893.00	150,362.00
Total Indirect Cost			150,362.00

F. Total Direct and Indirect Cost

	Funds Requested
Total Direct and Indirect Institutional Cost (D+E)	499,844.00

Figure 24-1 Sample budget for the first year of a 2-year study.

allotments for personnel to bring the budget in line, but caution is required here because you do not want to reduce their time to the point that they are not able to accomplish the proposed work.

- A second draft of the budget may still need some fine-tuning but should now be within the amounts allowed by the grantor. It is important to review every statement and every number in the budget to be sure they reflect the proposed research plan and make sense to you. Remember that while the finance person is the expert on numbers and salaries, you are the expert on the research plan, and you know what you need to accomplish to complete the study successfully.

- It is now time to write the budget justification if one is requested. This is simply an explanation of how you will use the funds that you have requested. Unless the instructions limit what you can say, a few words on the value of the contributions of the various members of the research team and consultants and the importance of travel or other expenses demonstrate your thoughtfulness in constructing the budget. Letters of agreement from proposed consultants are often requested.

Description of the Environment

Remember that the reviewers and funders are far less familiar with your work environment than you are. In fact, they may know virtually nothing about it. The type and amount of information about the environment that is requested by a funder varies widely, from several pages to just a few lines within the proposal. Most important is the extent to which the environment is supportive of your research. The following are some items that may be included:

- Accessibility to prospective participants: Letters of agreement or support from cooperating agencies or sites where the study will be conducted may be requested.

- Supportive infrastructure: A nursing research office or office of sponsored research and the availability of both pre-award and post-award assistance with adhering to the funder's guidelines, monitoring the budget, and so forth, is another indication of a research supportive environment.

- Availability of office space to maintain study documents and files in and sufficient computer hardware and software to facilitate your work are essentials.

- Library access, particularly searchable online databases and interlibrary loan services, needs to be readily available to the research team.

- Adequate laboratory space or services and animal facilities for those who are doing basic research using animal models may also be needed.

- Geographic and demographic characteristics of your community may also be of interest. Proximity to rural areas, access to ethnic enclaves, a high-volume emergency department, or a large neonatal intensive care unit are examples of what might be mentioned here. Some funders also ask about the size of your organization, numbers of patients (if a healthcare facility) or students, the type of organization, how it is governed, and the names of its officers and board of directors. This information generally is submitted only if requested.

Assurances

Some funders will provide grants only to nonprofit organizations, and so they will request what is called a certificate of 501(c) 3 status. Some require evidence of IRB approval of your proposed study at the time of the submission of the proposal although most will accept assurance that this has been applied for or will be done before the research begins. There are a number of other assurances related to protection of human subjects or animals, equal employment opportunities, and so forth that may be required. Your organization should be able to provide you with these.

SUGGESTIONS AND GUIDELINES FOR PREPARING APPLICATIONS FOR FUNDING

If there were space for only one line of advice regarding writing a research proposal for funding, it would be *follow the directions*. If, for example, the directions say eight pages are the maximum allowed, do not send them even one line more than eight pages. If font and spacing are specified, use the specified font and spacing. Why so rigid? You do not want to appear to do sloppy work, and you do not want the funder to send the proposal back unread. All of the work you have done to prepare the proposal is for naught if it is not even considered. Following are some additional suggestions:

1. *Write as clearly as possible.* For a moment, think of the poor reviewer who is reading your proposal at 3 a.m., eyes are burning; head is pounding from reading too long. It is the reviewer's responsibility to give your proposal due thought and consideration. It is your responsibility to provide the reviewer with the information needed to do so in as clear and readable a manner as possible.

2. *Choose your words carefully.* Careless use of terms may leave the unfortunate impression that you do not really know what you are writing about. An example would be referring to research questions when you are proposing to test several hypotheses. Another is using the term *significant* other than in reference to statistical significance. These little slips do not mean you are poorly informed, but they may suggest this to a critical reviewer.

3. *Use terms consistently.* This is not creative writing; it is scientific writing. Using three different terms for one idea suggests confusion, not sophistication. For example, use either the term *depression* or *depressive symptomatology* or *dysphoria*, but not all three, because there are differences in meaning, and it may seem that you are not aware of these differences unless you make that very clear.

4. *Emphasize the importance of your topic.* Capture the attention of the reviewer in the first paragraph, if not the first sentence. Include key statistics that emphasize the impact of the problem under study (Galvan, 2009).

5. *Let your passion for the subject show.* Your strong commitment to research, interest in the topic, and concern for the population of interest should be a subtext in your proposal. It is not directly stated but radiates from your writing. Proposal writing is serious writing, but the fact that you care about the outcomes can be conveyed to the reader.

6. *Keep science foremost in what is written.* It should be evident by now that proposals are not the place for personal anecdotes, cute cartoons, or excessive design elements (Singh, Cameron, & Duff, 2005). Instead, keep it clean, simple, and elegant. Leave some "white space" to aid the reader. For example, you could include a graph that illustrates the health concerns experienced by the population of interest such as a higher occupational risk for HIV-AIDS (see Figure 24-2 for an example). Use lists, figures, and tables where appropriate to break up the narrative (Harper, 2008), or put essential information such as the timeline for the proposed study in an easy-to-read table (see Figure 24-3).

7. *Reflect current thinking.* It is essential that your proposal refers to the most current, up-to-date research and theory on the topic. Any less than this will imply that you are not fully cognizant of the state of the field.

8. *Make everything fit together like pieces of a puzzle.* Congruence is essential. From the title to the data analysis, everything that is written should focus on the proposed topic of the research. Anything less than this suggests confusion to the reviewer.

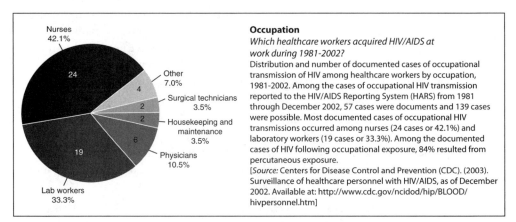

Figure 24-2 Use of a graph to illustrate an important point.

Source: National Institute for Occupational Safety and Health (NIOSH). Worker health chartbook, 2004. DHHS (NIOSH) Publication No. 2004-146. Retrieved July 14, 2010, from http://www.cdc.gov/niosh/docs/2004-146/pdfs/2004-146.pdf

TASK	| Year 1 | 1 2 3 4 5 6 7 8 9 10 11 12	| Year 2 | 1 2 3 4 5 6 7 8 9 10 11 12	| Year 3 | 1 2 3 4 5 6 7 8 9 10 11 12	Post
Convene Expert Panel	X			
Prepare Test Materials	X X (2,3)			
Hire & Train Research Assistants	X X (2,3)			
Contact Sites, Orient to Study Protocols	X X (1,2) ... X X (8,9)	X X (5,6)		
Random Sampling	X X (2,3) ... X X (9,10)	X X (6,7)		
Letter to Residents	X X (3,4) ... X X (11,12)	X X (7,8)		
Consents	X X X X X X X X X (4–12) — *Sites 1 & 2 & 3*	X X X X X X X X X X X X (1–12) — *Sites 4 & 5 & 6*	X X X X X (1–5)	
Schedule & Complete Testing	X X X X X X X X X (4–12)	X X X X X X X X X X X X (1–12)	X X X X X X X (1–7) — *Sites 7 & 8*	
Retest Subsample	X (11–12)	X X X X X X X X X X X X	X X X X X X X X (1–8)	
Data Input	X X X X X X X (6–12)	X X X X X X X X X X X X	X X X X X X X X (1–8)	
Preliminary Data Analysis		X X X X X (1–5)	X X X X X X X X (1–8)	
Reconvene Expert Panel			X (9)	
Final Data Analysis			X X X X (9–12)	
Final Report			X X X (10–12)	
Publication (postfunding)				X

Legend:

Site 1. W. Thompson Residence	Site 5. Grassy Point Nursing Center
Site 2. Live Oak Healthcare Center	Site 6. Hillyer Towers
Site 3. C.J. Smith Towers	Site 7. Sunset Arms Health Care Facility
Site 4. Pembroke Assisted Living	Site 8. Montgomery County Towers

Figure 24-3 Example of timeline for a large study.

9. *Seek a presubmission review.* You are encouraged to seek feedback from experienced researchers before submitting your proposal. These presubmission reviews may uncover gaps or errors or even problems that could be fatal flaws if allowed to remain in the proposal. Gitlin and Lyons (2008) provide some examples of fatal flaws: 1) the intervention requires so much time and staff involvement that it simply is not feasible, and (2) the design cannot be implemented because it requires random assignment to groups that could interfere with ongoing treatment (pp. 226–227). Another fatal flaw would be a mismatch between the stated hypotheses, data to be collected, and the analysis to be done.

   The following are a few other common flaws found in research proposals submitted for funding:

   • Inaccurate references: The reviewers are likely to be familiar with your source and will pick up errors if you do not.
   • Ignoring alternative viewpoints: If there are differing theories, be sure to acknowledge them.
   • Providing data that is not related to the proposed study: Keep everything that is clearly connected to your study. Eliminate anything else.
   • Poorly justified aims, hypotheses, method, measures, or analytic plans: Back up your proposed methodology with references, explanations, and rationales, but keep it brief (Yang, 2005).

10. *Anticipate technical challenges.* The majority of grant proposals are submitted online. In some cases you will have to preregister to be eligible to submit a proposal (Holtzclaw, Kenner, & Walden, 2008). You may have to spend some time learning how to upload documents and preparing them according to the specifications of the funder. It is best to practice ahead of time if possible, because you do not want to discover that you need an additional piece of software or additional document just before the deadline for submission.

11. *Fulfill the presubmission requirements.* Some funders ask for letters of intent, which are simply statements that you plan to submit a proposal and, usually, the topic of the proposal. Others ask for brief preproposals in which you state your topic and outline your plan for the study. These are screened by the funder, and only those with ideas of interest to the funder are invited to submit a full proposal.

All of the above are designed to persuade the reviewer that the study you are proposing to conduct is current, important, well designed, and can be done well by the research team within the proposed budget. Naturally, reviewer expectations are not as high for a pre-doctoral proposal as they are for a large, multisite study, but the essential expectations remain the same.

QUALITATIVE PROPOSALS: SPECIAL CONSIDERATIONS

One of the challenges to preparing a qualitative research application is that most recommended outlines for proposals and criteria for evaluation are based upon the quantitative paradigm. Reviewers may also be less familiar with the criteria for rigor in qualitative research (Locke, Spirduso, & Silverman, 2007; Marshall & Rossman, 2006). Here are several suggestions for addressing these challenges:

- Explain why qualitative research is the right approach to answering the research question posed. Provide a sound rationale, and show how useful the data obtained will be.

- Qualitative research involves a "series of choices" that are not familiar to quantitative researchers (Marshall & Rossman, 2006, p. 199). For example, because the plan for collecting data may be modified during the course of the study, which makes some reviewers uncomfortable, you can provide some examples of why this may occur and what course of action would be taken.

- Be sure to thoroughly address the ways in which trustworthiness (rigor or soundness) of the data will be established.

- Provide clear details about each phase of the data collection and analysis. Support these plans with liberal use of references to qualitative procedures.

Ungar (2006) also suggests using mixed methods and/or using more quantitatively oriented language and descriptive statistics to "dress up" a qualitative study to make it look more quantitative. Since qualitative research has gained far more recognition and respect in recent years, this not only should be unnecessary but might also backfire with a knowledgeable reviewer. A well-designed, solidly justified qualitative proposal to study a compelling topic should be able to stand on its own.

CONCLUSION

Writing proposals is clearly a challenging task, but the rewards are great. Even the most experienced and expert researchers are sometimes disappointed by the results of a grant review. Revision and resubmission of a proposal, unless strongly discouraged by the reviewers or funder, is an expected part of grant writing. As you gain experience, your grantsmanship skills will increase, as will your success.

REFERENCES

Devine, E. B. (2009). The art of obtaining grants. *American Journal of Health-System Pharmacy, 66*(6), 580–587.

DHHS. NIOSH Publication No. 2004-146. Retrieved April 30, 2010, from http://www.cdc.gov/niosh

Free Dictionary. (2009). Retrieved October 26, 2009, from http://www.thefreedictionary.com

Galvan, J. L. (2009). *Writing literature reviews: A guide for students of the social and behavioral sciences.* Glendale, CA: Pyrczak Publishers.
  ◇ A helpful guide that emphasizes and illustrates key points without a lot of narrative. Easy to use.

Gitlin, L. N., & Lyons, K. J. (2008). *Successful grant writing: Strategies for health and human service* (3rd Ed.). New York, NY: Springer.

Harper, P. J. (2008). Writing research proposals: Five rules. *HIV Nursing*, Summer, 15–17.

Holtzclaw, B. J., Kenner, C., & Walden, M. (2008). *Grant writing handbook for nurses.* Boston, MA: Jones and Bartlett.

   ✧ An informative book written especially for a nurse researcher audience.

Locke, L. F., Spirduso, W. W., & Silverman, S. J. (2007). *Proposals that work: A guide for planning dissertation and grant proposals.* Thousand Oaks, CA: Sage.

   ✧ You might find the proposal examples at the end of this book helpful.

Marshall, C., & Rossman, G. B. (2006). *Designing qualitative research.* Thousand Oaks, CA: Sage.

   ✧ These authors have written a helpful section on qualitative research proposals.

Singh, M. D., Cameron, C., & Duff, D. (2005). Writing proposals for research funds. *Canadian Association of Neuroscience Nurses AXONE, 26*(3), 26–30.

Ungar, M. (2006). "Too ambitious"—What happens when funders misunderstand the strengths of qualitative research design? *Qualitative Social Work, 5*(2), 261–277.

Yang, O. O. (2005). *Guide to effective grant writing: How to write an effective NIH grant application.* New York, NY: Kluwer Academic.

   ✧ They are scattered throughout the book, but Yang mentions many of the most common flaws found in research proposals, especially those submitted for funding.

CHAPTER 25

Evidence-Based Practice

Suppose you were a school nurse and a special needs teacher approached you with a request. Several parents of the autistic children in her class would like help in trying out a gluten-free diet for their children. You were somewhat skeptical, saying there is little evidence of a connection between gluten sensitivity and autism. However, if the diet is well balanced, it should not be harmful so you agreed to work with the parents "as an experiment." The school district's dietitian provided guidelines for gluten-free diets for school age children and spoke with the parents who were interested in trying the diet. All agreed that they would try the diet for 3 months and then assess their children's responses. At first, the parents were shocked by the number of food items that contained gluten and the cost of prepared gluten-free food products. However, they quickly began to test recipes and share them with each other. All five worked hard to follow the diet with their children, and no one dropped out.

At the end of the 3 months, the parents met with you, the special education teacher, and the district dietitian. All were encouraged by the progress their children had made and enthusiastic about continuing the gluten-free diet. You, on the other hand, remained skeptical.

Why was this? There were good reasons to remain skeptical. The following are a few of them:

- Only five children were involved in this "experiment." Further, while all were in the special education class, it was not established that they had all been accurately diagnosed as having autism.

- This really was not an experiment as there was no comparison group. How could anyone be sure that it was the diet that caused the improvement seen by the parents and the teacher? Perhaps the parents' enthusiasm motivated the teacher to try new behavioral approaches at the same time. Perhaps the parents were also being more consistent in their follow-through on these behavioral interventions at home because of the focus on their autistic child or because they were supporting each other much more than they had in the past.

- All of the enthusiastic comments about the improvement in the children were based upon the impressions of the teacher and the involved parents. They could be correct, but there could also be a lot of wishful thinking affecting their perception of the outcomes. There's little information available to tell you which it is.

From your perspective as a nurse researcher, the only conclusions that can be drawn from this "experiment" were that (1) at least some parents and teachers would be willing to try the gluten-free diet (in other words, that participants could be recruited into a study on this topic), (2) that the diet could be followed (adherence or compliance can be achieved), (3) that no apparent harm resulted, and (4) that there is a possibility that it may be of benefit, which should be further tested in a well-designed study. The addition of (1) a measure of child behavior, and (2) of a comparison group of children from the same class, and (3) permission to conduct the study from the appropriate oversight body would have transformed this experience into a pilot study. At this point, however, you are not able to recommend to other parents that they put their children on a gluten-free diet based solely upon this experience with five families.

WHY EVIDENCE-BASED PRACTICE?

The example of the gluten-free diet illustrates the difference between on-the-job experience and research-based evidence for the assessments and interventions that we use in practice every day. The recent emphasis on evidence-based practice comes from a recognition that healthcare practitioners' perceptions of the efficacy of their care may or may not be accurate and may be influenced by factors that the practitioners are not considering when informally evaluating the outcomes of the care they provide. The implementation of evidence-based practice is a means for reducing dependence on intuition, unsystematic clinical observation, ungrounded opinion, ritual, and tradition (Cullum, Ciliska, Haynes, & Marks, 2008; Melnyk & Fineout-Overholt, 2004). In fact, we are often surprised by evidence. For example, older patients in the community may not need a complete bath every day, but if they are hospitalized, especially if they are in an intensive care unit, then a skin cleansing with an antibacterial scrub solution can cut the incidence of sepsis dramatically (Climo, Sepkowitz, Auccotti et al., 2009). We have also learned that honey may be as effective as OTC cough medications (Paul, Beiler, McMonagle, Shaffer et al., 2007) or that surgical procedures assumed to be necessary may not lead to outcomes that are any better than nonsurgical treatment (Buchbinder, Osborne, Ebeling et al., 2009). For example, Buchbinder and associates (2009) compared the outcome of vertebroplasty to sham surgery and found that people in both groups experienced some improvement over time (i.e., diminished pain), but those on whom the actual surgical procedure was performed did not experience any appreciable increase in beneficial effect.

An example of premature enthusiasm for a treatment is the history of hormone replacement therapy (HRT) use in postmenopausal women. The results of large observational studies suggested that there was a cardiovascular benefit to long-term HRT, and many women were placed on HRT or kept on HRT primarily for this reason. The early studies had shown reduced cardiovascular disease-related mortality in women on HRT. It was thought that this was due to the lower cholesterol levels found in this group. However, later clinical trials of HRT told a different story: no benefit and possible risk of thrombosis in women who already had evidence of cardiovascular disease, and no benefit plus possible clotting problems in women with no evidence of existing cardiovascular disease (Cook &

DeMets, 2008, p. 1). What happened? To simplify a complex story, there were other differences between the women on HRT and those not on HRT in the observational studies that probably accounted for the differences in cardiovascular-related mortality rates. In other words, they were not comparable groups on factors that could affect cardiovascular health.

THE EVOLUTION OF EVIDENCE-BASED PRACTICE

The research utilization movement was the forerunner of evidence-based practice. Research utilization encourages and supports the application of research findings to clinical practice. It is the process used to inform clinical decision making (Estabrook, 2007). However, the findings that are applied may be from a single study, which is in contrast to the newer approach of evidence-based practice. The evidence-based practice movement emphasizes appraisal of all relevant studies and consideration of their applicability to a particular patient, setting, and situation (Melnyk & Fineout-Overholt, 2004).

In the literature, several different terms are used that are closely related. This movement began with *evidence-based medicine* (EBM), which Sackett and colleagues (1996) defined as follows:

> Evidence-based medicine is the conscientious, explicit, and judicious use of current test evidence in making decisions about the care of individual patients. The practice of evidence-based medicine means integrating individual clinical expertise with the best available external clinical evidence from systematic research. (p. 71)

This quickly morphed into *evidence-based health care* (EBH) as its leaders recognized the involvement of many other healthcare professionals and their contributions to our knowledge base of what constitutes effective care (Cullum et al., 2008; Popay & Williams, 1998).

In nursing, the term *evidence-based practice* (EBP) is used, but some prefer the term *evidence-based nursing* (EBN) to make it specific to nursing care. Ingersoll (2000) proposed a definition of evidence-based nursing practice that was designed to (1) encompass a broad spectrum of research designs, (2) not limit acceptable designs to randomized controlled trials (RCTs) or meta-analyses of RCT results, (3) emphasize theory-based research, (4) include groups of patients as well as individuals, and (5) recognize individual patient characteristics and preferences:

> Evidence-based nursing practice is the conscientious, explicit, and judicious use of theory-derived, research-based information in making decisions about care delivery to individuals or groups of patients and in consideration of individual needs and preferences. (p. 152)

There are several particularly important issues related to evidence-based practice that will be addressed in this chapter: the criteria used to judge the existing evidence for a particular health-related practice, the effect on healthcare policy, and the place of qualitative research findings in evidence-based analyses.

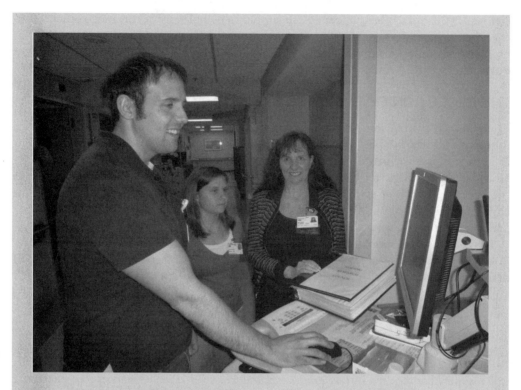

Dr. Marian Turkel, shown working with staff nurses Courtney Miller, RN, BSN, Clinical Scholar, and Steve Szablweski, RN, BSN, PCCN, Co-Chair Nursing Research-Evidence-Based Practice Council, who collaborated on a study entitled "Retrospective Chart Audit of Pain Management Practices" at Albert Einstein Hospital.

Source: Courtesy of Marian Turkel, RN, PhD, NEA-BC.

CRITERIA FOR EVIDENCE-BASED PRACTICE RECOMMENDATIONS

A considerable amount of effort and debate has gone into development of criteria for judging the strength of the evidence for and against a particular practice. A few examples will demonstrate the progression from relatively simple, straightforward criteria to complex sets of criteria and the use of quantitative meta-analysis (discussed in Chapter 6) to produce formal recommendations for practice and further research.

Basic Criteria

A review of interventions designed to prevent and/or treat child abuse done by Chaffin and Schmidt (2006) is a good example of a relatively simple, straightforward set of criteria. The criteria they used were as follows:

- Demonstrated efficacy in two or more well-designed, randomized controlled trials

- Comparison of the experimental intervention with either a no treatment or a standard treatment group

- Studies done by at least two different research teams

- The primary outcome or outcome of greatest importance, in this case occurrence or recurrence of child abuse, is measured directly, not just "softer" or peripheral outcomes such as change in presumed risk factors.

- Follow-up of future behavior (abuse occurrence or lack thereof) is long term, not just immediate or short term.

Note that these criteria, while generalizable, are especially suited to the particular issue of interest. Long-term follow-up (in terms of years, not just weeks or months), for example, may not be as relevant for some other interventions as it is for child abuse prevention and treatment.

Chaffin and Schmidt (2006) comment that practice in the field of child abuse prevention and treatment is still driven more by advocacy than by data (p. 63). In fact, some intervention strategies, such as Healthy Start, crisis intervention, and case-management based family preservation, have been repeatedly found to be ineffective in regard to the primary outcome.

One of the reasons practitioners continue to use them despite evidence that they are relatively ineffective is that today's active practitioners were not trained on the newer strategies and remain loyal to the strategies they learned even when they are shown to be ineffective. More effective interventions such as CBT (cognitive-behavioral therapy), PCIT (parent-child interaction therapy), and nurse-family partnership are available. The bottom line, according to Chaffin and Schmidt (2006), is that we need not only evidence of effectiveness but also strong dissemination of these results and strong systems to assure implementation.

Expanded Criteria

A number of sets of criteria for appraisal of research evidence can be found in the nursing literature (Brown, 2008; Cullum & Petherick, 2008). To a considerable extent, these are really guidelines for evaluating the design and implementation of the reported study or studies but with added considerations related to applicability to the patient and practice setting of interest. The following is an outline of the factors to be considered in appraising research evidence:

1. Topic: Is the study relevant to the topic of interest?

    You may find, for example, that while a study that is found in the search of the literature is on your general topic, such as breast cancer, it is not focused upon your specific interest, which might be immediate and long-term postoperative recovery after a mastectomy.

2. Quality: To what extent is the study well designed and well controlled?

The randomized clinical trial is often, although not always, held up as the gold standard against which relevant studies are appraised. This includes but is not limited to the following characteristics of the study:

a. Random selection and random assignment to treatment group
b. Use of a control group
c. Double blinding where possible
d. Use of outcome measures with established reliability and validity in similar populations
e. Handling of missing data
f. Follow-up of sufficient length of time
g. Appropriate analysis (for example, use of intent to treat analysis, inclusion of important covariates, addressing treatment adherence, withdrawals, and adverse events)

3. Results: Was the proposed intervention found effective?

The level of significance, confidence intervals, and effect size are generally considered important considerations.

4. Applicability: Are these results relevant to my practice?

Here, considerations of the characteristics of the sample and the setting within which the study took place are especially important. For example, many studies of pharmacological agents did not traditionally include children so dosages and safety margins for children were not known. Likewise, in the past, many studies omitted women or minorities, reducing their applicability to the general population. Further, studies done in one setting, such as acute care, may not be applicable to primary care or home care and vice versa.

Panel Reviews and Meta-Analyses

There is another level of complexity of appraisal that is exemplified by the work of expert panels for the National Guideline Clearinghouse (NGC, 2009) and the Cochrane Collaboration (2009). A Cochrane review includes the following sections:

• Summary in language that can be understood by nonprofessionals

• Abstract that summarizes each section of the review

• Background: Includes details of what is known and possible mechanisms through which the treatment under evaluation may work

• Aim of the review

• Criteria for selection of studies reviewed: This may include the type of study included (for example, randomized clinical trials) and excluded (for example, studies in which the method of participant selection is not clearly described), the population (for example, adults only), type of intervention (for example, certain antidepressants), and specific outcome measures (for example, the Hamilton and Montgomery-Asberg measures of depression)

- How the search for relevant studies was conducted

- Conduct of the review: Inclusion and exclusion criteria for the studies selected, assessment of the quality of the study, how data were extracted and analyzed, if any subsample results were analyzed, and so forth

- Description of the studies included

- Assessment of the quality of the included studies. The quality criteria may be quite extensive. They may include adequacy of the sample size, duration of the follow-up, randomization procedures, source of subjects, diagnostic criteria for selection of the subjects, exclusion criteria, and assessment of compliance with the treatment (Arroll, Elley, Fishman et al., 2009; Moncrieff, Churchill, Drummond, & McGuire, 2001). A quality rating may be reported for each of the studies included. You can see that these ratings are similar to the criteria listed in the previous section.

- Results

- Interpretation of the results

- Conclusions: Implications for practice and for research (Arroll et al., 2009; Cochrane Collaboration, 2009).

The topics addressed are wide ranging and include many of interest to nurses such as the effectiveness of antidepressant medications in primary care, absorbent products for urinary or fecal incontinence in men and women, acetaminophen for arthritis, breast stimulation for induction of labor, and breathing exercises for individuals with asthma (Arroll et al., 2009; Fader, Cottenden, & Getliffe, 2008; Holloway, 2004; Kavanagh, Kelly, & Thomas, 2005; Towheed, Maxwell, Judd, Catton, Hochberg, & Wells, 2006). Nurse researchers are included among the many expert reviewers who have contributed to these analyses.

Content of the Reviews

There are times when the reviewer finds few acceptable studies to appraise. For example, Fader, Cottenden, and Getliffe (2008) found only one published study comparing absorbent products (disposable pads, menstrual pads, washable pants, and so forth) for women with light urinary incontinence that met their criteria for inclusion. Other times, a more substantial number of eligible studies are found, and the reviewers are able to make some important recommendations concerning the intervention under study. For example, Arroll et al. (2009) found 14 eligible studies of tricyclic antidepressants (TCAs) and selective serotonin reuptake inhibitors (SSRIs) and noted that both evidenced effectiveness in treating depression in primary care settings, but the tricyclic antidepressants evidenced more adverse effects than did the selective serotonin reuptake inhibitors.

Kavanagh, Kelly, and Thomas (2005) found six eligible studies of breast stimulation to induce labor involving 719 women altogether. Three other studies were excluded because they did not report the outcomes of interest in the analysis, and one was excluded because subjects were not randomized. They also noted that double blinding is not possible in these studies because the women perform the breast stimulation procedure themselves. Only one of the trials included high-risk women and in this trial, four prenatal deaths (three in the breast stimulation group and one in the group receiving oxytocin) were reported. The study was stopped due to these deaths. The reviewers concluded that breast stimulation should only be used in low-risk women but that it could be beneficial for them given the reported 84% reduction in postpartum hemorrhage, a major cause of maternal deaths, in two of the trials that were evaluated.

Analyses Performed

When a substantial number of eligible studies are found, a meta-analysis on pooled data from all of the studies may be performed. Given the interventional nature of most of the topics under consideration, there are some particular analyses that are commonly performed and reported in these reviews. The terminology may seem complex at first. It may help to keep in mind that the goals are to assess the efficacy and safety of the intervention being appraised (Sackett, 1996; Sackett & Cook, 1994).

Once the quality of a study has been established, the usual analyses are done to determine significance, confidence intervals, and effect size. Once an intervention is found to evidence some benefit, the next question concerns the *clinical significance* of the effect (i.e., degree of efficacy) (Sackett & Cook, 1994; Guyatt, Jaeschker, & Cook, 1995). This may be expressed statistically in several different ways including absolute risk reduction, relative risk reduction, number needed to treat, and number needed to produce harm (the other side of number needed to treat to see benefit).

While we would like to think that treatment benefits everyone who receives it and rarely harms anyone, this is not necessarily the case. Relative risk (RR) is the ratio of the estimated probabilities of the risk given one treatment or situation versus the risk given another treatment or situation (Cook & DeMets, 2008, p. 48). Munro provides a simple example of the calculation of relative risk (2005, p. 305).

The data used by Munro were drawn from a study by Hawkins and colleagues (1996) of 3955 women, 220 of whom had low birth weight infants. The incidence of low birth weight infants was compared in those who smoked (746) and those who did not (2309). Of those who smoked, 76 had low birth weight infants. Of those who did not smoke, 144 had low birth weight infants. These raw numbers cannot be compared directly because they are derived from groups of different sizes: far less of the women smoked, so their group is smaller. The question of interest is the *relative risk*: what do these data indicate is the risk of having a low birth weight infant if one smokes versus if one does not smoke? Without smoking, the risk is 144 ÷ 2309 or .06 (i.e., about 1 out of 17, rounded); with smoking the risk is 76 ÷ 746 or .10 (i.e., about 1 out of 10). Clearly, the risk is greater if one smokes, but how much greater? To determine how much greater the risk is (i.e., the relative risk) divide .10 by .06, which equals 1.67 (rounded). Women who smoke have a 1.67 times greater risk of having a low birth weight infant (Munro, 2005). Note that this example does not address the effect of an active treatment in a clinical trial. Instead, it addresses the effect of a "natural experiment" in which the results of existing conditions are examined. This means that, as with the observational studies that first supported HRT, there may be other characteristics of the women who smoke that contribute to the higher relative risk of having a low birth weight infant.

Absolute risk reduction (ARR) is the difference in the rates expressed as percents of harmful outcomes in the experimental versus the control group. It is calculated by subtracting the percent who experienced harm in the group receiving the experimental treatment from the percent in the control or comparison group who experienced harm. If the experimental group experienced a 5% rate of harm such as readmission within a week of discharge from the hospital and the control group experienced a 15% rate of harm, the absolute risk reduction achieved would be 10% (15% minus 5% = 10%). Closely related is *relative risk reduction* (RRR), which is the difference in the rates of harmful outcomes experienced by the experimental group and the control or comparison group expressed as a proportion. It is calculated the same way as the ARR except that the result is then divided by the percent in the control group who experienced harm to produce a proportion (DiCenso, 2008; Sackett & Cook, 1994). To continue the hypothetical example, 10% would be divided by 15% to produce a relative risk ratio of .66. The *relative risk* for the experimental group was reduced by 66%. Relative risk reduction, then, tells us how much the treatment reduced the risk for an adverse outcome in the study or studies results evaluated (Guyatt, Jaeschker, & Cook, 1995, p. A-12).

Number needed to treat (NNT) is another useful statistic in describing the clinical significance of the study outcome. It is calculated by dividing the ARR into 1 to produce an estimate of the number of people who would need to receive this treatment in order to increase the number who receive a benefit (rather than harm) by one. In the hypothetical example regarding hospital readmission, the NNT would be $1 \div .10 = 10$, the number needed to have to prevent one additional hospital readmission. *Number needed to harm* (NNH) answers the question of how many people would need to receive the treatment to produce a harmful outcome for one additional person (DiCenso, 2008; Sackett & Cook, 1994).

Note that a dichotomous outcome measure needs to be created to use these statistics. This might be something like improvement/no improvement based on a predetermined cutoff score, response/no response to the treatment, or patient death versus survival. The hypothetical example used hospital readmission versus no readmission as the dichotomous outcome variable of interest.

Examples from the Cochrane reviews mentioned earlier may help to illustrate the use of these statistics. The use of breast stimulation to induce labor appeared to have both benefit and risk (Kavanagh, Kelly, & Thomas, 2005). When compared with no intervention, women who received the treatment had a relative risk (RR) of 0.65 to still be *not* in labor after 72 hours and a relative risk of 0.16 for postpartum hemorrhage.

Another example is the review of the use of tricyclic antidepressants (TCAs) or selective serotonin reuptake inhibitors (SSRIs) compared to placebo control. Pooled data showed a relative risk (RR) of 1.23 in favor of the TCAs and 1.28 in favor of the SSRIs compared with placebo. The median numbers needed to treat (NNTs) were 9 for the TCAs and 7 for the SSRIs. The numbers needed to harm (NNHs) (i.e., to cause side effects in one additional person) ranged from 4 to 30 for the TCAs and from 20 to 90 for the SSRIs (Arroll et al., 2009). It is evident from these data that more adverse events (operationalized as withdrawal due to side effects) could be expected from the use of TCAs than from the use of SSRIs given an equal number of individuals treated. While these calculations are very helpful in determining the value of a treatment, application to an individual patient or client requires consideration of the individual's condition or problem (e.g., mild, moderate, or severe), risk (low, moderate, or high), and other characteristics that might affect applicability of the results to an individual (Guyatt, Jaeschker, & Cook, 1995).

RESEARCH EVIDENCE AND HEALTHCARE POLICY

There has been some concern expressed that reimbursement for care will eventually be limited only to those treatments supported by evidence-based reviews (Ingersoll, 2000). On the other hand, evidence can be used to support beneficial changes as well. While it is not always the case that the development of healthcare policy is based upon research evidence, such evidence can have an important effect on policy as well as on practice. Flynn and colleagues (2008) provide an example of this impact:

> Members of the American Nephrology Nurses Association (ANNA) were concerned with the current regulation that allowed either an RN or LPN to fulfill the requirement that a nurse be present during dialysis. The association funded a study aimed at quantifying the relationship between staffing with RNs and incidence of adverse events in dialysis centers. They found that lower levels of RN staffing were related to a higher frequency of adverse events such as bleeding, hypotension, vascular access occlusion, and so forth. Leaders of ANNA brought this evidence to the attention of CMS (Centers for Medicare and Medicaid Services). The regulation was changed to require at least one RN to be present during dialysis treatment.

THE CONTRIBUTION OF QUALITATIVE RESEARCH TO EVIDENCE-BASED PRACTICE

You can see from the preceding discussion that in some instances, qualitative studies would be excluded from consideration based upon criteria for inclusion and exclusion. The gluten-free diet and HRT stories provide ample reason for seeking evidence from controlled trials. There has been much debate concerning the role of qualitative research in such reviews, with some qualitative researchers expressing deep concern about the impact on qualitative research should the evidence-based practice approach to appraisal of studies prevail.

Morse, for example, suggests that the Cochrane criteria be changed to accommodate high-quality qualitative studies (2006). There is also considerable concern that if such criteria are used to make funding decisions, it will become more difficult to obtain support for qualitative work. Morse makes these important points related to this concern:

1. Those who do only quantitative research are unlikely to understand how qualitative research is conducted and what constitutes rigor (trustworthiness) in qualitative research.

2. Many humanistically oriented questions are best addressed through qualitative research.

Popay and Williams (1998) describe a number of ways in which the results of qualitative research can contribute to our understanding of what constitutes effective practice. They suggest that qualitative research provides a unique and valuable contribution to explain why an intervention works, to explain unexpected results, and to generate hypotheses. Qualitative research can provide insights into people's behavior, including why they do or do not follow recommended regimens for self-care and preventive health. It can also highlight the effects of different settings and environments within which health care is provided. We know, for example, that the particular types of organizations within which nurses' function can affect their practice. Qualitative studies can highlight the impact of setting and patient approach on the outcomes of patient care.

Qualitative studies provide information that is different from that provided by quantitative studies. Each has its value, and each has its place in healthcare research. It is important that we recognize these different approaches for what they contribute to our knowledge base.

CONCLUSION

The ultimate goal of nursing research is to inform practice thereby benefiting those who receive our care. Slowly but surely we are building the research base that will inform nursing practice and strengthen that important connection between research and practice through increasing nurses' awareness of the value of the knowledge generated in clinical research. The use of such strategies as evidence-based practice reviews and guidelines will further the accomplishment of this goal.

REFERENCES

Arroll, B., Elley, C. R., Fishman, T., Goodyear-Smith, F. A., Kenealy, T., Blashki, G. et al. (2009). Antidepressants versus placebo for depression in primary care. *Cochrane Database of Systematic Review 2009*, 3. No: CD007954. doi: 10.1002/14651858.CD007954.

Brown, S. J. (2008). *Evidence-based nursing: The research-practice connection*. Sudbury, MA: Jones and Bartlett.

Buchbinder, R., Osborne, R. H., Ebeling, P. R., Wark, J. D., Mitchell, P., Wriedt, C. et al. (2009). A randomized trial of vertebroplasty for painful osteoporotic vertebral fractures. *New England Journal of Medicine, 361*, 557–568.

Chaffin, M., & Schmidt, S. (2006). An evidence-based perspective on interventions to stop or prevent child abuse. In J. R. Lutzker (Ed.), *Preventing violence: Research and evidence-based intervention strategies* (pp. 49–68). Washington, D.C: American Psychological Association.

Cochrane Collaboration. (2009). *What is a Cochrane review?* Retrieved April 30, 2010, from http://www2.cochrane.org/reviews/revstruc.htm

Cook, T. D., & DeMets, D. L. (2008). *Introduction to statistical methods for clinical trials.* Boca Raton, FL: Chapman & Hall/CRC.

Cullum, N., & Petherick, E. (2008). Evaluation of studies of treatment or prevention interventions. In N. Cullum, D. Ciliska, R. B. Haynes, & S. Marks (Eds.), *Evidence-based nursing: An introduction* (pp. 104–115). Oxford, UK: Blackwell.

Cullum, N., Ciliska, D., Haynes, R. B., & Marks, S. (2008). *Evidence-based nursing: An introduction.* Oxford, UK: Blackwell.

DiCenso, A. (2008). Number needed to treat: A clinically useful measure of the effects of nursing interventions. In N. Cullum, D. Ciliska, R. B. Haynes, & S. Marks, *Evidence-based nursing: An introduction* (pp. 121–129). Oxford, UK: Blackwell.
✧ Clear explanation of ARR, RRT, NNT, and NNH.

Estabrook, C. A. (2007). Prologue: A program of research in knowledge translation. *Nursing Research, 56*(4S), S4–S6.

Fader, M., Cottenden, A. M., & Getliffe, K. (2008). Absorbent products for moderate-heavy urinary and/or faecal incontinence in women and men. *Cochrane Database of Systematic Reviews 2008, 4.* No: CD0074808. doi: 10.1002/14651858.CD007408.

Flynn, L., Thomas-Hawkins, C., & Bodin, S. M. (2008). Using research to influence federal policy: The nephrology nurses' experience. In G. L. Dickson & L. Flynn (Eds.), *Nursing policy research: Turning evidence-based research into health policy* (pp. 343–353). New York, NY: Springer.

Guyatt, G. H., Jaeschker, R., & Cook, D. J. (1995). Applying the findings of clinical trials to individual patients. *American College of Physicians Journal Club, 122*(2), A12–A13.

Hawkins, J. W., Pearce, C. W., Kearny, M. H., Munro, B. H., Haggerty, L. A., Dwyer, J. et al. (1996). Abuse, women's self-care and pregnancy outcomes. Quoted in B. H. Munro (2005). *Statistical methods for healthcare research* (p. 304). Philadelphia, PA: Lippincott, Williams & Wilkins.

Holloway, E. A. (2004). Breathing exercises for asthma. *Cochrane Database of Systematic Reviews 2004, 1.* No: CD001277. doi: 10.1002/14651858.CD001277.pub2.

Ingersoll, G. L. (2000). Evidence-based nursing: What it is and what it isn't. *Nursing Outlook, 48,* 151–152.
✧ Source of the definition of EBN and brief review of many of the issues related to its prominence.

Kavanagh, J., Kelly, A. J., & Thomas, J. (2005). Breast stimulation for cervical ripening and induction of labour. *Cochrane Database of Systematic Reviews 2005, 3.* Art: CD003392. doi: 10.1002/14651858.CD003392.pub2.

Lazar, A. P., & Lazar, P. (1991). Dry skin, water, and lubrication. *Dermatologic Clinics, 9*(1), 45–51.

Lutzker, J. R. (2006). *Preventing violence: Research and evidence-based intervention strategies.* Washington, D.C: American Psychological Association.

Melnyk, B. M., & Fineout-Overholt, E. (2004). *Evidence-based practice in nursing and healthcare.* Philadelphia, PA: Lippincott, Williams & Wilkins.

Moncrieff, J., Churchill, R., Drummond, G., & McGuire, H. (2001). Development of a quality assessment instrument for trials of treatment for depression and neurosis. International *Journal of Methods in Psychiatric Research, 10,* 126–133.
✧ Includes a system for rating the quality of clinical trials.

Morse, J. M. (2006). It is time to revise the Cochrane Criteria. *Qualitative Health Research, 16*(3), 315–317.

Munro, B. H. (2005). *Statistical methods for healthcare research.* Philadelphia, PA: Lippincott, Williams & Wilkins.

Paul, I. M., Beiler, J., McMonagle, A., Shaffer, M. L., Duda, L., & Berlin, C. M. (2007). Effect of honey, dextromethorphan, and no treatment on nocturnal cough and sleep quality for coughing children and their parents. *Archives of Pediatric and Adolescent Medicine, 161*(12), 1140–1146.

Popay, J., & Williams, G. (1998). Qualitative research and evidence-based healthcare. *Journal of the Royal Society of Medicine, Suppl 35*(91), 32–37.

Popovich, K. J., Hota, B., Hayes, R., Weinstein, R. A., & Hayden, M. K. (2009). Effective routine patient cleansing with chlorhexidine gluconate for infection prevention in medical intensive care unit. *Infection Control and Hospital Epidemiology, 30*(10), 959–963.

Sackett, D. L. (1996). On some clinically useful measures of the effects of treatment. *Evidence-Based Medicine, 1,* 37–38.

Sackett, D. L., & Cook, R. J. (1994). Understanding clinical trials. *British Medical Journal, 309,* 7055–7056.

♦ Explains relative risk reduction and number needed to treat using treatment of hypertension as an example. You might have to read it more than once to thoroughly understand it, but this brief editorial also demonstrates how different an impression a clinician might get from research studies depending on the way the results are reported.

Towheed, T., Maxwell, L., Judd, M., Catton, J. M., Hochberg, M. C., & Wells, G. A. (2006). Acetaminophen for osteoarthritis. *Cochrane Database of Systematic Reviews 2006, 1.* No: CD004257. doi: 10.1002/14651858.CD004257.pub2.

CHAPTER 26

Developing a Program of Research

A program of research is a sequential "series of related studies aimed at addressing a particular knowledge gap" of importance to one's discipline (Pranulis, 1991, p. 274). The studies that make up a program of research have a consistent theme, such as comfort measures, grieving, infection control, postpartum depression (Beck, 1997), or childhood seizures (Austin, 2001). The studies should be progressive, building one upon the other, and increasing our understanding of a particular phenomenon. Many consider the development of a program of research to be the ideal way to build a research career as well as contributing to the "cumulative nature of science" (Conn, 2004, p. 594).

The opposite approach to deliberately building a program of research would be to conduct a number of discrete, unrelated studies on various topics. This is a more opportunistic, less planned approach to building a research portfolio.

For example, when HIV was first discovered and then recognized as a serious threat to the population's health, we had virtually no scientists who were knowledgeable about HIV or experienced in HIV-related research. Researchers in related fields had an opportunity to change the direction of their research without the painstaking building of preliminary studies on the same topic usually needed before funding could be obtained. A less successful opportunistic approach would be very scattered, doing a few small studies on such topics as emerging leaders in nursing, a study of pressure ulcer treatment, and another small study on art therapy. Despite an interest in all three areas, a new researcher would have difficulty demonstrating increasing skill and knowledge in any one area of research. In fact, going in several directions at once usually leads you right back to your starting point. In contrast, having a clear path to a long-term goal in mind, called a *research trajectory*, helps to guide your choices and maintain your focus as you build your research career.

THE VALUE OF BUILDING A PROGRAM OF RESEARCH

There are several reasons why a beginning researcher is encouraged to build a program of research:

- It enables you to develop expertise in your chosen area of research, developing much greater depth and breadth of knowledge and experience than would be possible if you worked on a great number of different topics.
- It increases the likelihood that you will be able to make a substantial contribution to our knowledge base and to nursing practice.

- It is also likely that your studies will be of a higher quality because you will have greater expertise if you are able to concentrate on one subject area that you will know very well.

- The depth and breadth of knowledge and experience also helps you see new connections, which are an important part of the process of discovery, and to combine data from several different studies for a secondary analysis.

LAUNCHING A PROGRAM OF RESEARCH

How do you begin developing a program of research? Because you cannot be sure where research will lead you, it's not possible to know *exactly* where your efforts will take you. In fact, Beck (1997) wrote that when you begin, you "cannot predict what future directions [your] program of inquiry will take" (p. 205). Nevertheless, there's much you can do to set some direction for your research:

- Choose an area of great interest to you. It is important to be passionate about your subject because you will be devoting a lot of time and energy to it if you hope to be successful.

- The subject you select should also be one that is important to the profession and has wide application to nursing practice. Examples would be prevention of nosocomial infection, reducing health disparities, or managing childhood asthma more effectively.

- Consider focusing your study on a persistent problem such as high levels of drug use, unprotected sex in adolescents, or low levels of adherence to dietary restrictions in overweight children.

- Be willing to drop a line of research that turns out to be a dead end. A new asthma treatment program that fails to reduce asthma symptoms would be an example.

- Begin with a small study. These first small studies are usually not funded and are likely to be your master's project and doctoral dissertation or part of your job in a clinical setting such as a quality improvement project.

- The goal of your first study should be to gain new insight into the subject of interest. It is likely but not necessarily going to be descriptive in nature. If little is known about the subject, you may consider beginning with a qualitative study. This decision should be based upon the subject of interest and the state of the science on that topic.

- A second small or medium-size study building upon the first study is the next step. This study may attract some internal funding (money from a small grant program for students or employees), a local organization that is devoted to promoting improvement of nursing care or interested in your chosen topic, or a nursing organization such as the American Psychiatric Nurses Association.

- This second study is often a pilot study in which you test your ideas and procedures before launching a large study.

- At this stage, you are likely to begin forming a research team. Forming a team allows you to combine the talents and expertise of several investigators. It might be a nursing team, combining the skills of a school nurse, pediatric nurse practitioner, and psych-mental health nurse, for example, or an interdisciplinary team with a pediatrician, child psychologist, dietitian, and epidemiologist or statistician. The combination depends on the type of study you propose, of course.

- It is time now for you to become involved in larger, more complex research studies, either as the lead investigator or as a co-investigator. These larger studies are usually supported by grants from a state or national agency such as the National Institutes of Health (NIH), a national organization such as the Parkinson's Foundation or American Cancer Society, a foundation interested in more general health concerns, or a gift from an interested donor. Your previous studies and publications on the subject will play a very important part in persuading a funder to support your research.

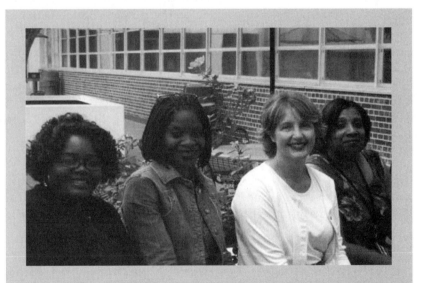

Dr. Shawn Kneipp with community and academic members of her CBPR research team working on a study to reduce health disparities in women receiving temporary assistance for needy families. Shown from left to right are: Deirdra Means (Research Assistant), Cynthia Allen (Study Coordinator), Shawn Kneipp, and Toni Watson (Research Assistant).

Source: Courtesy of Shawn Kneipp, PhD, ARNP.

- All along, it is important that you present the results of your work to local, regional, and national professional groups and publish the results in professional journals. You also need to attend the local and national conferences that focus on the health concerns of your population of interest. In addition, you may join research interest groups, become a reviewer for professional journals, join boards of related organizations, and become an advocate for your population of interest.

- As your program of research grows, you will probably add "branches," research that is related but not part of the main "trunk," building breadth now as well as depth. You may even begin to work with international collaborators (colleagues from other countries).

- You are now an established scholar and researcher, known nationally and internationally for your work and often called upon to share your expertise. While you continue your own work, you will also mentor new researchers, serve as a grant reviewer, and perhaps become a consultant. You will continue to develop your own expertise and build your program of research, adding new and creative lines of inquiry.

- Sound exciting? This is certainly a worthy career path within our profession, one that is rewarding both to you and to the people who are better served because of the knowledge gained through your research.

It is also a demanding career path. Passion for your area of research, commitment to excellence in your work, willingness to give it extra time and concentrated effort, and ability to delay gratification are all needed. Even the best researcher experiences delays, dead ends, and rejections along the way. You may want to read Austin's (2001) personal account of the ups and downs of developing a program of research as well as the following fictional example to help you decide if you want to pursue this path.

A FICTIONAL EXAMPLE

Let's consider now the story of Jolene Hayes, a fictional nurse whose personal struggles with overweight as a child inspired her research program and her decision to pursue a career in nursing research.

Jolene Hayes had been overweight as a child. Around the age of 8 or 9, her mother began buying "husky" sizes for her. By the age of 12, her mother was ordering her clothes online because most stores did not carry her size in the teen department.

Jolene loved computer games, preferring to stay indoors at the computer after school rather than joining neighborhood friends bicycling and skate boarding. As time went on, she found herself unable to keep up physically with others her age. They were faster and had more endurance on bike rides so she eventually stopped going along. Physical education was torture for her. She was mortified when the school nurse teacher and physical education teacher launched a Keep Fit program in her high school. The first day of the Keep Fit program was a weigh-in for all students. Jolene faked a stomach upset that day and stayed home almost every Thursday ("Keep Fit" Day) for the rest of that semester.

Jolene continued to struggle with her weight in college. There she learned much more about nutrition and weight loss programs. She began to get her weight under control and slowly but surely increased her physical activities, at first just walking more and eventually joining a gym.

Jolene began to select childhood nutrition and fitness as the topics for assigned clinical papers whenever possible. She became a pediatric nurse and entered a master's program to become a pediatric nurse practitioner. Her master's project was an after-school weight loss program for adolescent girls. When she returned to school to earn a doctoral degree, she focused her work on the effects of childhood obesity. Her goal was to help children avoid the emotional and physical stresses of being overweight. For her qualitative research course, Jolene conducted a small phenomenological study on the lived experience of overweight in school-age children. The children's stories broke her heart but also helped her realize that, while there were common themes, each had his or her own individual response to being overweight. Males and females had different concerns as well. Her doctoral dissertation continued this work and led to a new insight: that those who were morbidly obese had very different concerns and needs than those who had a less severe weight problem. She wrote several articles on the subject, including one published in *Nursing Research*. (Remember, this is a fictional example although based on real life experience.)

Based on her dissertation work, Jolene applied for a postdoctoral fellowship from the National Institute of Nursing Research. She took a cut in her pay as a pediatric nurse practitioner to devote her time to developing her research program. She took advanced courses in research methods, statistics, nutrition, and fitness. She completed several small studies and published five articles on morbid obesity in children. One of the studies was a pilot test of a creative new program to reduce weight and increase fitness in children with diabetes, funded by a $25,000 grant from the American Diabetes Association.

Upon completing her postdoc, Dr. Hayes accepted a dual appointment in a university medical center, dividing her time between teaching advanced pediatric nursing, pursuing her research, and seeing overweight children in the pediatric outpatient clinic. She encountered several colleagues who were interested in her research. Together, they collected more data in the pediatric outpatient clinic (as usual, following IRB guidelines) on morbidly obese children from several different ethnic groups. They found some culture-based differences in beliefs about diet and weight in children.

Dr. Hayes was fortunate to be employed in a dynamic academic health center that encouraged interdisciplinary research. In addition to working on her own research, she had several opportunities to work on large collaborative pediatric studies. This experience exposed her to more advanced research methodologies and many nationally known experts in the field. With her colleagues, she submitted a successful proposal for an investigator-initiated study to NINR for a large, multiethnic study of their Kid Fit program for morbidly obese school children.

She continued to focus on morbid obesity (still hating the term, by the way) in various age and ethnic groups and developed a program that attracted national attention. This led to a multimillion dollar grant from a large foundation to establish the program in schools across the country.

Dr. Jolene Hayes became a nationally known expert on morbid obesity in the pediatric population. She established a national center to study and treat overweight in children of all ages. Jolene had achieved her lifelong dream to help others avoid some of the pain she had experienced.

Looking back, Dr. Hayes thought about the 50 to 70 hours a week she worked on her research. She gave up a well-paying nurse practitioner position to engage in postdoctoral work. Along the way, she received 20 article rejections and 5 proposal rejections. Most of the articles and proposals were revised and resubmitted successfully; others were abandoned due to discouragement or to wisely deciding they were not of the quality expected by the reviewers. Jolene traveled extensively to present her work, meet with colleagues, and seek funding for her programs. She attended many evening meetings with parent groups and others interested in childhood overweight to share her expertise, raise funds for the center, and recruit study participants.

For Jolene, now Dr. Hayes, what was once a painful experience had become a rewarding career in nursing research.

REFERENCES

Austin, J. (2001). Developing a research program. *Journal of the American Psychiatric Nurses Association, 7*, 173–176.
⋄ A very readable personal account of a nurse researcher's ups and downs as she tries and eventually succeeds in launching her program of research.

Beck, C. T. (1997). Developing a research program using qualitative and quantitative approaches. *Nursing Outlook, 45*, 265–269.
⋄ See especially Box 1 in which Beck outlines 10 years of research on postpartum depression, and her description of this research on pp. 267–268 of the article.

Conn, V. S. (2004). Editorial: Building a research trajectory. *Western Journal of Nursing Research, 26*, 592–594.

National Institute for Nursing Research. *Executive summary*. Retrieved January, 14, 2009, from http://www.ninr.nih.gov/NR/rdonlyres/5AC1595B-08BF-4A6C-A08B-3B2B2FF82829/4750/ExecutiveSummary.pdf

Pranulis, M. F. (1991). Research programs in a clinical setting. *Western Journal of Nursing Research, 13*(2), 274–277.

The Belmont Report

The Belmont Report
Office of the Secretary
Ethical Principles and Guidelines for the Protection of Human Subjects of Research
The National Commission for the Protection of Human Subjects of
Biomedical and Behavioral Research
April 18, 1979

AGENCY: Department of Health, Education, and Welfare.

ACTION: Notice of Report for Public Comment.

SUMMARY: On July 12, 1974, the National Research Act (Pub. L. 93-348) was signed into law, there-by creating the National Commission for the Protection of Human Subjects of Biomedical and Behavioral Research. One of the charges to the Commission was to identify the basic ethical principles that should underlie the conduct of biomedical and behavioral research involving human subjects and to develop guidelines which should be followed to assure that such research is conducted in accordance with those principles. In carrying out the above, the Commission was directed to consider: (i) the boundaries between biomedical and behavioral research and the accepted and routine practice of medicine, (ii) the role of assessment of risk-benefit criteria in the determination of the appropriateness of research involving human subjects, (iii) appropriate guidelines for the selection of human subjects for participation in such research and (iv) the nature and definition of informed consent in various research settings.

The Belmont Report attempts to summarize the basic ethical principles identified by the Commission in the course of its deliberations. It is the outgrowth of an intensive four-day period of discussions that were held in February 1976 at the Smithsonian Institution's Belmont Conference Center supplemented by the monthly deliberations of the Commission that were held over a period of nearly four years. It is a statement of basic ethical principles and guidelines that should assist in resolving the ethical problems that surround the conduct of research with human subjects. By publishing the Report in the Federal Register, and providing reprints upon request, the Secretary intends that it may be made readily available to scientists, members of Institutional Review Boards, and Federal employees. The two-volume Appendix, containing the lengthy reports of experts and specialists who assisted the Commission in fulfilling this part of its charge, is available as

DHEW Publication No. (OS) 78-0013 and No. (OS) 78-0014, for sale by the Superintendent of Documents, U.S. Government Printing Office, Washington, D.C. 20402.

Unlike most other reports of the Commission, the Belmont Report does not make specific recommendations for administrative action by the Secretary of Health, Education, and Welfare.

Rather, the Commission recommended that the Belmont Report be adopted in its entirety, as a statement of the Department's policy. The Department requests public comment on this recommendation.

National Commission for the Protection of Human Subjects of Biomedical and Behavioral Research
Members of the Commission

Kenneth John Ryan, M.D., Chairman, Chief of Staff, Boston Hospital for Women.
Joseph V. Brady, Ph.D., Professor of Behavioral Biology, Johns Hopkins University.
Robert E. Cooke, M.D., President, Medical College of Pennsylvania.
Dorothy I. Height, President, National Council of Negro Women, Inc.
Albert R. Jonsen, Ph.D., Associate Professor of Bioethics, University of California at San Francisco.
Patricia King, J.D., Associate Professor of Law, Georgetown University Law Center.
Karen Lebacqz, Ph.D., Associate Professor of Christian Ethics, Pacific School of Religion.
***David W. Louisell, J.D., Professor of Law, University of California at Berkeley.
Donald W. Seldin, M.D., Professor and Chairman, Department of Internal Medicine, University of Texas at Dallas.
***Eliot Stellar, Ph.D., Provost of the University and Professor of Physiological Psychology, University of Pennsylvania.
***Robert H. Turtle, LL.B., Attorney, VomBaur, Coburn, Simmons & Turtle, Washington, D.C.
***Deceased.

Table of Contents

Ethical Principles and Guidelines for Research Involving Human Subjects

     1. Respect for Persons
     2. Beneficence
     3. Justice
  C. Applications
     1. Informed Consent
     2. Assessment of Risk and Benefits
     3. Selection of Subjects

ETHICAL PRINCIPLES & GUIDELINES FOR RESEARCH INVOLVING HUMAN SUBJECTS

Scientific research has produced substantial social benefits. It has also posed some troubling ethical questions. Public attention was drawn to these questions by reported abuses of human subjects in biomedical experiments, especially during the Second World War. During the Nuremberg War Crime Trials, the Nuremberg code was drafted as a set of standards for judging physicians and scientists who had conducted biomedical experiments on concentration camp prisoners. This code became the prototype of many later codes intended to assure that research involving human subjects would be carried out in an ethical manner.

The codes consist of rules, some general, others specific, that guide the investigators or the reviewers of research in their work. Such rules often are inadequate to cover complex situations; at times they come into conflict, and they are frequently difficult to interpret or apply. Broader ethical principles will provide a basis on which specific rules may be formulated, criticized and interpreted.

Three principles, or general prescriptive judgments, that are relevant to research involving human subjects are identified in this statement. Other principles may also be relevant. These three are comprehensive, however, and are stated at a level of generalization that should assist scientists, subjects, reviewers and interested citizens to understand the ethical issues inherent in research involving human subjects. These principles cannot always be applied so as to resolve beyond dispute particular ethical problems. The objective is to provide an analytical framework that will guide the resolution of ethical problems arising from research involving human subjects.

This statement consists of a distinction between research and practice, a discussion of the three basic ethical principles, and remarks about the application of these principles.

PART A: BOUNDARIES BETWEEN PRACTICE & RESEARCH

A. Boundaries Between Practice and Research

It is important to distinguish between biomedical and behavioral research, on the one hand, and the practice of accepted therapy on the other, in order to know what activities ought to undergo review for the protection of human subjects of research. The distinction between research and practice is blurred partly because both often occur together (as in research designed to evaluate a therapy) and partly because notable departures from standard practice are often called "experimental" when the terms "experimental" and "research" are not carefully defined.

For the most part, the term "practice" refers to interventions that are designed solely to enhance the well-being of an individual patient or client and that have a reasonable expectation of success. The purpose of medical or behavioral practice is to provide diagnosis, preventive treatment or therapy to particular individuals. By contrast, the term "research' designates an activity designed to test an hypothesis, permit conclusions to be drawn, and thereby to develop or contribute to generalizable knowledge (expressed, for example, in theories, principles, and statements of relationships). Research is usually described in a formal protocol that sets forth an objective and a set of procedures designed to reach that objective.

When a clinician departs in a significant way from standard or accepted practice, the innovation does not, in and of itself, constitute research. The fact that a procedure is "experimental," in the sense of new, untested or different, does not automatically place it in the category of research. Radically new procedures of this description should, however, be made the object of formal research at an early stage in order to determine whether they are safe and effective. Thus, it is the responsibility of medical practice committees, for example, to insist that a major innovation be incorporated into a formal research project.

Research and practice may be carried on together when research is designed to evaluate the safety and efficacy of a therapy. This need not cause any confusion regarding whether or not the activity requires review; the general rule is that if there is any element of research in an activity, that activity should undergo review for the protection of human subjects.

PART B: BASIC ETHICAL PRINCIPLES

B. Basic Ethical Principles

The expression "basic ethical principles" refers to those general judgments that serve as a basic justification for the many particular ethical prescriptions and evaluations of human actions. Three basic principles, among those generally accepted in our cultural tradition, are particularly relevant to the ethics of research involving human subjects: the principles of respect of persons, beneficence and justice.

1. Respect for Persons. Respect for persons incorporates at least two ethical convictions: first, that individuals should be treated as autonomous agents, and second, that persons with diminished autonomy are entitled to protection. The principle of respect for persons thus divides into two separate moral requirements: the requirement to acknowledge autonomy and the requirement to protect those with diminished autonomy.

An autonomous person is an individual capable of deliberation about personal goals and of acting under the direction of such deliberation. To respect autonomy is to give weight to autonomous persons' considered opinions and choices while refraining from obstructing their actions unless they are clearly detrimental to others. To show lack of respect for an autonomous agent is to repudiate that person's considered judgments, to deny an individual the freedom to act on those considered judgments, or to withhold information necessary to make a considered judgment, when there are no compelling reasons to do so.

However, not every human being is capable of self-determination. The capacity for self-determination matures during an individual's life, and some individuals lose this capacity wholly or in part because of illness, mental disability, or circumstances that severely restrict liberty. Respect for the immature and the incapacitated may require protecting them as they mature or while they are incapacitated.

Some persons are in need of extensive protection, even to the point of excluding them from activities which may harm them; other persons require little protection beyond making sure they undertake activities freely and with awareness of possible adverse consequence. The extent of protection afforded should depend upon the risk of harm and the likelihood of benefit. The judgment that any individual lacks autonomy should be periodically reevaluated and will vary in different situations.

In most cases of research involving human subjects, respect for persons demands that subjects enter into the research voluntarily and with adequate information. In some situations, however, application of the principle is not obvious. The involvement of prisoners as subjects of research provides an instructive example. On the one hand, it would seem that the principle of respect for persons requires that prisoners not be deprived of the opportunity to volunteer for research. On the other hand, under prison conditions they may be subtly coerced or unduly influenced to engage in research activities for which they would not otherwise volunteer. Respect for persons would then dictate that prisoners be protected. Whether to allow prisoners to "volunteer" or to "protect" them presents a dilemma. Respecting persons, in most hard cases, is often a matter of balancing competing claims urged by the principle of respect itself.

2. Beneficence. Persons are treated in an ethical manner not only by respecting their decisions and protecting them from harm, but also by making efforts to secure their well-being. Such treatment falls under the principle of beneficence. The term "beneficence" is often understood to cover acts of kindness or charity that go beyond strict obligation. In this document, beneficence is understood in a stronger sense, as an obligation. Two general rules have been formulated as complementary expressions of beneficent actions in this sense: (1) do not harm and (2) maximize possible benefits and minimize possible harms.

The Hippocratic maxim "do no harm" has long been a fundamental principle of medical ethics. Claude Bernard extended it to the realm of research, saying that one should not injure one person regardless of the benefits that might come to others. However, even avoiding harm requires learning what is harmful; and, in the process of obtaining this information, persons may be exposed to risk of harm. Further, the Hippocratic Oath requires physicians to benefit their patients "according to their best judgment." Learning what will in fact benefit may require exposing persons to risk. The problem posed by these imperatives is to decide when it is justifiable to seek certain benefits despite the risks involved, and when the benefits should be foregone because of the risks.

The obligations of beneficence affect both individual investigators and society at large, because they extend both to particular research projects and to the entire enterprise of research. In the case of particular projects, investigators and members of their institutions are obliged to give forethought to the maximization of benefits and the reduction of risk that might occur from the research investigation. In the case of scientific research in general, members of the larger society are obliged to recognize the longer term benefits and risks that may result from the improvement of knowledge and from the development of novel medical, psychotherapeutic, and social procedures.

The principle of beneficence often occupies a well-defined justifying role in many areas of research involving human subjects. An example is found in research involving children. Effective ways of treating childhood diseases and fostering healthy development are benefits that serve to justify research involving children—even when individual research subjects are not direct beneficiaries. Research also makes it possible to avoid the harm that may result from the application of previously accepted routine practices that on closer investigation turn out to be dangerous. But the role of the principle of beneficence is not always so unambiguous. A difficult ethical problem remains, for example, about research that presents more than minimal risk without immediate prospect of direct benefit to the children involved. Some have argued that such research is inadmissible, while others have pointed out that this limit would rule out much research promising great benefit to children in the future. Here again, as with all hard cases, the different claims covered by the principle of beneficence may come into conflict and force difficult choices.

3. Justice. Who ought to receive the benefits of research and bear its burdens? This is a question of justice, in the sense of "fairness in distribution" or "what is deserved." An injustice occurs when some benefit to which a person is entitled is denied without good reason or when some burden is imposed unduly. Another way of conceiving the principle of justice is that equals ought to be treated equally. However, this statement requires explication. Who is equal and who is unequal? What considerations justify departure from equal distribution? Almost all commentators allow that distinctions based on experience, age, deprivation, competence, merit and position do sometimes constitute criteria justifying differential treatment for certain purposes. It is necessary, then, to explain in what respects people should be treated equally. There are several widely accepted formulations of just ways to distribute burdens and benefits. Each formulation mentions some relevant property on the basis of which burdens and benefits should be distributed. These formulations are (1) to each person an equal share, (2) to each person according to individual need, (3) to each person according to individual effort, (4) to each person according to societal contribution, and (5) to each person according to merit.

Questions of justice have long been associated with social practices such as punishment, taxation and political representation. Until recently these questions have not generally been associated with scientific research. However, they are foreshadowed even in the earliest reflections on the ethics of research involving human subjects. For example, during the 19th and early 20th centuries the burdens of serving as research subjects fell largely upon poor ward patients, while the benefits of improved medical care flowed primarily to private patients. Subsequently, the exploitation of unwilling prisoners as research subjects in Nazi concentration camps was condemned as a particularly flagrant injustice. In this country, in the 1940's, the Tuskegee syphilis study used disadvantaged, rural black men to study the untreated course of a disease that is by no means confined to that population. These subjects were deprived of demonstrably effective treatment in order not to interrupt the project, long after such treatment became generally available.

Against this historical background, it can be seen how conceptions of justice are relevant to research involving human subjects. For example, the selection of research subjects needs to be scrutinized in order to determine whether some classes (e.g., welfare patients, particular racial and ethnic minorities, or persons confined to institutions) are being systematically selected simply because of their easy availability, their compromised position, or their manipulability, rather than for reasons directly related to the problem being studied. Finally, whenever research supported by public funds leads to the development of therapeutic devices and procedures, justice demands both that these not provide advantages only to those who can afford them and that such research should not unduly involve persons from groups unlikely to be among the beneficiaries of subsequent applications of the research.

PART C: APPLICATIONS

C. Applications

Applications of the general principles to the conduct of research leads to consideration of the following requirements: informed consent, risk/benefit assessment, and the selection of subjects of research.

1. Informed Consent. Respect for persons requires that subjects, to the degree that they are capable, be given the opportunity to choose what shall or shall not happen to them. This opportunity is provided when adequate standards for informed consent are satisfied.

While the importance of informed consent is unquestioned, controversy prevails over the nature and possibility of an informed consent. Nonetheless, there is widespread agreement that the consent process can be analyzed as containing three elements: information, comprehension and voluntariness.

Information. Most codes of research establish specific items for disclosure intended to assure that subjects are given sufficient information. These items generally include: the research procedure, their purposes, risks and anticipated benefits, alternative procedures (where therapy is involved), and a statement offering the subject the opportunity to ask questions and to withdraw at any time from the research. Additional items have been proposed, including how subjects are selected, the person responsible for the research, etc.

However, a simple listing of items does not answer the question of what the standard should be for judging how much and what sort of information should be provided. One standard frequently invoked in medical practice, namely the information commonly provided by practitioners in the field or in the locale, is inadequate since research takes place precisely when a common understanding does not exist. Another standard, currently popular in malpractice law, requires the practitioner to reveal the information that reasonable persons would wish to know in order to make a decision regarding their care. This, too, seems insufficient since the research subject, being in essence a volunteer, may wish to know considerably more about risks gratuitously undertaken than do patients who deliver themselves into the hand of a clinician for needed care.

It may be that a standard of "the reasonable volunteer" should be proposed: the extent and nature of information should be such that persons, knowing that the procedure is neither necessary for their care nor perhaps fully understood, can decide whether they wish to participate in the furthering of knowledge. Even when some direct benefit to them is anticipated, the subjects should understand clearly the range of risk and the voluntary nature of participation.

A special problem of consent arises where informing subjects of some pertinent aspect of the research is likely to impair the validity of the research. In many cases, it is sufficient to indicate to subjects that they are being invited to participate in research of which some features will not be revealed until the research is concluded. In all cases of research involving incomplete disclosure, such research is justified only if it is clear that (1) incomplete disclosure is truly necessary to accomplish the goals of the research, (2) there are no undisclosed risks to subjects that are more than minimal, and (3) there is an adequate plan for debriefing subjects, when appropriate, and for dissemination of research results to them. Information about risks should never be withheld for the purpose of eliciting the cooperation of subjects, and truthful answers should always be given to direct questions about the research. Care should be taken to distinguish cases in which disclosure would destroy or invalidate the research from cases in which disclosure would simply inconvenience the investigator.

Comprehension. The manner and context in which information is conveyed is as important as the information itself. For example, presenting information in a disorganized and rapid fashion, allowing too little time for consideration or curtailing opportunities for questioning, all may adversely affect a subject's ability to make an informed choice.

Because the subject's ability to understand is a function of intelligence, rationality, maturity and language, it is necessary to adapt the presentation of the information to the subject's capacities. Investigators are responsible for ascertaining that the subject has comprehended the information. While there is always an obligation to ascertain that the information about risk to subjects is complete and adequately comprehended, when the risks are more serious, that obligation increases. On occasion, it may be suitable to give some oral or written tests of comprehension.

Special provision may need to be made when comprehension is severely limited—for example, by conditions of immaturity or mental disability. Each class of subjects that one might consider as incompetent (e.g., infants and young children, mentally disable patients, the terminally ill and the comatose) should be considered on its own terms. Even for these persons, however, respect requires giving them the opportunity to choose to the extent they are able, whether or not to participate in research. The objections of these subjects to involvement should be honored, unless the research entails providing them a therapy unavailable elsewhere. Respect for persons also requires seeking the permission of other parties in order to protect the subjects from harm. Such persons are thus respected both by acknowledging their own wishes and by the use of third parties to protect them from harm.

The third parties chosen should be those who are most likely to understand the incompetent subject's situation and to act in that person's best interest. The person authorized to act on behalf of the subject should be given an opportunity to observe the research as it proceeds in order to be able to withdraw the subject from the research, if such action appears in the subject's best interest.

Voluntariness. An agreement to participate in research constitutes a valid consent only if voluntarily given. This element of informed consent requires conditions free of coercion and undue influence. Coercion occurs when an overt threat of harm is intentionally presented by one person to another in order to obtain compliance. Undue influence, by contrast, occurs through an offer of an excessive, unwarranted, inappropriate or improper reward or other overture in order to obtain compliance. Also, inducements that would ordinarily be acceptable may become undue influences if the subject is especially vulnerable.

Unjustifiable pressures usually occur when persons in positions of authority or commanding influence—especially where possible sanctions are involved—urge a course of action for a subject. A continuum of such influencing factors exists, however, and it is impossible to state precisely where justifiable persuasion ends and undue influence begins. But undue influence would include actions such as manipulating a person's choice through the controlling influence of a close relative and threatening to withdraw health services to which an individual would otherwise be entitle.

2. Assessment of Risks and Benefits. The assessment of risks and benefits requires a careful arrayal of relevant data, including, in some cases, alternative ways of obtaining the benefits sought in the research. Thus, the assessment presents both an opportunity and a responsibility to gather systematic and comprehensive information about proposed research. For the investigator, it is a means to examine whether the proposed research is properly designed. For a review committee, it is a method for determining whether the risks that will be presented to subjects are justified. For prospective subjects, the assessment will assist the determination whether or not to participate.

The Nature and Scope of Risks and Benefits. The requirement that research be justified on the basis of a favorable risk/benefit assessment bears a close relation to the principle of beneficence, just as the moral requirement that informed consent be obtained is derived primarily from the principle of respect for persons. The term "risk" refers to a possibility that harm may occur. However, when expressions such as "small risk" or "high risk" are used, they usually refer (often ambiguously) both to the chance (probability) of experiencing a harm and the severity (magnitude) of the envisioned harm.

The term "benefit" is used in the research context to refer to something of positive value related to health or welfare. Unlike, "risk," "benefit" is not a term that expresses probabilities. Risk is properly contrasted to probability of benefits, and benefits are properly contrasted with harms rather than risks of harm. Accordingly, so-called risk/benefit assessments are concerned with the probabilities and magnitudes of possible harm and anticipated benefits. Many kinds of possible harms and benefits need to be taken into account. There are, for example, risks of psychological harm, physical harm, legal harm, social harm and economic harm and the corresponding benefits. While the most likely types of harms to research subjects are those of psychological or physical pain or injury, other possible kinds should not be overlooked.

Risks and benefits of research may affect the individual subjects, the families of the individual subjects, and society at large (or special groups of subjects in society). Previous codes and Federal regulations have required that risks to subjects be outweighed by the sum of both the anticipated benefit to the subject, if any, and the anticipated benefit to society in the form of knowledge to be gained from the research. In balancing these different elements, the risks and benefits affecting the immediate research subject will normally carry special weight. On the other hand, interests other than those of the subject may on some occasions be sufficient by themselves to justify the risks involved in the research, so long as the subjects' rights have been protected. Beneficence thus requires that we protect against risk of harm to subjects and also that we be concerned about the loss of the substantial benefits that might be gained from research.

The Systematic Assessment of Risks and Benefits. It is commonly said that benefits and risks must be "balanced" and shown to be "in a favorable ratio." The metaphorical character of these terms draws attention to the difficulty of making precise judgments. Only on rare occasions will quantitative techniques be available for the scrutiny of research protocols. However, the idea of systematic, nonarbitrary analysis of risks and benefits should be emulated insofar as possible. This ideal requires those making decisions about the justifiability of research to be thorough in the accumulation and assessment of information about all aspects of the research, and to consider alternatives systematically. This procedure renders the assessment of research more rigorous and precise, while making communication between review board members and investigators less subject to misinterpretation, misinformation and conflicting judgments. Thus, there should first be a determination of the validity of the presuppositions of the research; then the nature, probability and magnitude of risk should be distinguished with as much clarity as possible. The method of ascertaining risks should be explicit, especially where there is no alternative to the use of such vague categories as small or slight risk. It should also be determined whether an investigator's estimates of the probability of harm or benefits are reasonable, as judged by known facts or other available studies.

Finally, assessment of the justifiability of research should reflect at least the following considerations: (i) Brutal or inhumane treatment of human subjects is never morally justified. (ii) Risks should be reduced to those necessary to achieve the research objective. It should be determined whether it is in fact necessary to use human subjects at all. Risk can perhaps never be entirely eliminated, but it can often be reduced by careful attention to alternative procedures. (iii) When research involves significant risk of serious impairment, review committees should be extraordinarily insistent on the justification of the risk (looking usually to the likelihood of benefit to the subject—or, in some rare cases, to the manifest voluntariness of the participation). (iv) When vulnerable populations are involved in research, the appropriateness of involving them should itself be demonstrated. A number of variables go into such judgments, including the nature and degree of risk, the condition of the particular population involved, and the nature and level of the anticipated benefits. (v) Relevant risks and benefits must be thoroughly arrayed in documents and procedures used in the informed consent process.

3. Selection of Subjects. Just as the principle of respect for persons finds expression in the requirements for consent, and the principle of beneficence in risk/benefit assessment, the principle of justice gives rise to moral requirements that there be fair procedures and outcomes in the selection of research subjects.

Justice is relevant to the selection of subjects of research at two levels: the social and the individual. Individual justice in the selection of subjects would require that researchers exhibit fairness: thus, they should not offer potentially beneficial research only to some patients who are in their favor or select only "undesirable" persons for risky research. Social justice requires that distinction be drawn between classes of subjects that ought, and ought not, to participate in any particular kind of research, based on the ability of members of that class to bear burdens and on the appropriateness of placing further burdens on already burdened persons. Thus, it can be considered a matter of social justice that there is an order of preference in the selection of classes of subjects (e.g., adults before children) and that some classes of potential subjects (e.g., the institutionalized mentally infirm or prisoners) may be involved as research subjects, if at all, only on certain conditions.

Injustice may appear in the selection of subjects, even if individual subjects are selected fairly by investigators and treated fairly in the course of research. Thus injustice arises from social, racial, sexual and cultural biases institutionalized in society. Thus, even if individual researchers are treating their research subjects fairly, and even if IRBs are taking care to assure that subjects are selected fairly within a particular institution, unjust social patterns may nevertheless appear in the overall distribution of the burdens and benefits of research. Although individual institutions or investigators may not be able to resolve a problem that is pervasive in their social setting, they can consider distributive justice in selecting research subjects.

Some populations, especially institutionalized ones, are already burdened in many ways by their infirmities and environments. When research is proposed that involves risks and does not include a therapeutic component, other less burdened classes of persons should be called upon first to accept these risks of research, except where the research is directly related to the specific conditions of the class involved. Also, even though public funds for research may often flow in the same directions as public funds for health care, it seems unfair that populations dependent on public health care constitute a pool of preferred research subjects if more advantaged populations are likely to be the recipients of the benefits.

One special instance of injustice results from the involvement of vulnerable subjects. Certain groups, such as racial minorities, the economically disadvantaged, the very sick, and the institutionalized may continually be sought as research subjects, owing to their ready availability in settings where research is conducted. Given their dependent status and their frequently compromised capacity for free consent, they should be protected against the danger of being involved in research solely for administrative convenience, or because they are easy to manipulate as a result of their illness or socioeconomic condition.

---

(1) Since 1945, various codes for the proper and responsible conduct of human experimentation in medical research have been adopted by different organizations. The best known of these codes are the Nuremberg Code of 1947, the Helsinki Declaration of 1964 (revised in 1975), and the 1971 Guidelines (codified into Federal Regulations in 1974) issued by the U.S. Department of Health, Education, and Welfare Codes for the conduct of social and behavioral research have also been adopted, the best known being that of the American Psychological Association, published in 1973.

(2) Although practice usually involves interventions designed solely to enhance the well-being of a particular individual, interventions are sometimes applied to one individual for the enhancement of the well-being of another (e.g., blood donation, skin grafts, organ transplants) or an intervention may have the dual purpose of enhancing the well-being of a particular individual, and, at the same time, providing some benefit to others (e.g., vaccination, which protects both the person who is vaccinated and society generally). The fact that some forms of practice have elements other than immediate benefit to the individual receiving an intervention, however, should not confuse the general distinction between research and practice. Even when a procedure applied in practice may benefit some other person, it remains an intervention designed to enhance the well-being of a particular individual or groups of individuals; thus, it is practice and need not be reviewed as research.

(3) Because the problems related to social experimentation may differ substantially from those of biomedical and behavioral research, the Commission specifically declines to make any policy determination regarding such research at this time. Rather, the Commission believes that the problem ought to be addressed by one of its successor bodies.

Source: U.S. Department of Health and Human Servicess. (1979). *The Belmont Report.* Retrieved July 15, 2010, from http://www.hhs.gov/ohrp/humansubjects/guidance/belmont.htm

The Nuremberg Code and the Declaration of Helsinki

THE NUREMBERG CODE

1. The voluntary consent of the human subject is absolutely essential.
   - This means that the person involved should have legal capacity to give consent; should be so situated as to be able to exercise free power of choice, without the intervention of any element of force, fraud, deceit, duress, over-reaching, or other ulterior form of constraint or coercion; and should have sufficient knowledge and comprehension of the elements of the subject matter involved as to enable him to make an understanding and enlightened decision. This latter element requires that before the acceptance of an affirmative decision by the experimental subject there should be made known to him the nature, duration, and purpose of the experiment; the method and means by which it is to be conducted; all inconveniences and hazards reasonably to be expected; and the effects upon his health or person which may possibly come from his participation in the experiment.
   - The duty and responsibility for ascertaining the quality of the consent rests upon each individual who initiates, directs or engages in the experiment. It is a personal duty and responsibility, which may not be delegated to another with impunity.

2. The experiment should be such as to yield fruitful results for the good of society, unprocurable by other methods or means of study, and not random and unnecessary in nature.

3. The experiment should be so designed and based on the results of animal experimentation and a knowledge of the natural history of the disease or other problem under study that the anticipated results will justify the performance of the experiment.

4. The experiment should be so conducted as to avoid all unnecessary physical and mental suffering and injury.

5. No experiment should be conducted where there is an a priori reason to believe that death or disabling injury will occur; except, perhaps, in those experiments where the experimental physicians also serve as subjects.

6. The degree of risk to be taken should never exceed that determined by the humanitarian importance of the problem to be solved by the experiment.

7. Proper preparations should be made and adequate facilities provided to protect the experimental subject against even remote possibilities of injury, disability, or death.

8. The experiment should be conducted only by scientifically qualified persons. The highest degree of skill and care should be required through all stages of the experiment of those who conduct or engage in the experiment.

9. During the course of the experiment the human subject should be at liberty to bring the experiment to an end if he has reached the physical or mental state where continuation of the experiment seemed to him to be impossible.

10. During the course of the experiment the scientist in charge must be prepared to terminate the experiment at any stage, if he has probably [sic] cause to believe, in the exercise of the good faith, superior skill and careful judgment required of him that a continuation of the experiment is likely to result in injury, disability, or death to the experimental subject.

Source: Trials of War Criminals Before the Nuremberg Military Tribunals Under Control Council Law No. 10, Vol. 2, pp. 181-182. Washington, DC: US Government Printing Office, 1949.

THE DECLARATION OF HELSINKI

(4) The "Declaration of Helsinki" states as follows:

RECOMMENDATIONS GUIDING PHYSICIANS IN BIOMEDICAL RESEARCH INVOLVING HUMAN SUBJECTS

Introduction

It is the mission of the physician to safeguard the health of the people. His or her knowledge and conscience are dedicated to the fulfillment of this mission.

The Declaration of Geneva of the World Medical Assembly binds the physician with the words, "The health of my patient will be my first consideration," and the International Code of Medical Ethics declares that, "A physician shall act only in the patient's interest when providing medical care which might have the effect of weakening the physical and mental condition of the patient."

The purpose of biomedical research involving human subjects must be to improve diagnostic, therapeutic and prophylactic procedures and the understanding of the aetiology and pathogenesis of disease.

In current medical practice most diagnostic, therapeutic or prophylactic procedures involve hazards. This applies especially to biomedical research.

Medical progress is based on research, which ultimately must rest in part on experimentation involving human subjects.

In the field of biomedical research a fundamental distinction must be recognized between medical research in which the aim is essentially diagnostic or therapeutic for a patient, and medical research, the essential object of which is purely scientific and without implying direct diagnostic or therapeutic value to the person subjected to the research.

Special caution must be exercised in the conduct of research, which may affect the environment, and the welfare of animals used for research must be respected.

Because it is essential that the results of laboratory experiments be applied to human beings to further scientific knowledge and to help suffering humanity, the World Medical Association has prepared the following recommendations as a guide to every physician in biomedical research involving human subjects. They should be kept under review in the future. It must be stressed that the standards as drafted are only a guide to physicians all over the world. Physicians are not relieved from criminal, civil and ethical responsibilities under the laws of their own countries.

I. Basic Principles

1. Biomedical research involving human subjects must conform to generally accepted scientific principles and should be based on adequately performed laboratory and animal experimentation and on a thorough knowledge of the scientific literature.

2. The design and performance of each experimental procedure involving human subjects should be clearly formulated in an experimental protocol which should be transmitted for consideration, comment and guidance to a specially appointed committee independent of the investigator and the sponsor provided that this independent committee is in conformity with the laws and regulations of the country in which the research experiment is performed.

3. Biomedical research involving human subjects should be conducted only by scientifically qualified persons and under the supervision of a clinically competent medical person. The responsibility for the human subject must always rest with a medically qualified person and never rest on the subject of the research, even though the subject has given his or her consent.

4. Biomedical research involving human subjects cannot legitimately be carried out unless the importance of the objective is in proportion to the inherent risk to the subject.

5. Every biomedical research project involving human subjects should be preceded by careful assessment of predictable risks in comparison with foreseeable benefits to the subject or to others. Concern for the interests of the subject must always prevail over the interests of science and society.

6. The right of the research subject to safeguard his or her integrity must always be respected. Every precaution should be taken to respect the privacy of the subject and to minimize the impact of the study on the subject's physical and mental integrity and on the personality of the subject.

7. Physicians should abstain from engaging in research projects involving human subjects unless they are satisfied that the hazards involved are believed to be predictable. Physicians should cease any investigation if the hazards are found to outweigh the potential benefits.

8. In publication of the results of his or her research, the physician is obliged to preserve the accuracy of the results. Reports of experimentation not in accordance with the principles laid down in this Declaration should not be accepted for publication.

9. In any research on human beings, each potential subject must be adequately informed of the aims, methods, anticipated benefits and potential hazards of the study and the discomfort it may entail. He or she should be informed that he or she is a liberty to abstain from participation in the study and that he or she is free to withdraw his or her consent to participation at any time. The physician should then obtain the subject's freely given informed consent, preferably in writing.

10. When obtaining informed consent for the research project the physician should be particularly cautious if the subject is in a dependent relationship to him or her or may consent under duress. In that case the informed consent should be obtained by a physician who is not engaged in the investigation and who is completely independent of this official relationship.

11. In case of legal incompetence, informed consent should be obtained from the legal guardian in accordance with national legislation. Where physical or mental incapacity makes it impossible to obtain informed consent, or when the subject is a minor, permission from the responsible relative replaces that of the subject in accordance with national legislation.

    Whenever the minor child is in fact able to give a consent, the minor's consent must be obtained in addition to the consent of the minor's legal guardian.

12. The research protocol should always contain a statement of the ethical considerations involved and should indicate that the principles enunciated in the present Declaration are complied with.

II. Medical Research Combined with Professional Care *(Clinical Research)*

1. In the treatment of the sick person, the physician must be free to use a new diagnostic and therapeutic measure, if in his or her judgment it offers hope of saving life, reestablishing health or alleviating suffering.

2. The potential benefits, hazards and discomfort of a new method should be weighed against the advantages of the best current diagnostic and therapeutic methods.

3. In any medical study, every patient—including those of a control group, if any— should be assured of the best proven diagnostic and therapeutic method.

4. The refusal of the patient to participate in a study must never interfere with the physician–patient relationship.

5. If the physician considers it essential not to obtain informed consent, the specific reasons for this proposal should be stated in the experimental protocol for transmission to the independent committee (I, 2).

6. The physician can combine medical research with professional care, the objective being the acquisition of new medical knowledge, only to the extent that medical research is justified by its potential diagnostic or therapeutic value for the patient.

III. Non-therapeutic Biomedical Research Involving Human Subjects *(Non-clinical Biomedical Research)*

1. In the purely scientific application of medical research carried out on a human being, it is the duty of the physician to remain the protector of the life and health of that person on whom biomedical research is being carried out.

2. The subjects should be volunteers—either healthy persons or patients for whom the experimental design is not related to the patient's illness.

3. The investigator or the investigating team should discontinue the research if in his/her or their judgment it may, if continued, be harmful to the individual.

4. In research on man, the interest of science and society should never take precedence over considerations related to the well-being of the subject.

[52 FR 8831, Mar. 19, 1987, as amended at 52 FR 23031, June 17, 1987; 56 FR 22113, May 14, 1991; 64 FR 401, Jan. 5, 1999; 67 FR 9586, Mar. 4, 2002]

Source: Foreign Clinical Studies Not Conducted Under an IND, 21 C.F.R. § 312.120 (2001).

Framingham Heart Study Consent Forms

BOSTON UNIVERSITY SCHOOLS OF MEDICINE,
PUBLIC HEALTH, DENTAL MEDICINE AND
THE BOSTON MEDICAL CENTER

RESEARCH CONSENT FORM
New Offspring Spouse Exam 2

H-22762- THE FRAMINGHAM HEART STUDY N01-HC-25195 1910G

Background
You are participating in the Framingham Heart Study (FHS) examination of New Offspring Spouses. This is an observational research study of relationships between risk factors, genetics, cardiovascular disease, and other health conditions. You are signing this consent form to cover your participation for all future exam cycles of the FHS. You may withdraw your participation from any single exam cycle or the whole study at any time. You will not be required to sign another consent form unless a new procedure is added. At each future exam cycle you will be provided an information sheet containing information about what will occur during that exam cycle.

Purpose
The purpose of this research study is to 1) investigate factors related to the development of heart and blood vessel diseases, lung and blood diseases, stroke, memory loss, cancer, and other major diseases and health conditions; and 2) examine DNA and its relationship to the risks of developing these diseases and other health conditions. THIS EXAMINATION DOES NOT TAKE THE PLACE OF A ROUTINE MEDICAL EXAMINATION BY YOUR PHYSICIAN.

What Happens In This Research Study
You will be one of approximately 103 subjects to be asked to participate in this study.

The research will take place at the following location(s): Boston University Medical Center.
Your research examination will take place at the FHS at 73 Mt. Wayte Avenue in Framingham, MA, or may take place in your home or other residence. The examination will take approximately 4 hours and will include the following:
1) History: An interview about your past and present medical status including: heart and lung illnesses, hospitalizations, emergency room visits, surgeries, physician visits, reproductive history, personal and family history, and health habits (including diet, exercise, prescription and non-prescription drug use, smoking and alcohol use).

2) Measurements and Procedures: A FHS physician will perform a physical examination. You will be asked to participate in standard measurements routinely done in your physician's office such as height, weight, blood pressure (including blood pressure in both arms and legs if you are 40 years old or older), and an electrocardiogram to measure your heart rate and regularity. Your lung function will be measured by breathing in and out of a machine. Some participants will be asked to inhale a bronchodilator medication (albuterol) used routinely in lung function testing, and then to repeat some of the tests. You will be asked in a recorded interview questions about your mood, memory, and mobility. Your hand grip strength, balance, and walking speed will be measured. You will also be asked to wear a small accelerometer to count your footsteps and measure your physical activity over the course of a week.
In the event that you may have a stroke, you would be examined during your hospitalization (if applicable) and at 3, 6, 12 and 24 months. The examination would include a neurological evaluation and an assessment of your ability to perform daily activities.

3) Blood and urine specimens: A technician will draw a sample of your blood (110 cc or about 7.5 tablespoons). You will be asked to take a standard glucose tolerance test which involves swallowing a sweet drink and taking a second blood sample two hours later (this test will not be given to anyone

NewOffspring Spouse Exam 2
Res.v12

BOSTON UNIVERSITY SCHOOLS OF MEDICINE,
PUBLIC HEALTH, DENTAL MEDICINE AND
THE BOSTON MEDICAL CENTER

RESEARCH CONSENT FORM
New Offspring Spouse Exam 2

H-22762- THE FRAMINGHAM HEART STUDY N01-HC-25195 1910G

known to have diabetes). You will be asked to give a sample of your urine. Both the blood and urine samples will be used to test for risk factors for the diseases and health conditions under investigation. You may choose to withdraw your blood samples from future use and the samples will be destroyed after your request is received. If you choose to withdraw your samples, you should call the lab manager of the FHS at (508) 935-3477.

Genetic Studies: You will be asked if a sample of the blood you have donated may be used to obtain genetic material (for example DNA) for research. Genetic research will include the detailed description of the building blocks of DNA and thus may identify genetic conditions that have important health and treatment implications for you. Neither your name nor clinic number appears on the sample.
Data and DNA will be distributed to the FHS researchers and other qualified researchers interested in the genetics of heart and blood vessel diseases, lung and blood diseases, stroke, memory loss, cancer, and other major diseases and health conditions. The researchers will be given the DNA without any personally identifying information. Knowledge from the research on your DNA may be used to develop new tests or medicines for the diseases and conditions under investigation. Your DNA will not be sold to any person, institution, or company for financial gain or commercial profit. Neither you nor your heirs will gain financially from discoveries made using the information and/or specimens that you provide.

4) Vascular function testing: You will be asked to participate in an experimental test of blood vessel function that takes about 15 minutes. Arterial tonometry tests blood vessel (artery) stiffness by carefully recording the blood pressure waveform. A technician will perform the arterial waveform evaluation using a tonometer (a flat sensor, which, when pressed lightly on the skin over the artery records a waveform). The blood vessels in the neck (carotid), arm (brachial and radial), and groin (femoral) will be studied by tonometry. You will also be asked to lie on a long, narrow sensor placed between your shoulder blades. The sensor warms your skin and uses infrared light to detect the timing of arrival of blood flow to the skin of your back. We use this information to evaluate the stiffness of your aorta, which is the largest artery in your body. You will also be asked to wear electrocardiographic leads to measure your heart rhythm.

5) Medical Records: You will be asked to sign a release form to allow the FHS staff to obtain and review copies of your hospital, cancer registry, and medical records. These copies will be reviewed by the FHS physician investigators. The medical release form is considered valid to obtain these records, and will be valid until canceled by you.

You may be contacted later to obtain additional health information or be invited to participate in other FHS health-related studies. You will be asked to give your social security number for the purpose of locating you in the future; you may choose to decline this request. You may be asked to come back for another exam. With your permission, a summary letter of routine test results from this exam will be sent to you and your physician. Any questions you have regarding your rights as a research subject can be directed to the Office of the Institutional Review Board of Boston Medical Center at (617) 638-7207. The FHS is a medical research project sponsored by the National Institutes of Health. It is authorized under 42USC 285b-3. The system of records which applies to the Framingham Heart Study is documented in the Federal Register: September 26, 2002 (Vol. 67, No. 1879) pages 60776-60780.

NewOffspring Spouse Exam 2
Res.v12

BOSTON UNIVERSITY SCHOOLS OF MEDICINE,
PUBLIC HEALTH, DENTAL MEDICINE AND
THE BOSTON MEDICAL CENTER

RESEARCH CONSENT FORM
New Offspring Spouse Exam 2

H-22762- THE FRAMINGHAM HEART STUDY N01-HC-25195 1910G

Risks and Discomforts

The test procedures and their risks and discomforts are listed below:
- The Blood Draw. Minimal bruising, pain, or bleeding may occur.
- The Lung Function Test: This involves a very low level of risk. On rare occasions a person taking a lung function test may feel lightheaded or may faint. The primary risk involved is injury from falling. Participants asked to inhale the medication called albuterol, used during lung function testing, may notice an increase in heart rate (pulse) or symptoms of jitteriness or shakiness (tremors).

Possible general discomforts include: headaches or feeling hungry if you have not eaten before the examination and fatigue or chill during the visit. We do not expect any unusual risk or injury to occur as a result of participation. There are no known risks if you are, or may become, pregnant. In the unlikely event that during examination procedures you should require medical care, first aid will be available.

There may be unknown risks/discomforts involved. Study staff will update you in a timely way on any new information that may affect your health, welfare, or decision to stay in this study

Potential Benefits

You will receive no direct benefit from your participation in this study. However, your participation may help the investigators better understand the causes and prevention of cardiovascular disease and other medical conditions, including potential genetic factors.

Alternatives

Your alternative is to not participate in the study.

Subject Costs and Payments

You will not be charged for any part of the examination. If the examination uncovers any medical problems that require medical diagnosis or treatment, you will be so advised and that information will be provided to the physician or clinic of your choice. In the event that your physician decides that follow up clinical tests or treatments are necessary, payment must be provided by you or your third party payer, if applicable (for example, health insurance or Medicare). No special arrangements will be made by the FHS for compensation or for payment of treatment solely because of your participation in this study. This does not waive any of your legal rights. Costs that you might incur the day of your participation include, but are not limited to, loss of work, and transportation (gas, tolls, etc.). You will not receive payment for your participation. However, if necessary, we will provide transportation to the clinic and your return home at no cost.

Confidentiality

Information obtained about you will be treated as confidential; a code number will be assigned to you and your data. The codes will only be provided to qualified investigators. The risk in providing this sample is minimal. Your samples will be kept until they are not of scientific value. You will not be routinely informed of results of the research performed upon your genetic samples, although with your permission you may be informed of some findings about genetics, cardiovascular disease or other health conditions generated from DNA analyses, directly or through publication in newsletters. Genetic tests may be developed as a result of the analysis of samples in the FHS.

NewOffspring Spouse Exam 2
Res v12

BOSTON UNIVERSITY SCHOOLS OF MEDICINE,
PUBLIC HEALTH, DENTAL MEDICINE AND
THE BOSTON MEDICAL CENTER

RESEARCH CONSENT FORM
New Offspring Spouse Exam 2

H-22762- THE FRAMINGHAM HEART STUDY N01-HC-25195 1910G

When study results are published, your name and other identifying information will not be revealed. Information from this study and from your medical record may be reviewed and photocopied by the state and federal regulatory agencies, such as the Office of Human Research Protection, as applicable, and the Institutional Review Board of Boston University Medical Center. To help us further protect your privacy, the investigators have obtained a Confidentiality Certificate from the Department of Health and Human Services (DHHS). With this Certificate, the investigators cannot be forced (for example by court subpoena) to disclose research information that may identify you in any Federal, State, or local civil, criminal, administrative, legislative, or other proceedings. Disclosure will be necessary, however, upon request of DHHS for audit or program evaluation purposes.

A Confidentiality Certificate does not prevent you or a member of your family from voluntarily releasing information about yourself or your involvement in this research. If an insurer or employer learns about your participation, and obtains your consent to receive research information, then the investigator may not use the Certificate of Confidentiality to withhold this information. This means that you and your family must also actively protect your own privacy. Finally, you should understand that the investigator is not prevented from taking steps, including reporting to authorities, to prevent serious harm to yourself or others. Please check the appropriate box above each of the following statements:

1) |___| YES |___| NO (Office Code 0)
I agree to participate in the FHS clinic examination and studies of the factors contributing to heart and blood vessel diseases, lung and blood diseases, stroke, memory loss, cancer, and other major diseases and health conditions.

2) |___| YES |___|NO (Office Code 3)
I agree to provide a blood sample from which genetic material (DNA and other components) can be obtained. I agree to allow my data and blood samples to be used in the genetic studies of factors contributing to heart and blood vessel diseases, lung and blood diseases, stroke, memory loss, cancer, and other diseases and health conditions.

3) |___| YES |___| NO (Office Code 12)
I agree to allow my data and blood samples to be used in genetic studies of reproductive conditions, and mental health conditions such as alcohol use and depressive symptoms.

4) |___| YES |___| NO (Office Code 4)
I agree to allow researchers from commercial companies to have access to my DNA and genetic data which may be used to develop new lab tests or treatments that could benefit many people. (You or your heirs will not benefit financially from this, nor will your DNA be sold to anyone.)

5) |___| YES |___| NO (Office Code 30)
I agree to allow the FHS to release the findings of non-genetic tests and examinations to my physician, clinic, or hospital.

6) |___| YES |___| NO (Office Code 31)
If a genetic condition is identified that may have important health and treatment implications for me, I agree to allow the FHS to notify me, and then with my permission to notify my physician.

NewOffspring Spouse Exam 2
Res.v12

BOSTON UNIVERSITY SCHOOLS OF MEDICINE,
PUBLIC HEALTH, DENTAL MEDICINE AND
THE BOSTON MEDICAL CENTER

RESEARCH CONSENT FORM
New Offspring Spouse Exam 2

H-22762- THE FRAMINGHAM HEART STUDY N01-HC-25195 1910G

Subject's Rights

By consenting to participate in this study you do not waive any of your legal rights. Giving consent means that you have heard or read the information about this study and that you agree to participate. You will be given a copy of this form to keep.

If at any time you withdraw from this study you will not suffer any penalty or lose any benefits to which you are entitled.

You may obtain further information about your rights as a research subject by calling the Office of the Institutional Review Board of Boston University Medical Center at 617-638-7207. If this study is being done outside the United States you can ask the investigator for contact information for the local Ethics Board.

The investigator or a member of the research team will try to answer all of your questions. If you have questions or concerns at any time, or if you need to report an injury while participating in this research, contact PHILIP A. WOLF, MD, or DANIEL LEVY, MD, at (508) 872-6562.

Compensation for Research Related Injury

If you think that you have been injured by being in this study, please let the investigator know right away. If your part in this study takes place at Boston Medical Center, you can get treatment for the injury at Boston Medical Center. If your part in the study is not at Boston Medical Center, ask the investigator where treatment for injury would be available locally. You and your insurance company will be billed for this treatment. Some research sponsors may offer a program to cover some of the treatment costs which are not covered by your insurance. You should ask the research team if such a program is available.

Right to Refuse or Withdraw

Taking part in this study is voluntary. You have the right to refuse to take part in this study. If you decide to be in the study and then change your mind, you can withdraw from the research. Your participation is completely up to you. Your decision will not affect your being able to get health care at this institution or payment for your health care. It will not affect your enrollment in any health plan or benefits you can get.

If you choose to take part, you have the right to stop at any time. If there are any new findings during the study that may effect whether you want to continue to take part, you will be told about them as soon as possible.

The investigator may decide to discontinue your participation without your permission because he/she may decide that staying in the study will be bad for you, or the sponsor may stop the study.

BOSTON UNIVERSITY SCHOOLS OF MEDICINE,
PUBLIC HEALTH, DENTAL MEDICINE AND
THE BOSTON MEDICAL CENTER

RESEARCH CONSENT FORM
New Offspring Spouse Exam 2

H-22762- THE FRAMINGHAM HEART STUDY N01-HC-25195 1910G

Protection of Subject Health Information

You have certain rights related to your health information. These include the right to know who will get your health information and why they will get it. If you choose to be in this research study, we will get information about you as explained below.

HEALTH INFORMATION ABOUT YOU THAT MIGHT BE USED OR GIVEN OUT DURING THIS RESEARCH:
- Information from your hospital or office health records at BUMC/BMC or elsewhere. This information is reasonably related to the conduct and oversight of the research study. If health information is needed from your doctors or hospitals outside of BUMC/BMC, you will be asked to give permission for these records to be sent to the researcher.
- New health information from tests, procedures, visits, interviews, or forms filled out as part of this research study.

WHY HEALTH INFORMATION ABOUT YOU MIGHT BE USED OR GIVEN OUT TO OTHERS
The reasons we might use or share your health information are:
- To do the research described here
- To make sure we do the research according to certain standard set by ethics, law, and quality groups

PEOPLE AND GROUPS THAT MAY USE OR GIVE OUT YOUR HEALTH INFORMATION
1. PEOPLE OR GROUPS WITHIN BUMC/BMC
- Researchers involved in this research study
- The BUMC Institutional Review Board that oversees this research

2. PEOPLE OR GROUPS OUTSIDE BUMC/BMC
- People or groups that we hire to do certain work for us, such as data storage companies, or laboratories.
- Federal and state agencies if they are required by law or involved in research oversight. Such agencies may include the U.S. Department of Health and Human Services, the Food and Drug Administration, the National Institutes of Health, the Massachusetts Department of Public Health.
- Organizations that make sure hospital standards are met
- The sponsor(s) of the research study, and people or groups it hires to help them do the research
- Other researchers that are part of this research study
- A group that oversees the research information and safety of this study
- Government agencies in other countries
- Other:
Some people or groups who get your health information might not have to follow the same privacy rules that we follow. We share your health information only when we must. We ask anyone who gets it from us to protect your privacy. However, once the information leaves BUMC, we cannot promise that it will be kept private.

In most cases any health data that is being given out to others is identified by a unique study number

NewOffspring Spouse Exam 2
Res.v12

BOSTON UNIVERSITY SCHOOLS OF MEDICINE,
PUBLIC HEALTH, DENTAL MEDICINE AND
THE BOSTON MEDICAL CENTER

RESEARCH CONSENT FORM
New Offspring Spouse Exam 2

H-22762- THE FRAMINGHAM HEART STUDY N01-HC-25195 1910G

and not with your name. So, although in some cases it is possible to link your name to the study data, this is not usually done.

TIME PERIOD FOR USING OR GIVING OUT YOUR HEALTH INFORMATION
Because research is an ongoing process, we cannot give you an exact date when we will either destroy or stop using or sharing your health information.

YOUR PRIVACY RIGHTS
- You have the right not to sign this form that allows us to use and give out your health information for research. If you don't sign this form, you can't be in the research. This is because we need to use the health information to do the research.
- You have the right to withdraw your permission to use or share your health information in this research study. If you want to withdraw your permission, you must write a letter to the researchers in charge of this research study.

If you withdraw your permission, you will not be able to take back information that has already been used or shared with others. This includes information used or shared to do the research study or to be sure the research is safe and of high quality. If you withdraw your permission, you cannot continue to be in the study.

- You have the right to see and get a copy of your health information that is used or shared for research. However, you may only get this after the research is finished. To ask for this information, please contact the person in charge of this research study.

IF RESEARCH RESULTS ARE PUBLISHED OR USED TO TEACH OTHERS
The results of this research study may be published in a medical book or journal, or used to teach others. However, your name or other identifying information will not be used for these purposes without your specific permission.

Signing this consent form indicates that you have read this consent form (or have had it read to you), that your questions have been answered to your satisfaction, and that you voluntarily agree to participate in this research study. You will receive a copy of this signed consent form.

_____|_____   _____
Subject (Signature and Printed Name)   Date

_____|_____   _____
Person Obtaining Consent (Signature and Printed Name)   Date

NewOffspring Spouse Exam 2
Res.v12

BOSTON UNIVERSITY SCHOOLS OF MEDICINE,
PUBLIC HEALTH, DENTAL MEDICINE AND
THE BOSTON MEDICAL CENTER

RESEARCH CONSENT FORM
CTADD Exam 2 - Offsite

H-22762- THE FRAMINGHAM HEART STUDY N01-HC-25195 1910G

Background

The Computed Tomography (CT) Study is an observational research study designed to identify the relationship between calcium deposits in your arteries, fat deposits, and lung function with other health conditions. You are being asked to participate in this study because you are a woman over the age of 40 or a man over the age of 35 and are enrolled in the research study entitled the Framingham Heart Study. The study is sponsored by the National Institutes of Health (NIH) and is conducted in collaboration with the Massachusetts General Hospital (MGH).

The CT scan that you will undergo is very similar to the one that you had previously. However, there are a few differences. The CT machine is newer and stronger. Instead of two scans of the chest, we will only perform one. You will also undergo a CT scan of your abdomen similar to the one that you had previously.

Purpose

The purpose of this research study is to investigate the role of calcium deposits in your arteries, fat deposits, and lung function in the development of 1) heart and blood vessel diseases, lung and blood diseases, stroke, memory loss, joint disease, bone loss, cancer, and other major diseases and health conditions; and 2) metabolic conditions including diabetes and high cholesterol; and 3) to examine the role of inherited factors (genes) in calcification of the arteries, fat deposits, and lung function.

What Happens In This Research Study

You will be one of approximately 2900 subjects to be asked to participate in this study.

The research will take place at the following location(s): Boston University Medical Center.
Your CT examination will take place at the PARC Center, located at 40 Second Avenue, Suite 120 (CT/MRI Services) in Waltham, MA at Massachusetts General Hospital West or at 80 Everett Avenue, Chelsea, MA 02150 at Mass General Imaging Chelsea. The examination will take approximately 30 minutes and will include the following Computed Tomography scan taking about 15 minutes:

1) The CT Scan

A Computed Tomography (CT) scan will be performed for research purposes. This is an x-ray done to measure the amount of calcium in the arteries of your heart and abdomen, fat in the abdomen, liver, and around the heart, and lung function.

One scan of your chest and one scan of your abdomen will be performed. For this scan, you will lie on a table with just your torso (not your head) inside the doughnut shaped CT scanner. You will be asked to remain still and hold your breath for about 20-30 seconds during the scan.

2) Pregnancy Test (for some women only)

Most women under the age of 55 will be asked to provide a urine sample for a pregnancy test within 24 hours before the CT scan. Women who are not pregnant after undergoing the pregnancy test will proceed with the CT scan. If the pregnancy test is positive, you will be referred to your physician for follow up and the scan will not be performed.

This CT scan will not be done on women who are pregnant, or who have been breast feeding for less

CTADD Exam 2 - Offsite

BOSTON UNIVERSITY SCHOOLS OF MEDICINE,
PUBLIC HEALTH, DENTAL MEDICINE AND
THE BOSTON MEDICAL CENTER

RESEARCH CONSENT FORM
CTADD Exam 2 - Offsite

H-22762- THE FRAMINGHAM HEART STUDY N01-HC-25195 1910G

than six months.

3) Results
When the CT scan is read the amount of calcium in your arteries is given a score. At present, it is the opinion of experts that the scores of the amount of coronary calcium detected by CT scanner are not usually used to make clinical decisions. Therefore, the results of the calcium tests or of genetic research that results from the CT scanning tests will not routinely be reported to your physician. However, markedly abnormal levels of calcium deposits in your arteries will be reported to your physician. If you don't have a doctor, you can be referred if you so desire.

In addition, your images will be reviewed for the presence of other findings. In the event that this reading will detect potential medical problems that require further diagnostic testing or treatment, you will be notified and a letter will be sent to you and your physician or the clinic that you choose with your permission.

Because a complete clinical evaluation of the CT scan images for all possible abnormalities in the chest and abdomen will not be performed, some clinically important findings may not be discovered.

You will be asked to sign an additional medical release form giving permission to MGHW or MGH Chelsea to release your CT information to the Framingham Heart Study Investigators.

The results of your CT scans will be shared with the Framingham Heart Study investigators. To ensure confidentiality, a code number will be assigned to all subjects and any other potentially identifying information will not be used on any information provided by subjects. When study results based on subject information are published, names and other potentially identifying information will not be revealed. Only the code numbers will be provided to qualified investigators studying the information.

Any questions you have regarding your rights as a research subject may be directed to the Office of the Institutional Review Board of Boston Medical Center at (617) 638-7207. The Framingham Heart Study is a medical research project sponsored by the National Institutes of Health. It is authorized under 42USC 285b-3. The system of records which applies to the Framingham Heart Study is documented in the Federal Register: September 26, 2002 (Vol. 67, No. 1879) pages 60776-60780.
Risks and Discomforts
As a result of your participation in this study, you will be exposed to radiation from a CT scan of your chest and abdomen. The amount of radiation to which you will be exposed is 6 milliSieverts (mSv). A mSv is a unit of measure of radiation dose. This amount of radiation is approximately equal to 12% of the amount of radiation to which a person who works with radiation can be exposed each year.

We do not expect an unusual risk or injury to occur as a result of your participation. However, there may be unknown risks/discomforts involved. Study staff will update you in a timely way on any new information that may affect your health, welfare, or decision to stay in this study. In the unlikely event that during examination procedures you should require medical care, first aid will be available.

CTADD Exam 2 - Offsite

BOSTON UNIVERSITY SCHOOLS OF MEDICINE,
PUBLIC HEALTH, DENTAL MEDICINE AND
THE BOSTON MEDICAL CENTER

RESEARCH CONSENT FORM
CTADD Exam 2 - Offsite

H-22762- THE FRAMINGHAM HEART STUDY N01-HC-25195 1910G

There may be unknown risks/discomforts involved. Study staff will update you in a timely way on any new information that may affect your health, welfare, or decision to stay in this study

Potential Benefits

You will receive no direct benefit from your participation in this study. However, your participation may help the investigators better understand the causes of heart disease, and prevention of cardiovascular disease and other medical conditions involving the heart, including the possibility of genetic linkages. These studies may also lead to the development of new methods of prevention and treatment of these diseases.

Alternatives

Your alternative is to not participate in the study.

Subject Costs and Payments

You will not be charged for the scan. If the research evaluation of the CT scan examination uncovers markedly abnormal levels of calcium deposits in your arteries or any medical problems that require medical diagnosis or treatment, you will be so advised and that information will be provided to the physician or clinic that you choose.

In the event that your physician decides that follow up clinical tests or treatments are necessary, payment must be provided by you or your third party payer, if applicable (for example, health insurance or Medicare). No special arrangements will be made by the Framingham Heart Study for compensation or for payment of treatment solely because of your participation in this study. This does not waive any of your legal rights.

Costs that you might incur the day of your participation include, but are not limited to, loss of work, and transportation (gas, tolls, etc.). You will not receive payment for your participation. However, if necessary, we will provide transportation from the Framingham Heart Study to and from the center at no cost.

Confidentiality

Any information we obtain about you during this study will be treated as strictly confidential to the full extent permitted by applicable law. To ensure confidentiality, a code number will be assigned to you and any of your potentially identifying information. The code numbers will be provided only to qualified investigators.

You will not be informed of the results of the research including the genetic research that may arise from the CT scan, although genetic tests may be developed as a result of the combined analysis of data in the Framingham Heart Study.

When study results based on your information are published, your name and any other potentially identifying information (i.e. code numbers) will not be revealed. You will be kept informed through periodic publications from the Framingham Heart Study of any new information of findings about CT testing or genetic findings related to CT testing, which may be of importance to you and/or your family.

CTADD Exam 2 - Offsite

BOSTON UNIVERSITY SCHOOLS OF MEDICINE,
PUBLIC HEALTH, DENTAL MEDICINE AND
THE BOSTON MEDICAL CENTER

RESEARCH CONSENT FORM
CTADD Exam 2 - Offsite

H-22762- THE FRAMINGHAM HEART STUDY N01-HC-25195 1910G

To help us further protect your privacy, the investigators have obtained a Confidentiality Certificate from the Department of Health and Human Services (DHHS). With this Certificate, the investigators cannot be forced (for example by court subpoena) to disclose research information that may identify you in any Federal, State, or local civil, criminal, administrative, legislative, or other proceedings. Disclosure will be necessary, however, upon request of DHHS for audit or program evaluation purposes. You should understand that a Confidentiality Certificate does not prevent you or a member of your family from voluntarily releasing information about yourself or your involvement in this research. Note however, that if an insurer or employer learns about your participation, and obtains your consent to receive research information, then the investigator may not use the Certificate of Confidentiality to withhold this information. This means that you and your family must also actively protect your own privacy. Finally, you should understand that the investigator is not prevented from taking steps, including reporting to authorities, to prevent serious harm to yourself or others.

Please check the appropriate box that you agree with:

|___| YES |___| NO I agree to allow the Framingham Heart Study to release the findings from CT scan to my physician, clinic, or hospital.

Subject's Rights
By consenting to participate in this study you do not waive any of your legal rights. Giving consent means that you have heard or read the information about this study and that you agree to participate. You will be given a copy of this form to keep.

If at any time you withdraw from this study you will not suffer any penalty or lose any benefits to which you are entitled.

You may obtain further information about your rights as a research subject by calling the Office of the Institutional Review Board of Boston University Medical Center at 617-638-7207.

The investigator or a member of the research team will try to answer all of your questions. If you have questions or concerns at any time, or if you need to report an injury while participating in this research, contact DR. CAROLINE FOX at (508) 872-6562.

Compensation for Research Related Injury
If you think that you have been injured by being in this study, please let the investigator know right away. If your part in this study takes place at Boston Medical Center, you can get treatment for the injury at Boston Medical Center. If your part in the study is not at Boston Medical Center, ask the investigator where treatment for injury would be available locally. You and your insurance company will be billed for this treatment. Some research sponsors may offer a program to cover some of the treatment costs which are not covered by your insurance. You should ask the research team if such a program is

CTADD Exam 2 - Offsite

BOSTON UNIVERSITY SCHOOLS OF MEDICINE,
PUBLIC HEALTH, DENTAL MEDICINE AND
THE BOSTON MEDICAL CENTER

RESEARCH CONSENT FORM
CTADD Exam 2 - Offsite

H-22762- THE FRAMINGHAM HEART STUDY N01-HC-25195 1910G

available.

Right to Refuse or Withdraw

Taking part in this study is voluntary. You have the right to refuse to take part in this study. If you decide to be in the study and then change your mind, you can withdraw from the research. Your participation is completely up to you. Your decision will not affect your being able to get health care at this institution or payment for your health care. It will not affect your enrollment in any health plan or benefits you can get.

If you choose to take part, you have the right to stop at any time. If there are any new findings during the study that may effect whether you want to continue to take part, you will be told about them as soon as possible.

The investigator may decide to discontinue your participation without your permission because he/she may decide that staying in the study will be bad for you, or the sponsor may stop the study.

Signing this consent form indicates that you have read this consent form (or have had it read to you), that your questions have been answered to your satisfaction, and that you voluntarily agree to participate in this research study. You will receive a copy of this signed consent form.

_____   _____
Subject (Signature and Printed Name)   Date

_____   _____
Person Obtaining Consent (Signature and Printed Name)   Date

CTADD Exam 2 - Offsite

BOSTON UNIVERSITY SCHOOLS OF MEDICINE,
PUBLIC HEALTH, DENTAL MEDICINE AND
THE BOSTON MEDICAL CENTER

RESEARCH CONSENT FORM
Blood Draw Consent for Cell Line Creation

H-22762- THE FRAMINGHAM HEART STUDY N01-HC-25195 1910G

Background

A cell line is a frozen sample of specially processed white cells from your blood that allows the Framingham Heart Study to grow more white cells and get more DNA from them in future as needed for research projects.

Purpose

A cell line will be created from a blood sample you provide in order to study the cause and prevention of cardiovascular disease and other health conditions, including the possibility of how genetic factors influence health status.

What Happens In This Research Study

You will be one of approximately 150 subjects to be asked to participate in this study.

All or part of the research in this study will take place at the following location(s): Boston University Medical Center.
Your research blood draw will take place at the Framingham Heart Study located at 73 Mount Wayte Avenue in Framingham, MA, or the place where you reside. A laboratory technician will draw a sample of your blood (16 cc or about 1 tablespoon) for the preparation of DNA (genetic material) and for the creation of a living sample of white blood cells (cell line).

Risks and Discomforts

Minimal bruising, pain, or bleeding may occur as a result of the blood draw. A latex allergy can occur from the gloves worn by the technician. If you have a known latex allergy, inform the technician and he/she will use another form of protection.

There may be unknown risks/discomforts involved. Study staff will update you in a timely way on any new information that may affect your health, welfare, or decision to stay in this study

Potential Benefits

You will receive no direct benefit from your participation in this study. However, your participation may help the investigators better understand the cause and prevention of cardiovascular disease and other health conditions, including the possibility of how genetic factors influence health status.

Alternatives

Your alternative is to not participate in the study.

Subject Costs and Payments

You will not be charged for the examination. If the examination finds any medical problems requiring medical diagnosis or treatment, you will be so advised and that information will be provided to the physician or clinic that you choose.

In the event that your physician decides that follow up clinical tests or treatments are necessary, payment must be provided by you or your third party payer, if applicable (for example, health insurance or Medicare). No special arrangements will be made by the Framingham Heart Study for compensation or for payment of treatment solely because of your participation in this study. This does not waive any of your legal rights.

Blood Draw Consent for Cell Line Creation
Res.v10

BOSTON UNIVERSITY SCHOOLS OF MEDICINE,
PUBLIC HEALTH, DENTAL MEDICINE AND
THE BOSTON MEDICAL CENTER

RESEARCH CONSENT FORM
Blood Draw Consent for Cell Line Creation

H-22762- THE FRAMINGHAM HEART STUDY N01-HC-25195 1910G

Costs that you might incur the day of your participation include, but are not limited to, transportation costs (gas, tolls, etc). You will not receive payment for your participation. However, if necessary, we will provide transportation to the clinic and your return home at no cost.

Confidentiality

Information obtained during this study will be treated as strictly confidential. A code number will be assigned to you and to your personally identifying information. Cell lines will be stored at a central site. Files linking names to samples will be kept locked and accessible only to the Framingham Heart Study (FHS) data managers. The coded samples will be stored securely and kept until no longer of scientific value. The risk in providing this sample is minimal.

Data and DNA will be distributed to the FHS researchers and other qualified researchers interested in the genetics of heart and blood vessel diseases, lung and blood diseases, stroke, memory loss, joint disease, bone loss, deafness, cancer, and other major diseases and health conditions. The researchers will be given the DNA without any personally identifying information. Information gained from research on your DNA may be used for the development of diagnostic procedures or new treatments for major diseases. Your DNA will not be sold to any person, institution, or company for financial gain or commercial profit. However, neither you nor your heirs will gain financially from discoveries made using the information and/or specimens that you provide.

When study results are published, your name and any other identifying information will not be revealed. You will be informed through periodic publications from the FHS of some findings about genetics, cardiovascular disease or other health conditions generated from the DNA analyses.

To help us further protect your privacy, the investigators have obtained a Confidentiality Certificate from the Department of Health and Human Services (DHHS). With this Certificate, the investigators cannot be forced (for example by court subpoena) to disclose research information that may identify you in any Federal, State, or local civil, criminal, administrative, legislative, or other proceedings. Disclosure will be necessary, however, upon request of DHHS for audit or program evaluation purposes. You should understand that a Confidentiality Certificate does not prevent you or a member of your family from voluntarily releasing information about yourself or your involvement in this research. Note however, that if an insurer or employer learns about your participation, and obtains your consent to receive research information, then the investigator may not use the Certificate of Confidentiality to withhold this information. This means that you and your family must also actively protect your own privacy. Finally, you should understand that the investigator is not prevented from taking steps, including reporting to authorities, to prevent serious harm to yourself or others.

You may choose to withdraw your blood samples and your samples would be destroyed after the request is received. If you choose to withdraw your samples, you should call the Framingham Heart Study at (508) 935-3477 and ask for the lab manager.

The FHS is a medical research project sponsored by the National Institutes of Health. It is authorized under 42USC 285b-3. The system of records which applies to the FHS is documented in the Federal

Blood Draw Consent for Cell Line Creation
Res v10
_____
Last Amendment: 1/21/2009 **Approval valid from April 07, 2009 through April 06, 2010. Chair Initials: J. W.**   Page 2

BOSTON UNIVERSITY SCHOOLS OF MEDICINE,
PUBLIC HEALTH, DENTAL MEDICINE AND
THE BOSTON MEDICAL CENTER

RESEARCH CONSENT FORM
Blood Draw Consent for Cell Line Creation

H-22762- THE FRAMINGHAM HEART STUDY N01-HC-25195 1910G

Register: September 26, 2002 (Vol. 67, No. 1879) pages 60776-60780.

Please check the appropriate box beside the statement you agree with:

1) |___| YES |___| NO (Office Code 1)
I agree to allow a cell line to be made from my blood to provide a renewable supply of DNA. (A cell line is
a frozen sample of specially processed white cells from your blood that allows us to grow more white
cells and obtain more DNA from them as needed for future research projects).

Subject's Rights
By consenting to participate in this study you do not waive any of your legal rights. Giving consent
means that you have heard or read the information about this study and that you agree to participate.
You will be given a copy of this form to keep.

If at any time you withdraw from this study you will not suffer any penalty or lose any benefits to which
you are entitled.

You may obtain further information about your rights as a research subject by calling the Office of the
Institutional Review Board of Boston University Medical Center at 617-638-7207.

The investigator or a member of the research team will try to answer all of your questions. If you have
questions or concerns at any time, or if you need to report an injury while participating in this research,
contact PHILIP A. WOLF, MD, or DANIEL LEVY, MD, at (508) 872-6562.

Compensation for Research Related Injury
If you think that you have been injured by being in this study, please let the investigator know right away.
If your part in this study takes place at Boston Medical Center, you can get treatment for the injury at
Boston Medical Center. If your part in the study is not at Boston Medical Center, ask the investigator
where treatment for injury would be available locally. You and your insurance company will be billed for
this treatment. Some research sponsors may offer a program to cover some of the treatment costs
which are not covered by your insurance. You should ask the research team if such a program is
available.

Right to Refuse or Withdraw
Taking part in this study is voluntary. You have the right to refuse to take part in this study. If you decide
to be in the study and then change your mind, you can withdraw from the research. Your participation is
completely up to you. Your decision will not affect your being able to get health care at this institution or
payment for your health care. It will not affect your enrollment in any health plan or benefits you can get.

If you choose to take part, you have the right to stop at any time. If there are any new findings during the
study that may affect whether you want to continue to take part, you will be told about them as soon as

Blood Draw Consent for Cell Line Creation
Res v10

BOSTON UNIVERSITY SCHOOLS OF MEDICINE,
PUBLIC HEALTH, DENTAL MEDICINE AND
THE BOSTON MEDICAL CENTER

RESEARCH CONSENT FORM
Blood Draw Consent for Cell Line Creation

H-22762- THE FRAMINGHAM HEART STUDY N01-HC-25195 1910G

possible.

The investigator may decide to discontinue your participation without your permission because he/she may decide that staying in the study will be bad for you, or the sponsor may stop the study.

Signing this consent form indicates that you have read this consent form (or have had it read to you), that your questions have been answered to your satisfaction, and that you voluntarily agree to participate in this research study. You will receive a copy of this signed consent form.

_____   _____
Subject (Signature and Printed Name)   Date

_____   _____
Person Obtaining Consent (Signature and Printed Name)   Date

Blood Draw Consent for Cell Line Creation
Resv10

BOSTON UNIVERSITY SCHOOLS OF MEDICINE,
PUBLIC HEALTH, DENTAL MEDICINE AND
THE BOSTON MEDICAL CENTER

RESEARCH CONSENT FORM
Generation III Exam 2

H-22762- THE FRAMINGHAM HEART STUDY N01-HC-25195 1910G

Background

You are participating in the Framingham Heart Study Generation III. The Framingham Heart Study (FHS) is an observational study to find relationships between risk factors, genetics, heart and blood vessel disease, and other health conditions over three generations. You are signing this consent form to cover your participation for all future exam cycles of the FHS. You may withdraw your participation from any single exam cycle or the whole study at any time. You will not be required to sign another consent form unless a new procedure is added. At each future exam cycle you will be provided an information sheet containing information about what will occur during that exam cycle.

Purpose

The purpose of this research is to 1) investigate factors related to the development of heart and blood vessel diseases, lung and blood diseases, stroke, memory loss, cancer, and other major diseases and health conditions; and 2) examine DNA and its relationship to the risks of developing these diseases and other health conditions. THIS EXAMINATION DOES NOT TAKE THE PLACE OF A ROUTINE MEDICAL CHECK UP BY YOUR PHYSICIAN.

What Happens In This Research Study

You will be one of approximately 4010 subjects to be asked to participate in this study.

All or part of the research in this study will take place at the following location(s): Boston University Medical Center.
Your research examination will take place at the FHS at 73 Mt. Wayte Avenue in Framingham, MA, or may take place in your home or other residence. The examination will take approximately 4 hours and will include the following:

1) History: An interview about your past and present medical status including: heart and lung illnesses, hospitalizations, emergency room visits, surgeries, physician visits, reproductive history, personal and family history, and health habits (including diet, exercise, prescription and non-prescription drug use, smoking and alcohol use).

2) Measurements and Procedures: A FHS physician will perform a physical examination. You will be asked to participate in standard measurements routinely done in your physician's office such as height, weight, blood pressure (including blood pressure in both arms and legs if you are 40 years old or older), and an electrocardiogram to measure your heart rate and regularity. Your lung function will be measured by breathing in and out of a machine. Some participants will be asked to inhale a bronchodilator medication (albuterol) used routinely in lung function testing, and then to repeat some of the tests. You will be asked in a recorded interview questions about your mood, memory, and mobility. Your hand grip strength, balance, and walking speed will be measured. You will also be asked to wear a small accelerometer to count your footsteps and measure your physical activity over the course of a week.

In the event that you may have a stroke, you would be examined during your hospitalization (if applicable) and at 3, 6, 12 and 24 months. The examination would include a neurological evaluation and an assessment of your ability to perform daily activities.

3) Blood and urine specimens: A technician will draw a sample of your blood (110 cc or about 7.5

Generation III Exam 2
Res. v12

BOSTON UNIVERSITY SCHOOLS OF MEDICINE,
PUBLIC HEALTH, DENTAL MEDICINE AND
THE BOSTON MEDICAL CENTER

RESEARCH CONSENT FORM
Generation III Exam 2

H-22762- THE FRAMINGHAM HEART STUDY N01-HC-25195 1910G

tablespoons). You will be asked to take a standard glucose tolerance test which involves swallowing a sweet drink and taking a second blood sample two hours later (this test will not be given to anyone known to have diabetes). You will be asked to give a sample of your urine. Both the blood and urine samples will be used to test for risk factors for the diseases and health conditions under investigation. You may choose to withdraw your blood samples from future use and the samples will be destroyed after your request is received. If you choose to withdraw your samples, you should call the lab manager of the FHS at (508) 935-3477.

Genetic Studies: You will be asked if a sample of the blood you have donated may be used to obtain genetic material (for example DNA) for research. Genetic research will include the detailed description of the building blocks of DNA and thus may identify genetic conditions that have important health and treatment implications for you. Neither your name nor clinic number appears on the sample. Data and DNA will be distributed to the FHS researchers and other qualified researchers interested in the genetics of heart and blood vessel diseases, lung and blood diseases, stroke, memory loss, cancer, and other major diseases and health conditions. The researchers will be given the DNA without any personally identifying information. Knowledge from the research on your DNA may be used to develop new tests or medicines for the diseases and conditions under investigation. Your DNA will not be sold to any person, institution, or company for financial gain or commercial profit. Neither you nor your heirs will gain financially from discoveries made using the information and/or specimens that you provide.

4) Vascular function testing: You will be asked to participate in an experimental test of blood vessel function that takes about 15 minutes. Arterial tonometry tests blood vessel (artery) stiffness by carefully recording the blood pressure waveform. A technician will perform the arterial waveform evaluation using a tonometer (a flat sensor, which, when pressed lightly on the skin over the artery records a waveform). The blood vessels in the neck (carotid), arm (brachial and radial), and groin (femoral) will be studied by tonometry. You will also be asked to lie on a long, narrow sensor placed between your shoulder blades. The sensor warms your skin and uses infrared light to detect the timing of arrival of blood flow to the skin of your back. We use this information to evaluate the stiffness of your aorta, which is the largest artery in your body. You will also be asked to wear electrocardiographic leads to measure your heart rhythm.

5) Medical Records: You will be asked to sign a release form to allow the FHS staff to obtain and review copies of your hospital, cancer registry, and medical records. These copies will be reviewed by the FHS physician investigators. The medical release form is considered valid to obtain these records, and will be valid until canceled by you.

You may be contacted later to obtain additional health information or be invited to participate in other FHS health-related studies. You will be asked to give your social security number for the purpose of locating you in the future; you may choose to decline this request. You may be asked to come back for another exam. With your permission, a summary letter of routine test results from this exam will be sent to you and your physician. Any questions you have regarding your rights as a research subject can be directed to the Office of the Institutional Review Board of Boston Medical Center at (617) 638-7207. The FHS is a medical research project sponsored by the National Institutes of Health. It is authorized under 42USC 285b-3. The system of records which applies to the Framingham Heart Study is

Generation III Exam 2
Res v12

BOSTON UNIVERSITY SCHOOLS OF MEDICINE,
PUBLIC HEALTH, DENTAL MEDICINE AND
THE BOSTON MEDICAL CENTER

RESEARCH CONSENT FORM
Generation III Exam 2

H-22762- THE FRAMINGHAM HEART STUDY N01-HC-25195 1910G

documented in the Federal Register: September 26, 2002 (Vol. 67, No. 1879) pages 60776-60780.

Risks and Discomforts

The tests and their risks and discomforts are listed below:
- The Blood Draw. Minimal bruising, pain, or bleeding may occur.
- The Lung Function test: This involves a very low level of risk. On rare occasions, a person taking a lung function test may feel lightheaded or may faint. The primary risk involved is injury from falling. Participants asked to inhale the medication called albuterol, used during lung function testing, may notice an increase in heart rate (pulse) or symptoms of jitteriness or shakiness (tremors).

Possible general discomforts include headaches or feeling hungry if you have not eaten before the examination and fatigue and chill during the visit. We do not expect any unusual risk or injury to occur as a result of participation. In the unlikely event that during the examination you should require medical care, first aid will be available.

There may be unknown risks/discomforts involved. Study staff will update you in a timely way on any new information that may affect your health, welfare, or decision to stay in this study

Potential Benefits

You will receive no direct benefit from your participation in this study. However, your participation may help the investigators better understand the causes and prevention of cardiovascular disease and other medical conditions, including the potential of genetic factors..

Alternatives

Your alternative is to not participate in the study.

Subject Costs and Payments

You will not be charged or paid for any part of the examination. If the examination finds medical problems that require tests or treatments, you will be so advised and that information will be provided to the physician or clinic that you choose. If your physician decides that follow up tests or treatments are necessary, payment must be provided by you or a third party payer (for example, health insurance or Medicare). No special arrangement will be made by the Framingham Heart Study for compensation or payment solely because of your participation in this study. This does not waive any of your legal rights. Costs that you may incur the day of your participation include, but are not limited to, loss of work, and transportation (gas, tolls, etc.). You will not receive payment for your participation.

Confidentiality

Information obtained about you will be treated as confidential; a code number will be assigned to you and your data. The codes will only be provided to qualified investigators. The risk in providing this sample is minimal. Your samples will be kept until they are not of scientific value. You will not be routinely informed of results of the research performed upon your genetic samples, although with your permission you may be informed of some findings about genetics, cardiovascular disease or other health conditions generated from DNA analyses, directly or through publication in newsletters. Genetic tests may be developed as a result of the analysis of samples in the FHS.

When study results are published, your name and other identifying information will not be revealed.

Generation III Exam 2
Res. v12

BOSTON UNIVERSITY SCHOOLS OF MEDICINE,
PUBLIC HEALTH, DENTAL MEDICINE AND
THE BOSTON MEDICAL CENTER

RESEARCH CONSENT FORM
Generation III Exam 2

H-22762- THE FRAMINGHAM HEART STUDY N01-HC-25195 1910G

Information from this study and from your medical record may be reviewed and photocopied by state and federal regulatory agencies, such as the Office of Human Research Protection, as applicable, and the Institutional Review Board of Boston University Medical Center. To help us further protect your privacy, the investigators have obtained a Confidentiality Certificate from the Department of Health and Human Services (DHHS). With this Certificate, the investigators cannot be forced (for example by court subpoena) to disclose research information that may identify you in any Federal, State, or local civil, criminal, administrative, legislative, or other proceedings. Disclosure will be necessary, however, upon request of DHHS for audit or program evaluation purposes.

A Confidentiality Certificate does not prevent you or a member of your family from voluntarily releasing information about yourself or your involvement in this research. If an insurer or employer obtains your participation, and obtains your consent to receive research information, then the investigator may not use the Certificate of Confidentiality to withhold this information. This means that you and your family must also actively protect your own privacy. Finally, you should understand that the investigator is not prevented from taking steps, including reporting to authorities, to prevent serious harm to yourself or others. Please check the appropriate box above each of the following statements:

1) |___| YES |___| NO (Office Code 0)
I agree to participate in the FHS clinic examination and studies of the factors contributing to heart and blood vessel diseases, lung and blood diseases, stroke, memory loss, cancer, and other major diseases and health conditions.

2) |___| YES |___| NO (Office Code 3)
I agree to provide a blood sample from which genetic material (DNA and other components) can be obtained. I agree to allow my data and blood samples to be used in the genetic studies of factors contributing to heart and blood vessel diseases, lung and blood diseases, stroke, memory loss, cancer, and other diseases and health conditions.

3) |___| YES |___| NO (Office Code 12)
I agree to allow my data and blood samples to be used in genetic studies of reproductive conditions, and mental health conditions such as alcohol use and depressive symptoms.

4) |___| YES |___| NO (Office Code 4)
I agree to allow researchers from commercial companies to have access to my DNA and genetic data which may be used to develop new lab tests or treatments that could benefit many people. (You or your heirs will not benefit financially from this, nor will your DNA be sold to anyone.)

5) |___| YES |___| NO (Office Code 30)
I agree to allow the FHS to release the findings of non-genetic tests and examinations to my physician, clinic, or hospital.

6) |___| YES |___| NO (Office Code 31)
If a genetic condition is identified that may have important health and treatment implications for me, I agree to allow the FHS to notify me, and then with my permission to notify my physician.

Generation III Exam 2
Res. v12

BOSTON UNIVERSITY SCHOOLS OF MEDICINE,
PUBLIC HEALTH, DENTAL MEDICINE AND
THE BOSTON MEDICAL CENTER

RESEARCH CONSENT FORM
Generation III Exam 2

H-22762- THE FRAMINGHAM HEART STUDY N01-HC-25195 1910G

Subject's Rights

By consenting to participate in this study you do not waive any of your legal rights. Giving consent means that you have heard or read the information about this study and that you agree to participate. You will be given a copy of this form to keep.

If at any time you withdraw from this study you will not suffer any penalty or lose any benefits to which you are entitled.

You may obtain further information about your rights as a research subject by calling the Office of the Institutional Review Board of Boston University Medical Center at 617-638-7207. If this study is being done outside the United States you can ask the investigator for contact information for the local Ethics Board.

The investigator or a member of the research team will try to answer all of your questions. If you have questions or concerns at any time, or if you need to report an injury while participating in this research, contact PHILIP A. WOLF, MD, or DANIEL LEVY, MD, at (508) 872-6562.

Compensation for Research Related Injury

If you think that you have been injured by being in this study, please let the investigator know right away. If your part in this study takes place at Boston Medical Center, you can get treatment for the injury at Boston Medical Center. If your part in the study is not at Boston Medical Center, ask the investigator where treatment for injury would be available locally. You and your insurance company will be billed for this treatment. Some research sponsors may offer a program to cover some of the treatment costs which are not covered by your insurance. You should ask the research team if such a program is available.

Right to Refuse or Withdraw

Taking part in this study is voluntary. You have the right to refuse to take part in this study. If you decide to be in the study and then change your mind, you can withdraw from the research. Your participation is completely up to you. Your decision will not affect your being able to get health care at this institution or payment for your health care. It will not affect your enrollment in any health plan or benefits you can get.

If you choose to take part, you have the right to stop at any time. If there are any new findings during the study that may affect whether you want to continue to take part, you will be told about them as soon as possible.

The investigator may decide to discontinue your participation without your permission because he/she may decide that staying in the study will be bad for you, or the sponsor may stop the study.

Generation III Exam 2
Res. v12

BOSTON UNIVERSITY SCHOOLS OF MEDICINE,
PUBLIC HEALTH, DENTAL MEDICINE AND
THE BOSTON MEDICAL CENTER

RESEARCH CONSENT FORM
Generation III Exam 2

H-22762- THE FRAMINGHAM HEART STUDY N01-HC-25195 1910G

Protection of Subject Health Information

You have certain rights related to your health information. These include the right to know who will get your health information and why they will get it. If you choose to be in this research study, we will get information about you as explained below.

HEALTH INFORMATION ABOUT YOU THAT MIGHT BE USED OR GIVEN OUT DURING THIS RESEARCH:
- Information from your hospital or office health records at BUMC/BMC or elsewhere. This information is reasonably related to the conduct and oversight of the research study. If health information is needed from your doctors or hospitals outside of BUMC/BMC, you will be asked to give permission for these records to be sent to the researcher.
- New health information from tests, procedures, visits, interviews, or forms filled out as part of this research study.

WHY HEALTH INFORMATION ABOUT YOU MIGHT BE USED OR GIVEN OUT TO OTHERS
The reasons we might use or share your health information are:
   - To do the research described here
   - To make sure we do the research according to certain standard set by ethics, law, and quality groups

PEOPLE AND GROUPS THAT MAY USE OR GIVE OUT YOUR HEALTH INFORMATION
1. PEOPLE OR GROUPS WITHIN BUMC/BMC
- Researchers involved in this research study
- The BUMC Institutional Review Board that oversees this research

2. PEOPLE OR GROUPS OUTSIDE BUMC/BMC
- People or groups that we hire to do certain work for us, such as data storage companies, or laboratories.
- Federal and state agencies if they are required by law or involved in research oversight. Such agencies may include the U.S. Department of Health and Human Services, the Food and Drug Administration, the National Institutes of Health, the Massachusetts Department of Public Health.
- Organizations that make sure hospital standards are met
- The sponsor(s) of the research study, and people or groups it hires to help them do the research
- Other researchers that are part of this research study
- A group that oversees the research information and safety of this study
- Government agencies in other countries
- Other:
Some people or groups who get your health information might not have to follow the same privacy rules that we follow. We share your health information only when we must. We ask anyone who gets it from us to protect your privacy. However, once the information leaves BUMC, we cannot promise that it will be kept private.

In most cases any health data that is being given out to others is identified by a unique study number
Generation III Exam 2
Res. v12

BOSTON UNIVERSITY SCHOOLS OF MEDICINE,
PUBLIC HEALTH, DENTAL MEDICINE AND
THE BOSTON MEDICAL CENTER

RESEARCH CONSENT FORM
Generation III Exam 2

H-22762- THE FRAMINGHAM HEART STUDY N01-HC-25195 1910G

and not with your name. So, although in some cases it is possible to link your name to the study data, this is not usually done.

TIME PERIOD FOR USING OR GIVING OUT YOUR HEALTH INFORMATION
Because research is an ongoing process, we cannot give you an exact date when we will either destroy or stop using or sharing your health information.

YOUR PRIVACY RIGHTS
- You have the right not to sign this form that allows us to use and give out your health information for research. If you don't sign this form, you can't be in the research. This is because we need to use the health information to do the research.
- You have the right to withdraw your permission to use or share your health information in this research study. If you want to withdraw your permission, you must write a letter to the researchers in charge of this research study. If you withdraw your permission, you will not be able to take back information that has already been used or shared with others. This includes information used or shared to do the research study or to be sure the research is safe and of high quality. If you withdraw your permission, you cannot continue to be in the study.
- You have the right to see and get a copy of your health information that is used or shared for research. However, you may only get this after the research is finished. To ask for this information, please contact the person in charge of this research study.

IF RESEARCH RESULTS ARE PUBLISHED OR USED TO TEACH OTHERS
The results of this research study may be published in a medical book or journal, or used to teach others. However, your name or other identifying information will not be used for these purposes without your specific permission.

Signing this consent form indicates that you have read this consent form (or have had it read to you), that your questions have been answered to your satisfaction, and that you voluntarily agree to participate in this research study. You will receive a copy of this signed consent form.

_____   _____
Subject (Signature and Printed Name)   Date

_____   _____
Person Obtaining Consent (Signature and Printed Name)   Date

Generation III Exam 2
Res. v12

Last Amendment: 1/21/2009 **Approval valid from April 07, 2009 through April 06, 2010. Chair Initials: J. W.**   Page 7

Note: Consent forms in longitudinal studies are revised from time to time and several recent versions of the FHS consent forms are posted on our website, www.framinghamheartstudy.org.
Source: Used with permission of the Framingham Heart Study, National Heart, Lung, and Blood Institute, Boston University.

Index

Note: Italicized page locators indicate a figure; tables are noted with a *t*.